Fundamentals of Oncologic PET/CT

Fundamentals of Oncologic PET/CT

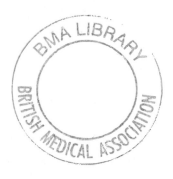

GARY A. ULANER, MD, PhD, FACNM
Associate Member, Department of Radiology
Memorial Sloan Kettering Cancer Center;
Associate Professor, Department of Radiology
Weill Cornell Medical School
New York, New York

ELSEVIER

ELSEVIER

1600 John F. Kennedy Blvd.
Ste 1800
Philadelphia, PA 19103-2899

FUNDAMENTALS OF ONCOLOGIC PET/CT   ISBN: 978-0-323-56869-2

Notices

Knowledge and best practice in this field are constantly changing. As new research and experience broaden our understanding, changes in research methods, professional practices, or medical treatment may become necessary.

Practitioners and researchers must always rely on their own experience and knowledge in evaluating and using any information, methods, compounds, or experiments described herein. In using such information or methods they should be mindful of their own safety and the safety of others, including parties for whom they have a professional responsibility.

With respect to any drug or pharmaceutical products identified, readers are advised to check the most current information provided (i) on procedures featured or (ii) by the manufacturer of each product to be administered, to verify the recommended dose or formula, the method and duration of administration, and contraindications. It is the responsibility of practitioners, relying on their own experience and knowledge of their patients, to make diagnoses, to determine dosages and the best treatment for each individual patient, and to take all appropriate safety precautions.

To the fullest extent of the law, neither the Publisher nor the authors, contributors, or editors, assume any liability for any injury and/or damage to persons or property as a matter of products liability, negligence or otherwise, or from any use or operation of any methods, products, instructions, or ideas contained in the material herein.

Library of Congress Cataloging-in-Publication Data or Control Number: 2018940042

Content Strategist: Russell Gabbedy
Content Development Specialist: Angie Breckon
Publishing Services Manager: Julie Eddy
Senior Project Manager: Rachel E. McMullen
Design Direction: Maggie Reid

Printed in China

Last digit is the print number: 9   8   7   6   5   4   3   2   1

To Robert Henderson, the teacher who taught me to love PET/CT.
And to my wife, Alena; son, Ilya; and expectant daughter,
who have taught me how to love everything else.

Preface

Positron emission tomography/computed tomography (PET/CT) is a rapidly growing modality which has made a tremendous impact in the care of patients with cancer. Its success can be attributed to the sum of PET/CT being more than its individual parts. PET dramatically improves the sensitivity of cancer detection over CT, while CT makes PET more specific and increases reader confidence. Thus, practitioners of PET/CT need to master two complementary but very different imaging modalities. This "fundamentals" text emphasizes the integration of PET and CT findings to optimize the interpretation of oncologic PET/CT. Physicians experienced in PET will find the discussion of the corresponding CT valuable. Likewise, physicians experienced in CT will learn the value of PET.

Many PET texts are designed around diagnoses. This text is designed around organ systems. There is a chapter on lung cancer which shows images of lung cancer. I demonstrate PET and CT findings in the lung, and then offer guidance on how to best determine if the findings represent primary lung cancer, lung metastases, or benign lung lesions that must be distinguished from malignancy. This approach parallels how radiologists and nuclear medicine physicians confront challenging imaging studies every day.

I hope you find my approach educational and beneficial to your medical practice.

Gary A. Ulaner, MD, PhD, FACNM

Contents

CHAPTER 1

Introduction to FDG PET/CT

18F-flourodeoxyglucose positron emission tomography/ computed tomography (FDG PET/CT) provides noninvasive metabolic and anatomic imaging. The radioisotope, flouride-18, has a short half-life allowing for imaging with limited patient dose. Fluoride-18 is used to chemically replace a hydroxyl group on glucose, and the resultant FDG is taken up into cells analogous to glucose. As tumor cells often uptake more glucose than normal tissues, FDG allows effective imaging of tumors.

The majority of this textbook focuses on hybrid FDG PET/CT for oncology. More than 1.7 million PET examinations are performed each year in the United States. There are several interesting facts about these PET examinations.

1 Greater than 95% of PET scans are performed with FDG as the radiotracer.

2 95% of PET scans are performed for oncology (3% for cardiology, 2% for neurology).

3 Greater than 95% of PET scans are performed as hybrid PET/CT studies. (Data from IMV 2015 PET Imaging Market Summary Report, http:// www.imvinfo.com/index.aspx?sec=pet&sub=dis&ite mid=200083.)

Let's look at each point.

1. Greater than 95% of PET scans are performed with FDG as the radiotracer.

   FDG is by far the most commonly used radiotracer for PET imaging. There are other PET radiotracers that are U.S. Food and Drug Administration (FDA) approved for imaging, and many more which are not FDA approved, but the vast majority of PET scans are currently performed with FDG as the tracer. Thus the majority of this book focuses on the interpretation of FDG PET. The final chapter introduces other radiotracers with strong potential for increased utilization in the future.

2. 95% of PET scans are performed for oncology.

   There are important applications of PET for cardiology and neurology; however, the vast majority of PET examinations are performed to evaluate patients with malignancy. Thus this book focuses on oncologic FDG PET.

3. Greater than 95% of PET scans are performed as hybrid PET/CT studies.

   There are several reasons for this. First, PET scans are easier to interpret when they are corrected for attenuation. A PET camera counts 511 keV photons that are received by its detectors, but this is not the number of photons that are actually emitted. Many photons are attenuated while passing through the body before they reach the camera. In general, the deeper the photons originate within the body, the more tissue they need to pass through, and the more attenuation occurs. Thus the camera sees a greater percentage of the photons that originate near the body surface, less from those that originate deeper within the body. We can create an image from the number of photons actually detected by the PET camera. This is called the nonattenuation corrected image (Fig. 1.1).

   Notice how the surface of the body appears to have more counts than areas deeper in the body. For example, the superficial portion of the liver (arrow) appears to have more counts than the deeper portions of the liver in the nonattenuation corrected image (see Fig. 1.1). However, we know that in a normal liver, the number of photons emitted from the liver cells should be about equal. This limits visualization of the deeper structures in the body.

   When we "correct" for attenuation, the FDG images appear the way we are used to seeing them (Fig. 1.2).

   Now the liver appears homogeneous in the attenuation corrected image (see Fig. 1.2). How is this attenuation correction done? The PET/CT camera uses the data from CT photon attenuation as a map to "correct" for attenuation of the photons created by

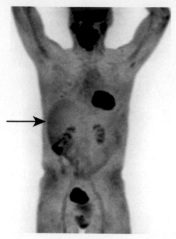

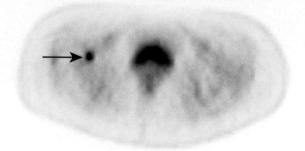

FIG. 1.3 **Axial FDG PET through the pelvis in a patient with breast cancer.** There is an FDG focus in the right pelvis *(arrow)*. The midline FDG avidity is urine in the bladder.

FIG. 1.1 **Nonattenuated corrected maximum intensity projection image from an FDG PET scan.** *Arrow* points at the liver surface, which appears to have more photon counts than the deeper portions of the liver.

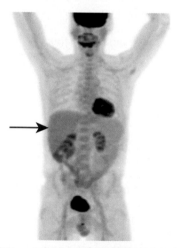

FIG. 1.2 **Attenuated corrected maximum intensity projection image from the same FDG PET scan as Fig. 1.1.** *Arrow* points at the liver surface, which after attenuation correction appears to have the same photon counts as the deeper portions of the liver.

positron annihilation. In general, the attenuation corrected image is much easier to interpret. How does a PET-only camera correct for attenuation? A PET-only camera uses a transmission positron source. Thus both PET-only and PET/CT cameras can effectively correct for attenuation. However, the CT scan takes only seconds to acquire on a PET/CT, but the transmission data may take 30 minutes to acquire

on a PET-only camera. Thus the use of hybrid PET/CT allows much faster patient throughput than a PET-only camera.

Second, the CT component of a PET/CT allows for lesion localization. Sometimes it is difficult to determine where a PET focus is in the body (Fig. 1.3). Fig. 1.3 depicts a patient with breast cancer. There is an FDG focus in the right pelvis. What this FDG focus represents depends on where this focus is. If it is within a bone, then it is suspicious for an osseous metastasis. However, if it is outside the bone in a muscle, then it is probably physiologic muscle and is benign. The ability to fuse the FDG PET and CT images (Fig. 1.4) allows for localization of the FDG focus to the bone, and thus the FDG focus is suspicious for osseous metastasis. This biopsy was proven to be an osseous metastasis.

Third, the CT component of a PET/CT helps with lesion characterization. The corresponding findings on the CT of a PET/CT can help determine what an FDG focus represents (Fig. 1.5). In Fig. 1.5, a patient with lymphoma has an FDG-avid focus in the right inguinal region, which at first glance is suspicious for an FDG-avid lymph node. However, look at the corresponding CT image. The lesion is lower in attenuation than expected for a lymphoma node. The Hounsfield units of this lesion are 0, equal to water. This CT finding would be unusual for a lymphoma node and thus prompts further investigation. The same patient in sagittal projection is shown in Fig. 1.6. On the sagittal PET image, there is again an FDG focus in the right inguinal region; however, on the sagittal CT image, the bladder can be seen to be herniating through an inguinal hernia. The FDG focus in the right inguinal region is due to is a benign bladder hernia, rather than nodal lymphoma. This

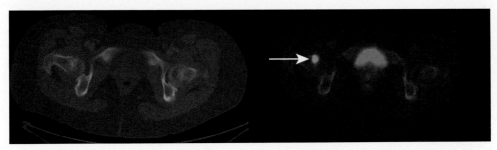

FIG. 1.4 **Axial CT and fused FDG PET/CT that correspond with Fig. 1.3.** The FDG focus in the right pelvis localizes to the right femur *(arrow)* and is suspicious for an osseous metastasis. Biopsy proved this was an osseous metastasis.

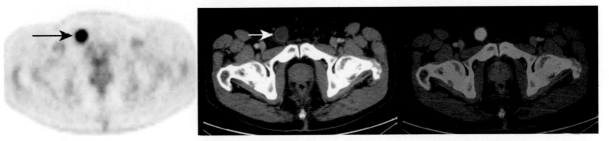

FIG. 1.5 **Axial FDG PET, CT, and fused FDG PET/CT through the pelvis of a patient with lymphoma.** The FDG-avid focus on the PET-only image *(arrow)* is at first glance suspicious for a malignant node. However, on the corresponding CT image, the lesion has attenuation equal to water *(short arrow)*. This is unusual for a lymphoma node and prompts further evaluation.

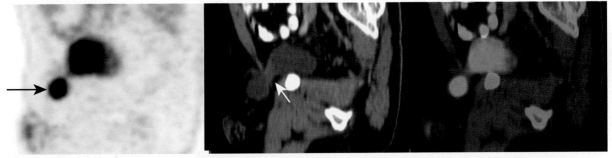

FIG. 1.6 **Sagittal FDG PET, CT, and fused FDG PET/CT through the pelvis of the same patient as Fig. 1.5.** The FDG focus in the right inguinal region is again seen on the PET-only images *(arrow)*. The sagittal CT image demonstrates the herniation of the bladder through an inguinal hernia *(short arrow)*. The CT helps characterize the FDG focus in the right inguinal region as a benign bladder hernia, rather than malignancy.

explains the Hounsfield units of 0 on CT. The FDG "lesion" is actually only urine within a herniated bladder. The CT component of the PET/CT was instrumental in characterizing the PET finding and preventing misdiagnosis.

Given the advantages for (1) rapid attenuation correction, (2) lesion localization, and (3) lesion characterization, almost all PET scans are performed as hybrid PET/CT scans. Thus this book focuses on hybrid PET/CT.

In summary, the vast majority of PET scans currently performed are hybrid FDG PET/CT for oncology, and thus the majority of this book focuses on these examinations. This content will cover organ system by organ system throughout the body, emphasizing how to integrate FDG PET and CT findings to arrive at the best interpretation of FDG PET/CT studies. My goal is to provide you with an organized, systematic approach to reading oncologic FDG PET/CT.

CHAPTER 2

FDG PET/CT Performance and Reporting

PERFORMING FDG PET/CT

Patients need to be prepared for 18F-flourodeoxyglucose (FDG) positron emission tomography/computed tomography (PET/CT) in order to optimize the distribution of FDG in the body. Patients should avoid exercise starting the day before the examination in order to prevent muscular FDG uptake. Patients should not consume food or liquids other than unflavored water for at least 4 hours prior to administration of FDG, in order to prevent insulinemia and FDG uptake in muscles and fat. Hydration with a liter of water in the hours before the scan will help dilute excreted FDG in the urine, both reducing patient radiation exposure and artifacts. The patient should be kept warm, starting before FDG administration, in order to prevent FDG-avid brown fat. Blood glucose level is measured before FDG administration, as a glucose level greater than 200 mg/dL may alter FDG biodistribution. FDG is administered intravenously with the patient sitting or lying comfortably, and the patient should remain in this position to minimize muscular uptake. If possible, the patient should remain silent to prevent FDG uptake in vocal musculature, particularly for patients with cancer in the head/neck. The patient should void before being positioned on the PET/CT scanner to remove excreted FDG in the urine. PET/CT imaging usually begins about 60 minutes after FDG administration. The extent of FDG uptake in tissues changes with time; thus it is important to keep the uptake times relatively similar in order to best compare studies. The patient is positioned comfortably on a PET/CT scanner for the examination, which may take 30 to 60 minutes, depending on the field of view and number of minutes per bed position. The typical field of view is the mid-skull to mid-thigh. Additional views of the neck, brain, or extremities may be obtained in selected patients. See Box 2.1 for a list of these maneuvers. Following imaging, CT images are reconstructed and used to create an attenuation map in order to attenuation correct the PET images. CT, nonattenuation corrected PET, and attenuation corrected PET images are produced. The attenuation corrected PET images are usually fused to the CT images to allow evaluation of fused PET/CT images. All images are displayed in multiplanar reconstructions.

QUANTIFYING FDG AVIDITY WITH STANDARDIZED UPTAKE VALUES

FDG avidity is increasingly being quantitated, in order to have numerical values for comparisons. Quantitation of FDG avidity is most commonly performed with standardized uptake values (SUV), a measurement of tracer uptake in a lesion normalized to a distribution volume. There are many different formulas of SUV, depending on how the SUV is normalized (weight, lean body mass [LBM], body surface area), and how the region of interest (ROI) is analyzed (SUVmax, SUVmean, SUVpeak, etc.). Most commonly, SUVmax is reported, which is the SUV normalized for body weight for the most FDG-avid voxel within a ROI. SUV normalized for LBM is called SUL, as is recommended by several organizations. SUL provides less variation in the calculated value than SUV normalized for body weight. However, SUVmax is so highly reproducible and easy to calculate that it is currently the most commonly utilized measure of FDG avidity in clinical practice. SUVmax is calculated as SUVmax = tracer uptake in ROI / (injected activity / patient weight). This provides a number (2, 10, 20, etc.) that conveys a sense of the relative extent of FDG uptake in a lesion.

It is important to remember that calculated SUV values are "semiquantitative." If you perform an FDG PET/CT in the same patient on two consecutive days, you may get slightly different SUV values, despite the lesion truly being the same. This is because the amount of FDG uptake in a lesion is dependent on multiple biologic and technical factors (Box 2.2). For example, higher blood glucose levels may reduce FDG uptake in tumors and a long FDG uptake time (time between FDG injection and image acquisition) often results in increased FDG uptake. To minimize variations in SUV because of these biologic and technical factors, a number of guidelines are suggested for the performance on FDG PET/CT (Box 2.3). These biologic and technical factors often result in a 10% to 20% difference in SUV, even if there is no change in the tumor.

BOX 2.1
Basic Preparation and Performance of FDG PET/CT

1. Avoid exercise starting the day before the FDG PET/CT.
2. No food or liquids other than water starting at least 4 hours before the FDG PET/CT.
3. Hydration with a liter of water in the hours before FDG administration.
4. Keep patient warm starting before FDG administration.
5. Measure blood glucose level before FDG administration.
6. Administer FDG intravenously while patient sits or lies comfortably and quietly.
7. Patient should void before being placed on PET/CT scanner.
8. Position patient comfortably on scanner for the relatively long image acquisition. Imaging begins about 60 minutes following FDG administration.

BOX 2.3
Guidelines for Performing FDG PET/CT to Minimize Variability Between Scans

A. Patients should fast a minimum of 4 hours before FDG administration
B. Measured serum glucose should be ≤200 mg/dL.
C. Patients may be on oral hypoglycemic mediations, but not insulin
D. PET scan should be obtained 50–70 minutes after FDG administration, and uptake time on follow-up scans should be within 15 minutes of the baseline scan
E. Scans should be performed on well-calibrated and well-maintained scanners
F. Scans for the same patient should be obtained on the same scanner
G. Scans should be performed with the same administered FDG dose (±20%)
H. Same method of performed and reconstructing the scans should be used

BOX 2.2
Some Factors That Influence Standardized Uptake Value

A. Biologic factors
   1. Patient weight
   2. Blood glucose level
   3. Insulin
   4. FDG uptake time
   5. Lesion size (partial volume effects, see Chapter 23)
B. Technical factors
   1. Variability in different scanners
   2. Variation in calibration of scanners
   3. Variability in reconstruction methods
   4. Motion

REPORTING FDG PET/CT EXAMINATIONS
Structured Reports

There are multiple methods to report an oncologic FDG PET/CT examination. The report is often challenging, given the large field of view of oncologic FDG PET/CT scans, often extending from the mid-skull to the mid-thigh, as well as the importance of both FDG PET and CT findings. Presented here is an example of structured PET/CT reporting. The organ system–based outline takes a little while to get used to, but many oncologists and surgeons who

order PET/CT examinations find it useful. If a physician is interested in an analysis of a specific organ, he or she knows exactly where in the report to look. This saves a lot of time for physicians reading the reports. And it ends up saving radiologists a lot of time, too. When dictating a follow-up study, the radiologist can more easily find what he or she needs from the prior report. Again, practitioners not used to a structured report may struggle with it initially, but many who use it come to see its advantages and adapt it for their own purposes. An example of a structured report is demonstrated in Box 2.4.

A few components to notice in the structured FDG PET/CT report:

1. Contrast. Oral and intravenous contrast agents are not required, but often very helpful for interpretation of FDG PET/CT. Most of our FDG PET/CT examinations are performed with low-dose CT component (40–100 mA depending on patient size, 120 kV) with oral contrast (e.g., Omnipaque 300, 30 mL mixed into 1000 mL of water or other sugar-free aqueous diluent) but not intravenous (IV) contrast. A few exceptions:
   a. Pediatric patients (<18 years) are usually not given oral contrast.
   b. When the referring physician orders both an FDG PET/CT and a contrast enhanced CT, the two examinations are combined into one, with a full dose CT scan (variable mA up 400 depending on patient size, 120 kV) performed with both oral

BOX 2.4
Standard Normal Oncologic FDG PET/CT Structured Report for an Examination From Mid-Skull to Mid-Thighs

BODY FDG PET/CT

CLINICAL STATEMENT: [ ]
RADIOPHARMACEUTICAL: [ ] mCi FDG.
TECHNIQUE: Following intravenous injection of FDG and an approximately [ ] minute uptake period, CT and PET images from the mid-skull to the upper thighs were acquired on the [ ] PET/CT with the patient in the fasted state. [ ] contrast material was administered. Plasma glucose at the time of this test: [ ] mg/dL. The SUV are normalized to patient body weight and indicate the highest activity concentration (SUVmax) in a given disease site.
STUDIES USED FOR CORRELATION: [ ]
FINDINGS:
HEAD/FACE: Physiologic FDG uptake is seen in the visualized regions of the brain, extraocular muscles, large salivary glands, and oropharynx.
NECK: Physiologic FDG uptake is seen in neck muscles.
CHEST: Physiologic FDG avidity is seen in mediastinal blood pool and myocardium.
LUNGS: No abnormal uptake.
PLEURA/PERICARDIUM: No abnormal uptake.
THORACIC NODES: No abnormal uptake.
HEPATOBILIARY: No abnormal uptake. Liver background SUV mean, as a reference for comparing FDG studies, is [ ].
SPLEEN: No abnormal uptake.
PANCREAS: No abnormal uptake.
ADRENAL GLANDS: No abnormal uptake.
KIDNEYS/URETERS/BLADDER: Excreted activity is seen.
ABDOMINOPELVIC NODES: No abnormal uptake.
BOWEL/PERITONEUM/MESENTERY: No abnormal uptake.
PELVIC ORGANS: No abnormal uptake.
BONES/SOFT TISSUES: No abnormal uptake.
OTHER FINDINGS: None.

IMPRESSION:
Since [Date]

SUV, Standardized uptake values.
Used with permission from Memorial Sloan Kettering Cancer Center.

TABLE 2.1
MSKCC Lexicon of Diagnostic Certainty MSKCC 2010

Consistent with	>90%
Suspicious/Probable	~75%
Possible	~50%
Less likely	~25%
Unlikely	<10%

Used with permission of MSKCC, 2010.

and IV contrast (Omnipaque 300 mg iodine/mL, 150 mL delivered via power injector at 2 cc/s).

2. Plasma glucose. Elevated blood glucose may lead to endogenous production of insulin. Insulin may drive FDG into muscles, resulting in suboptimal imaging. To prevent this, we do not administer FDG to a patient until plasma glucose is under 200 mg/dL. There are multiple ways to manage elevated blood glucose levels. Hydration and subcutaneous insulin are possible methods to help lower glucose levels.

3. Liver background. The liver background is used to compare the intensity of liver uptake in the prior study to that of the current study. Small differences are not significant. However, if the current liver background in an SUV is 4, but the prior liver background demonstrates an SUV of 2, this tips us off that the measurement of lesions may not be comparable.

Conveying Diagnostic Certainty

Another reporting issue to consider is how to deal with uncertainty. Sometimes you are not 100% sure what you are looking at! It this scenario I find it useful to use a standard system to describe the confidence of your interpretation. The Memorial Sloan Kettering Cancer Center (MSKCC) Lexicon of Diagnostic Certainty is given in Table 2.1.

For example, Fig. 2.1 demonstrates a tiny FDG avid focus in the right pelvis in a patient with treated cervical cancer. The corresponding CT demonstrates a small soft tissue nodule near the colon. This was new from the prior scan, and there were no other findings of concern. Could this be a metastasis? Yes. Could this be benign? Sure, but less likely. A new FDG-avid soft tissue nodule in the pelvis of a patient with cervical cancer is suspicious for a metastasis. Thus, a reasonable approach to this finding is to dictate in the impression, "FDG-avid small soft tissue nodule in the pelvis of a patient with cervical

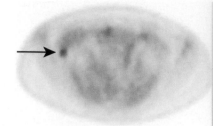 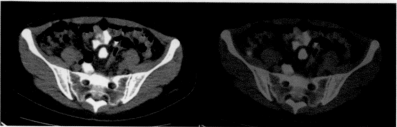

FIG. 2.1 **Axial FDG PET, CT, and Fused FDG PET/CT of a Patient with Treated Cervical Cancer.** The FDG-avid subcentimeter soft tissue nodule in the right pelvis *(arrow)* is new from prior imaging, and thus "suspicious" for metastasis in the MSKCC Lexicon of Diagnostic Certainty. On follow-up this lesion grew and was then biopsy-proven to be a metastasis.

cancer is suspicious for a metastasis." This is probably more helpful than a descriptive sentence such as "FDG-avid small soft tissue nodule in the pelvis," which leaves it up to the person reading the report to determine what it is. Using a system to convey your level of confidence helps the person reading your report, and encourages you to take a stand for what a finding represents. In this case, the follow-up scan demonstrated growth of the nodule and pathology and then confirmed it was a metastasis.

PET Findings Versus CT Findings

A potential pitfall in PET/CT reports is not being clear about whether you are referring to the PET or the CT. A PET/CT report may say, "Unchanged lymph node with increased FDG avidity." This is a contradiction. Is the lymph node unchanged or is there increased FDG avidity? What the radiologist meant to say was, "Unchanged size of a lymph node with increased FDG avidity."

Reference Lesions

There are often many PET and CT findings to describe in an FDG PET/CT report. This can lead to reports that are overly long and less focused in the important issues. One potential way to clarify reports is to use a topic sentence and examples. Compare the following two "thoracic nodes" sections:

THORACIC NODES:
Hypermetabolic left axillary lymph nodes measure up to 1.1 × 1.1 cm at the most superficial location, SUV 7.4. A deeper left axillary node measures 1.7 × 0.9 cm with SUV 5.8. Additional smaller hypermetabolic left axillary nodes are present. Hypermetabolic left supraclavicular lymph node measuring 1.8 × 1.2 cm, SUV 6.8. Enhancing 0.9 × 0.9 cm left supraclavicular node and adjacent smaller left supraclavicular nodes measuring up to 0.7 × 0.6 cm; however, diffuse hypermetabolism

in the supraclavicular and infraclavicular regions related to brown fat limits evaluation of FDG uptake in the supraclavicular lymph nodes.

Versus

THORACIC NODES:
FDG avid axillary and supraclavicular nodal metastases, seen among brown fat. Reference Lesions:
1. Left axillary node, 1.1 × 1.1 cm, SUV 7.4.
2. Left supraclavicular node, 1.8 × 1.2 cm, SUV 6.8.

Which example is easier to read and understand? The topic sentence with "reference lesions" (or "examples," or whatever you want to call them) is a technique that helps de-clutter and clarify reports. Many physicians have found this "reference lesion" system to be faster and more clear than the free text example above.

SUGGESTED READINGS

Boellaard R, et al: FDG PET/CT: EANM procedure guidelines for tumour imaging: version 2.0, *Eur J Nucl Med Mol Imaging* 42:328–354, 2015. PMID: 25452219.

Delbeke D, et al: Procedure guideline for tumor imaging with 18F-FDG PET/CT 1.0, *J Nucl Med* 47:885–895, 2006. PMID: 16644760.

Hillner BE, et al: Impact of positron emission tomography/computed tomography and positron emission tomography (PET) alone on expected management of patients with cancer: initial results from the National Oncologic PET Registry, *J Clin Oncol* 26:2155–2161, 2008. PMID: 18362365.

Subramaniam RM, et al: Impact on patient management of [18F]-fluorodeoxyglucose-positron emission tomography (PET) used for cancer diagnosis: analysis of data from the National Oncologic PET Registry, *Oncologist* 21:1079–1084, 2016. PMID: 27401896.

Thie JA, et al: Understanding the standarized uptake value, its methods, and implications for usage, *J Nucl Med* 45:1431–1434, 2004. PMID:15347707.

CHAPTER 3

Skeleton on FDG PET/CT

When approaching interpretation of osseous lesions on 18F-fluorodeoxyglucose positron emission topography/computed tomography (FDG PET/CT), it may be useful to use a 2 × 2 box divided into quadrants based on presence or absence of FDG avidity and malignant versus benign (Fig. 3.1). Malignancy is often FDG avid, and thus FDG PET helps to identify malignancy that is otherwise difficult to appreciate. However, it is important to remember that not all malignancy is FDG avid, and not everything that is FDG avid is malignant. The combination of the FDG PET and CT findings often allows us to properly identify a finding as benign or malignant.

FDG-AVID CANCER
Metastases

The upper right-hand corner of the 2 × 2 box is where FDG PET provides tremendous value. FDG PET often provides superior evaluation of osseous metastases than anatomic imaging such as CT and even magnetic resonance (MR). CT requires substantial alterations in the structure of bone before the lytic or sclerotic changes allow for identification of osseous malignancy. Thus FDG PET has higher sensitivity for detection of osseous malignancy than CT in most cases.

Fig. 3.2 demonstrates a patient with invasive ductal breast cancer. The patient was initially stage IIIB (locally advanced breast cancer [LABC]). LABC would be treated with neoadjuvant chemotherapy and surgery. FDG PET/CT demonstrates unsuspected distant metastases in approximately 30% of locally advanced ductal breast cancer. The identification of these previously unsuspected distant metastases increases the patient's stage to IV (metastatic disease) and changes the treatment strategy from neoadjuvant chemotherapy and surgery to palliative systemic therapy. An example of this is seen in Fig. 3.2. FDG PET/CT identified a previously unsuspected osseous metastasis, dramatically altering this patient's course of treatment. There was no definite corresponding abnormality on CT, thus the FDG PET demonstrated CT occult malignancy. Some may suggest that the osseous

lesion could have been detected by 99m-technetium methylene diphosphonate (MDP) bone scan; however, in this case a bone scan had been recently performed and failed to identify the osseous metastasis. This is a demonstration of how FDG PET/CT may replace the use of CT with bone scan for systemic staging of patients with breast cancer.

It is not uncommon for FDG PET to identify CT occult osseous metastases. Thus round foci of FDG avidity within a bone, without a CT correlate, should be considered suspicious for osseous metastases until proven otherwise (Fig. 3.3). Even small FDG-avid foci within the bone without CT correlate are significant (Fig. 3.4).

In addition to early detection of osseous metastases, FDG PET greatly adds to the follow-up of osseous metastases. It may be very difficult to determine whether osseous disease is increasing, decreasing, or unchanged on anatomic imaging, whereas FDG PET more accurately demonstrates the extent of active malignancy (Fig. 3.5).

Lymphoma

Similar as for osseous metastases, FDG PET often provides greater sensitivity for detection of osseous lymphoma than does anatomic imaging. After the diagnosis of lymphoma, common staging studies include FDG PET/CT and bone marrow biopsy. Bone marrow biopsy is usually performed in the posterior pelvis and may detect osseous lymphomatous involvement in the absence of focal FDG avidity. However, bone marrow biopsy samples only one specific osseous site, and thus body imaging with FDG PET may demonstrate foci suspicious for lymphomatous involvement in the absence of positive bone marrow biopsy. In this case, FDG PET/CT may provide localization for a potential biopsy site to pathologically document osseous lymphoma. Some studies have suggested that focal osseous FDG avidity that is suspicious for osseous lymphoma may be taken as evidence of osseous lymphoma without pathologic proof. After diagnosis, FDG PET/CT provides valuable information about response to therapy in osseous lymphoma, similar to other sites of lymphomatous involvement. The Lugano Criteria state that (for initially

	Malignant	Benign
FDG avidity +	FDG-avid cancer	FDG avid but not cancer
FDG avidity −	Not FDG avid but cancer	Not FDG avid and not cancer

FIG. 3.1 This 2 × 2 box defines categories of osseous lesions on FDG PET/CT by FDG avidity and malignant/benign.

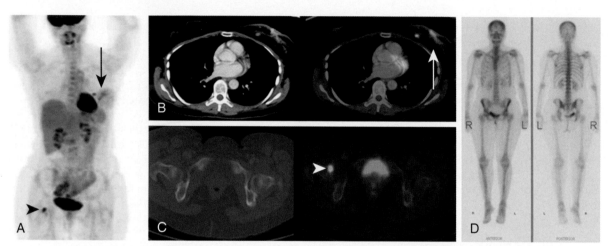

FIG. 3.2 FDG PET Identifies a Previously Unsuspected Osseous Metastasis in a Patient with Newly Diagnosed Locally Advanced Invasive Ductal Breast Cancer. (A) FDG PET maximum intensity projection demonstrates FDG avidity overlying the left chest *(arrow)* and a focus in the right lower pelvis *(arrowhead)*. (B) Axial CT and fused FDG PET/CT images through the chest demonstrate FDG avidity and correspond with multifocal breast opacities on CT, representing the patient's primary locally advanced breast malignancy *(arrow)*. (C) Axial CT and fused PET/CT images demonstrate the FDG focus in the right pelvis corresponds to the right femoral head *(arrowhead)*, without CT correlate. Biopsy of this lesion demonstrated an osseous metastasis and increased this patient's stage to IV (metastatic disease). (D) Anterior and posterior whole-body planar MDP bone scan images failed to demonstrate the osseous metastasis.

FDG-avid lymphoma) posttreatment reduction of FDG avidity to less than liver background represents a complete response to treatment, whereas residual FDG avidity greater than liver background is suspicious for residual active lymphoma.

Multiple Myeloma

Traditional staging of multiple myeloma was performed with skeletal survey radiographs; however, the use of FDG PET/CT and whole-body MR is increasing. The 2014 International Myeloma Working Group Consensus now includes FDG PET/CT criteria for diagnosis of multiple myeloma. Interestingly, it is not the presence of FDG-avid osseous lesions, but rather the presence of osteolytic osseous lesions on the CT component that is used to make the diagnosis of myeloma. Osseous

FDG avidity needs to correlate with a lytic lesion on CT, signal abnormality on MR, or biopsy-proven myeloma to be used for myeloma diagnosis. At diagnosis, multiple myeloma demonstrates a range of FDG avidity, extending from not appreciably avid to markedly FDG avid. For myeloma with appreciable FDG avidity at diagnosis, follow-up FDG PET/CT can be used to demonstrate treatment response. Changes in FDG avidity following treatment on FDG PET usually occur more rapidly than do changes apparent on CT or MR anatomic imaging.

Primary Osseous Sarcomas

FDG PET has little value in the diagnosis of primary osseous sarcomas, such as osteosarcoma or Ewing sarcoma. These sarcomas are far better diagnosed by

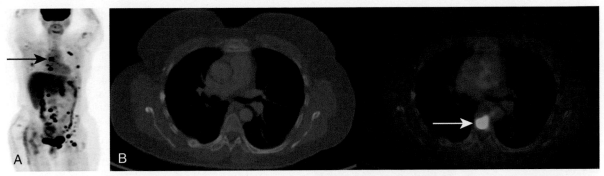

FIG. 3.3 FDG PET Identifies Previously Unsuspected Widespread Osseous Metastases in a Patient with Ductal Breast Cancer. (A) FDG PET maximum intensity projection (MIP) demonstrates multiple FDG-avid foci, for example in the mid-thorax *(arrow)*. (B) Axial CT and fused FDG PET/CT images demonstrate the focus in the mid-thorax localizes to a vertebral body *(arrow)*, without CT correlate. Similar findings were found for the other FDG-avid foci. These represent previously unsuspected widespread osseous metastatic disease.

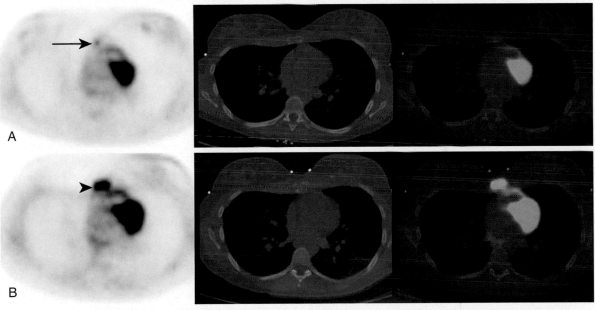

FIG. 3.4 Small FDG-avid Osseous Focus Is an Early Metastasis. (A) Axial FDG PET, axial CT, and fused FDG PET images demonstrate a small focus of FDG avidity which localizes to the sternum *(arrow)*, without CT correlate. This was called suspicious for osseous metastasis, although this was the only suspicious finding and there was no change in patient management. (B) Axial FDG PET, axial CT, and fused FDG PET images 6 months later demonstrate an increased FDG-avid osseous metastasis *(arrowhead)* now with a lytic correlate on CT.

radiograph, CT, or MR imaging. FDG PET/CT could be used for systemic staging of osseous sarcomas because sites of osseous metastases may be detected by whole-body imaging. Lung metastases, a common site of metastatic disease from primary sarcomas, are probably better evaluated by dedicated chest CT imaging than by FDG PET/CT because dedicated chest CT imaging can be performed with breath-hold, which increases the ability to detect small pulmonary lesions. The CT component of FDG PET/CT is typically performed during

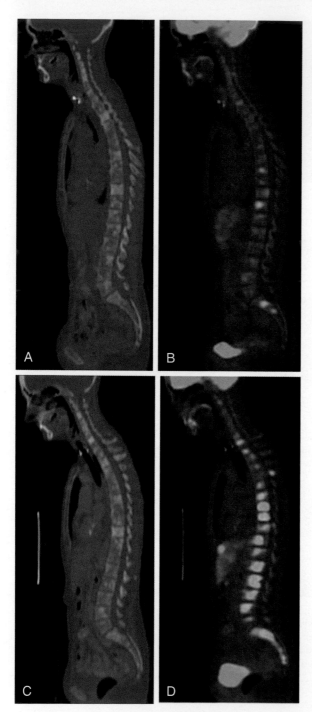

FIG. 3.5 **Increased Osseous Metastases Better Demonstrated on FDG PET and CT.** (A) Baseline sagittal CT and (B) sagittal fused FDG PET/CT demonstrate several FDG-avid osseous metastases with more extensive non–FDG-avid osseous sclerotic lesions. (C) Follow-up sagittal CT and (D) sagittal fused FDG PET/CT. No change can be appreciated on the follow-up CT; however, follow-up FDG PET demonstrates markedly increased FDG-avid osseous malignancy, as well as a new focus of hepatic malignancy.

free breathing, for the CT component to be registered to the FDG PET component (which may take 20 to 30 minutes to acquire so breath-hold is not possible), which limits visualization of small pulmonary lesions.

NOT FDG AVID AND NOT CANCER

The lower left-hand corner of the 2 × 2 box demonstrates an additional area of value for FDG PET. Following treatment, it is often more difficult to determine the extent of treatment response on anatomic imaging compared with FDG PET. Indeed, treatment response cannot be confused with new malignancy on CT. For example, in Fig. 3.6, a patient with breast cancer at baseline demonstrates FDG-avid osseous lesions that are occult on CT. Following treatment, the FDG-avid foci resolve, but there are new sclerotic osseous lesions on the CT. Because osseous metastases in patients with breast cancer may be lytic or sclerotic on CT, the appearance of new sclerotic osseous lesions on the follow-up examination could be mistaken for new osseous metastases on the CT. However, the correlating FDG PET data demonstrate that the osseous metastases have been successfully treated, and the new sclerotic lesions on CT are due to treatment response rather than to new osseous malignancy.

It is important to remember that osseous lesions often become more sclerotic on CT following successful treatment, and this should not be confused with disease progression. Fig. 3.7 demonstrates a patient with initially lytic osseous lesions that become more sclerotic following treatment. Perhaps the most confusing scenario is when the osseous malignancy is initially sclerotic and the lesions become larger or more sclerotic following treatment (Fig. 3.8). Whether the osseous metastases are lytic, sclerotic, or occult on CT, changes in FDG avidity on FDG PET are almost always more valuable in determining treatment response than are changes on CT.

Another scenario in which FDG PET can provide superior assessment of treatment response is following

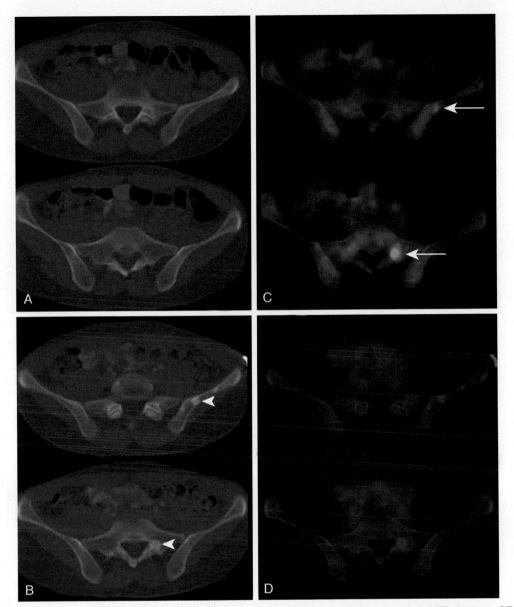

FIG. 3.6 **Treatment Response in Osseous Metastases Better Visualized by FDG PET than on CT.**
(A) Two axial CT images from a patient with breast cancer at baseline. (B) Two axial CT images at follow-up demonstrate new sclerotic osseous lesions *(arrowheads)*. The new osseous lesions could be interpreted as new osseous metastases. (C) Two axial FDG PET images from this patient at baseline. This patient has FDG-avid osseous metastases *(arrows)* which are occult on CT. (D) Two axial FDG PET images at follow-up demonstrate that the FDG-avid osseous metastases resolved following treatment. The new sclerotic osseous lesions seen on PET/CT are a treatment response, not new osseous malignancy.

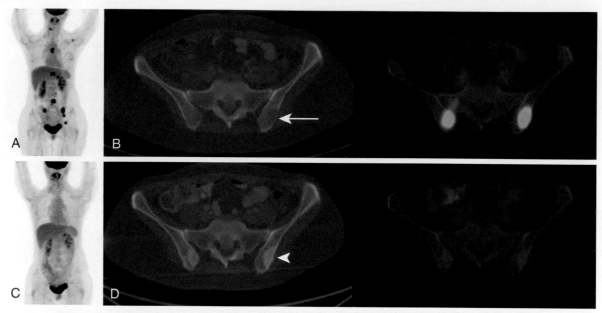

FIG. 3.7 Treatment Response in Osseous Metastases. (A) Axial maximum intensity projection (MIP) demonstrates multiple FDG-avid lesions. (B) Axial CT and fused PET/CT images demonstrate these foci localize to lytic osseous metastases on CT *(arrow)*. (C) Axial MIP following treatment demonstrates resolution of the FDG-avid lesions. (D) Axial CT and fused PET/CT images demonstrate resolution of FDG-avid sclerotic osseous lesions, as well as increased sclerosis of the previously lytic osseous lesions *(arrowhead)*. The increased sclerosis of the osseous lesions on CT is a treatment response.

interventional procedures such as ablations (Fig. 3.9). Following an ablation, the treated lesion on anatomic imaging is often larger than the original malignancy. This is because a rim of tissue around the malignancy is also ablated to increase the likelihood that the margins of the tumor have been killed. The resulting CT lesion following an ablation may be confused with increased malignancy, particularly if the history of an interval ablation was not provided. On the other hand, the resolution of FDG avidity within the lesion on FDG PET more accurately depicts successful treatment.

NOT FDG AVID BUT CANCER

The lower left-hand corner of the 2 × 2 box is an area of concern for correct interpretation of FDG PET/CT. Because FDG PET often demonstrates malignancy that may not be apparent on CT, it is sometimes forgotten that not all malignancy is FDG avid. It is the opinion of the author that it is still the responsibility of the interpreting physician to evaluate the CT component of FDG PET/CT for evidence of malignancy that is not apparent on the FDG PET. For the skeleton, that means being aware that some histologies of malignancy are

more likely to produce non–FDG-avid osseous metastases, such as lobular breast cancers. Lobular breast cancer is a histology of malignancy that is clinically and molecularly distinct from the more common ductal breast cancers. Lobular breast cancers are more difficult to visualize on all current imaging modalities, including mammogram, ultrasound, MR, and FDG PET. However, the reaction to the malignancy in bone may produce osseous lesions that are not apparent on FDG PET. Thus the appearance of new osseous lesions on CT following a diagnosis of malignancy may represent osseous metastases, even if lacking FDG avidity (Fig. 3.10).

FDG AVID BUT NOT CANCER

The lower left-hand corner of the 2 × 2 box is another area of concern for correct interpretation of FDG PET/CT. There are many causes of FDG avidity in the skeleton which do not represent malignancy. These need to be recognized as benign because, overall, calling it malignancy may have adverse effects on patient care, as well as reduce confidence in FDG PET/CT as an imaging modality for referring physicians. It may be impossible to describe all of the potential causes of benign FDG

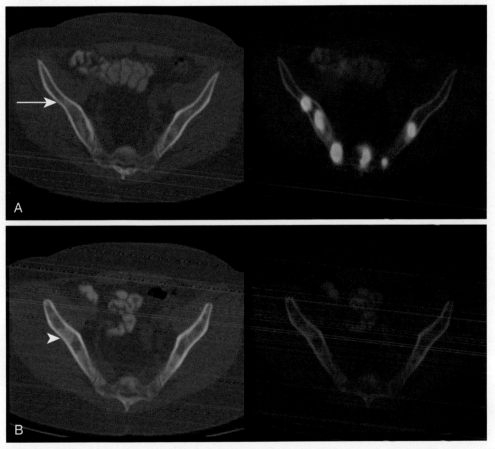

FIG. 3.8 **Treatment Response in Osseous Metastases Better Visualized by FDG PET than on CT.**
(A) Axial CT and axial fused PET/CT images from a patient with breast cancer at baseline demonstrate multiple FDG-avid sclerotic osseous metastases *(arrow)*. (B) Axial CT and axial fused PET/CT images following treatment demonstrate increased sclerosis of the osseous lesions on CT *(arrowhead)*. This could represent increased malignancy or decreased malignancy with treatment response, and these two possibilities are very difficult to distinguish on CT. The corresponding FDG PET data demonstrate resolution of the FDG-avid lesions and are far more clear in demonstrating successful treatment response.

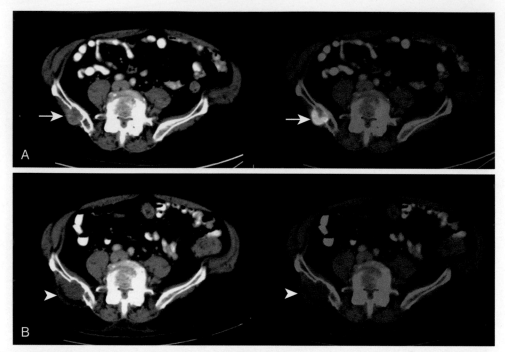

FIG. 3.9 Ablation Response in Osseous Metastases Better Visualized by FDG PET than on CT. (A) Axial CT and axial fused PET/CT images from a patient with breast cancer at baseline demonstrate an FDG-avid osseous metastasis with adjacent soft tissue mass *(arrows)*. This mass was causing pain, and thus the patient was referred for CT-guided ablation of the mass by interventional radiology. (B) Axial CT and axial fused PET/CT images following the ablation. A CT performed the same day as the FDG PET was interpreted as an increased metastasis, probably because the interpreting radiologist was unaware of the interval ablation. On the FDG PET/CT, the mass may have increased in size, but the FDG avidity resolved *(arrowheads)*, demonstrating successful treatment response and prompting investigation into an interval procedure. The medical record confirmed an interval ablation. The rim of mildly FDG avidity surrounding the ablation is a common finding on FDG PET following ablations and represents damaged tissue at the ablation margin.

avidity in the skeleton, but many of the most common and the most commonly mistaken causes of benign osseous FDG avidity are described next.

Granulocyte Colony-Stimulating Factors

Patients with malignancy may suffer from bone marrow suppression, which may be treated with bone marrow–stimulating agents such as colony-stimulating factors. The use of colony-stimulating factors causes homogenously increased FDG avidity within bone marrow. Even if the history of colony-stimulating factor use is not provided, the appearance of bone marrow repopulation needs to be distinguished from osseous malignancy on FDG PET/CT (Fig. 3.11). One clue is a homogeneous appearance of increased FDG, without CT correlate. Another clue is the presence of increased FDG avidity in the spleen, which also repopulates in response to colony-stimulating factors. FDG-avid bone marrow

repopulation usually lasts longer than the FDG-avid splenic repopulation area, so FDG-avid bone marrow repopulation may be seen without corresponding findings in the spleen. How long colony-stimulating factors produce changes on FDG PET depends on the colony-stimulating factor used. Short-acting colony-stimulating factors such as filgrastim (Neupogen) may result in FDG-avid bone marrow repopulation that lasts 1 to 2 weeks. Longer-acting colony-stimulating factors such as pegfilgrastim (Neulasta) may result in FDG-avid bone marrow repopulation that lasts 1 to 2 months. Particularly problematic is the possibility of an FDG-avid malignancy that underlies FDG-avid bone marrow repopulation. It may be difficult, if not impossible, to evaluate for the underlying FDG-avid malignancy. One possibility for improving the evaluation of underlying malignancy is adjusting the FDG PET window level. If malignancy is more FDG avid than the bone marrow

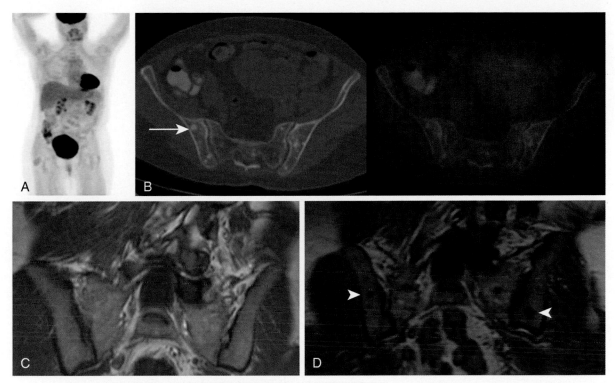

FIG. 3.10 Non–FDG-avid Osseous Metastases. (A) Axial maximum intensity projection (MIP) in a patient with lobular breast cancer following mastectomy, but before systemic therapy, does not demonstrate any FDG avidity suspicious for malignancy. (B) Axial CT and fused PET/CT images demonstrate multiple sclerotic osseous lesions with background FDG avidity *(arrow)*. These sclerotic osseous lesions could be multiple bone islands, such as in a patient with osteopoikilosis; however, not FDG-avid osseous metastases need to be considered. Coronal magnetic resonance (MR) images of the sacrum before (C) and after (D) the diagnosis breast cancer demonstrate that the osseous lesions are new *(arrowheads)*, and thus suspicious for metastases. Biopsy confirmed non–FDG-avid osseous metastases. Recognizing the potential for non–FDG-avid osseous metastases helped appropriately stage this patient.

repopulation, then adjusting the FDG PET to a higher maximum window level may help to visualize the underlying FDG-avid malignancy (Fig. 3.12).

Degenerative Changes

Common sources of benign FDG avidity involving the skeleton are degenerative changes. Degenerative changes may recruit inflammatory cells which result in the visualization of focal FDG avidity on FDG PET. Fortunately, the CT component of an FDG PET/CT can be used to help distinguish benign FDG-avid osseous degenerative changes from FDG-avid malignancy. First, FDG-avid foci in osseous structures on both sides of a joint probably represent a joint-centered, rather than a bone-centered, process. Joint-centered FDG avidity is more commonly benign. Of course, FDG PET and CT images need to be evaluated to make sure registration

is good and there is no misregistration between the FDG PET and CT images. Second, CT findings that correlate with degenerative processes (joint space narrowing, osteophyte, subchondral cysts) can be used to help recognize a lesion as benign and degenerative. Common sites of FDG-avid degenerative changes are the hip (Fig. 3.13), spine (Figs. 3.14 and 3.15), and even sternomanubrial joint (Fig. 3.16). For the spine and sternomanubrial joint, axial images may be misleading. Comparison with sagittal images may help to better classify FDG-avid findings.

An important guideline to remember, bone-centered FDG avidity, even without a CT correlate, is often malignant. Joint-centered FDG avidity is usually benign, and consider benign etiologies such as degenerative changes and inflammatory arthropathies. Of course, rare

Text continued on p. 23

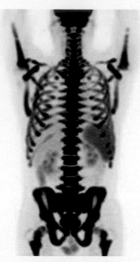

FIG. 3.11 **FDG-avid Bone Marrow Repopulation Resulting from the Use of Colony-Stimulating Factors.** Axial maximum intensity projection (MIP) demonstrates diffuse increased FDG avidity in the bone marrow and spleen in a patient who recently received Neupogen. The presence of FDG-avid bone marrow repopulation limits evaluation of underlying FDG avid malignancy.

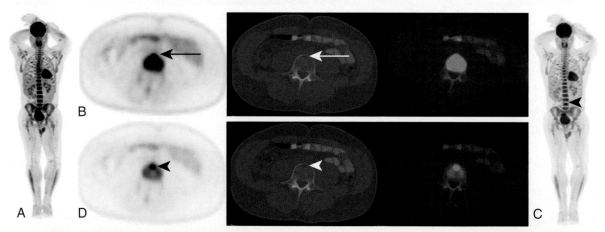

FIG. 3.12 **Altering the PET Window Level to Help Evaluate for FDG-avid Osseous Malignancy Underlying FDG-avid Bone Marrow Repopulation in a Patient with Multiple Myeloma.** (A) Axial maximum intensity projection (MIP), set with an upper limit of 5 (all FDG avid foci within standardized uptake value maximum of 5 or greater appear black) demonstrates homogenous widespread FDG avidity in the bone marrow. This patient had recently received colony-stimulating factors, resulting in the bone marrow repopulation. This could make it difficult to evaluate for underlying FDG-avid osseous malignancy. (B) Axial PET, CT, and fused PET/CT images demonstrate a lytic lesion in the L4 vertebral body. FDG-avid bone marrow repopulation makes it difficult to determine if this is a site of active malignancy *(arrows)*. (C) Axial MIP, set with an upper limit of 10, demonstrates a more focal area of FDG avidity in the L4 vertebral body *(arrowhead)*, greater than the FDG-avid bone marrow repopulation. (D) Axial PET, CT, and fused PET/CT images demonstrate this FDG focus corresponds to the lytic lesion *(arrowheads)*. In this example, changing the PET window level was able to distinguish the FDG-avid osseous malignancy because in this case the FDG-avid malignancy was more avid than the benign bone marrow repopulation.

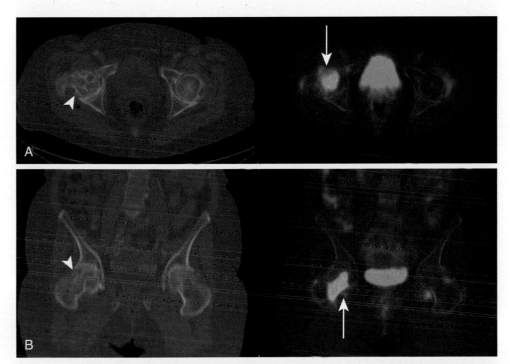

FIG. 3.13 **Benign FDG-avid Degenerative Changes in the Hip.** (A) Axial CT and fused PET/CT, as well as (B) coronal CT and fused PET/CT, demonstrate FDG avidity overlying the right femoral head *(arrows)* and corresponding to lucent changes on CT. These findings would first raise suspicion for osseous metastasis. However, the CT images demonstrate joint space narrowing and osteophytes *(arrowheads)*, which represent degenerative changes. The lucent changes in the right femoral head are actually subchondral cysts, part of the spectrum of degenerative changes. The fact that this patient has a head/neck malignancy (base of tongue squamous cell carcinoma), which almost always metastasizes to the lung before other distant metastatic sites, further increases confidence in the diagnosis. Benign degenerative FDG avidity can be confused with FDG-avid osseous metastases.

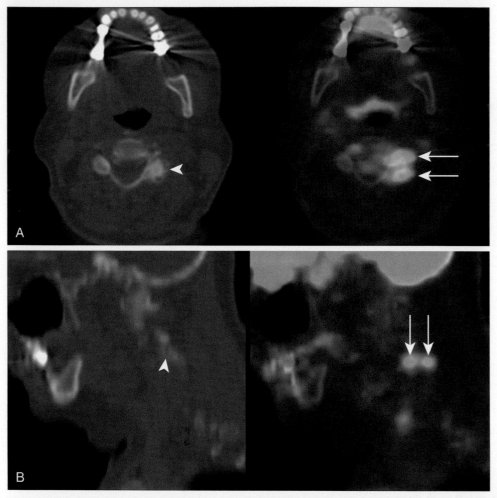

FIG. 3.14 (A) Axial CT and fused PET/CT, as well as (B) sagittal CT and fused PET/CT, demonstrate foci of FDG avidity in the cervical spine *(arrows)*, corresponding with mixed sclerotic/lucent changes on CT *(arrowhead* in A). However, note on the sagittal images of the FDG-avid foci are on both sides of a facet joint CT *(arrowhead* in B). Joint-centered FDG avidity is usually benign, as in this case of degenerative changes. The mixed sclerotic/lucent changes on CT are benign degenerative changes in the cervical spine. Again, benign degenerative FDG avidity can be confused with FDG-avid osseous metastases. Comparison with sagittal images may help to reclassify FDG-avid findings in the spine.

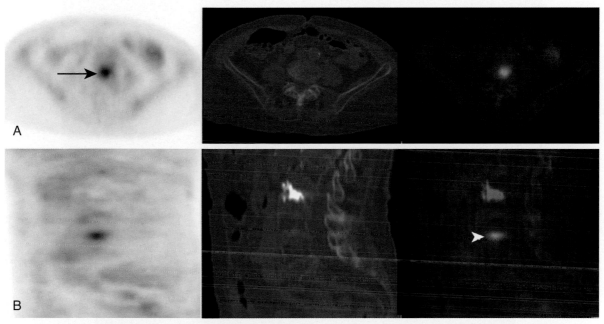

FIG. 3.15 Benign FDG-avid Degenerative Changes in the Spine. (A) Axial PET, CT, and fused PET/CT through the lumbar spine demonstrates an FDG-avid focus overlying the region of the lumbar vertebra *(arrow)*. (B) Sagittal PET, CT, and fused PET/CT demonstrate that the FDG avidity localizes to the intervertebral disk *(arrowhead)*, rather than a vertebra. Joint-centered FDG avidity is usually benign. The fact that this patient has a head/neck malignancy (buccal squamous cell carcinoma), which almost always metastasizes to the lung before other distant metastatic sites, further increases confidence in the diagnosis. Be careful that benign degenerative FDG avidity is not mistaken for FDG-avid osseous metastases. Comparison with sagittal images may help interpretation of FDG-avid findings in the spine.

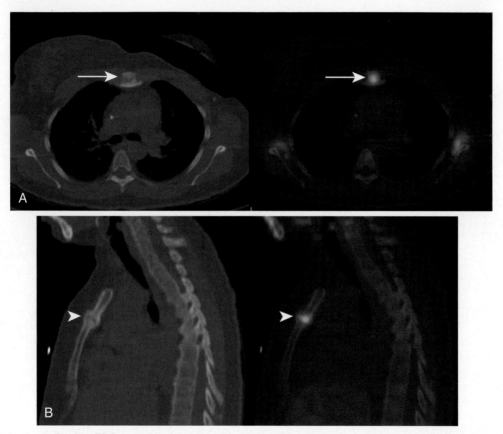

FIG. 3.16 **Benign FDG-avid Degenerative Changes in the Sternomanubrial Joint.** (A) Axial CT and fused PET/CT demonstrates an FDG-avid focus overlying the sternum, possibly corresponding with a sclerotic lesion on CT *(arrows)*. (B) Sagittal CT and fused PET/CT demonstrate that the FDG avidity localizes to the sternomanubrial joint *(arrowheads)*, rather than the sternum. Joint-centered FDG avidity is usually benign. Benign degenerative FDG avidity can be mistaken for FDG-avid osseous metastases. Comparison with sagittal images may help to reclassify FDG-avid findings in the spine.

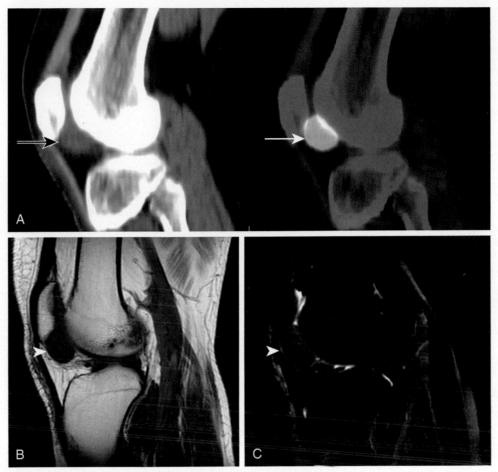

FIG. 3.17 **FDG-avid Pigmented Villonodular Synovitis (PVNS).** (A) Sagittal CT and fused PET/CT demonstrates an FDG-avid soft tissue mass in the knee joint *(arrows)*. (B) Sagittal T1 and (C) sagittal T2 fat-saturated
magnetic resonance (MR) images demonstrate the mass has low T1 and T2 signal *(arrowheads)*, consistent
with PVNS.

joint-centered neoplasms, such as pigmented villonodular synovitis (PVNS), need to be excluded (Fig. 3.17). PVNS is an idiopathic overgrowth of the synovium with potential for local aggressive growth. PVNS may be FDG avid and should be included in the differential of FDG-avid joint masses.

Inflammatory Diseases

Multiple inflammatory arthropathies may be FDG avid and confused with malignancy. Rheumatoid arthritis is associated with symmetric joint space narrowing, marginal erosions, osteopenia, and subluxations. Active inflammation associated with arthritis may be FDG avid. Likewise, rheumatoid-related arthropathies such as systemic lupus erythematosus, scleroderma, or

dermatomyositis may have FDG-avid arthropathy. The seronegative spondyloarthropathies such as psoriasis (Fig. 3.18), reactive arthritis, ankylosing spondylitis, and arthritis associated with inflammatory bowel disease have all been shown to demonstrate FDG-avid joint-centered abnormalities. Septic arthritis may be particularly FDG avid, with clinical features such as fever and elevated white cell counts leading to the diagnosis. A key feature of these inflammatory arthropathies is that the FDG avidity is joint centered, which helps to distinguish these benign etiologies from bone-centered malignancies.

Fractures

Fractures elicit an inflammatory response that is often FDG avid. It is difficult to predict how long a benign

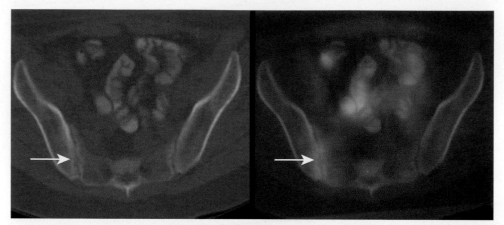

FIG. 3.18 Benign FDG-avid Inflammation Associated with Psoriatic Arthritis. Axial CT and fused PET/CT through the pelvis demonstrates FDG avidity in the region of the right sacroiliac joint *(arrows)*. The corresponding CT demonstrates loss of cortex and erosions on both sides of the joint, consistent with a benign joint-centered process in this patient with known psoriasis.

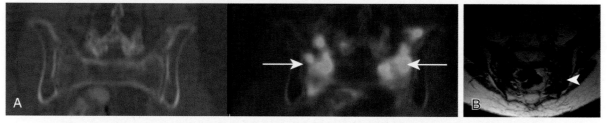

FIG. 3.19 Benign FDG Avidity Associated with Bilateral Sacral Insufficiency Fractures. (A) Coronal CT and fused PET/CT through the pelvis demonstrates bilateral sacral FDG avidity *(arrows)*. No other notable FDG avidity was apparent on the FDG PET/CT scan. (B) T1-weighted magnetic resonance (MR) imaging demonstrates the preservation of high T1 signal fat within the areas of FDG avidity *(arrowhead)*, which highly favors benign sacral insufficiency fracture, rather than osseous malignancy which would replace the high T1-signal marrow fat.

fracture will remain FDG avid. Fractures at sites where the fracture edges may rub against each other, such as rib fractures, may remain FDG avid for long periods. It is sometimes also difficult to distinguish a benign fracture from a more ominous malignant pathologic fracture. Some clues that may help to make this distinction include the corresponding CT finding, morphology of the FDG avidity (linear vs. rounded), and location of fracture. Multiple adjacent rib fractures are almost always benign and traumatic in etiology, as would be seen on an MDP bone scan. Bilateral sacral FDG avidity, without additional osseous foci, should raise the possibility of benign sacral insufficiency fractures (Fig. 3.19). A linear morphology of the FDG avidity favors a benign compression fracture in a vertebra (Fig. 3.20) because most osseous malignancies grow as a round tumor focus. More difficult to recognize are less common forms of fracture, such as Hill-Sachs fractures (Fig. 3.21).

Often, it takes correlation of PET findings, CT findings, and the clinical scenario to best distinguish benign FDG-avid fractures from FDG-avid osseous malignancy. Magnetic resonance imaging (MRI) may be useful in distinguishing benign from pathologic fractures because the preservation of high T1-signal intensity fat within a fractured bone may help to exclude a marrow-replacing malignancy.

Bone Infarcts (Avascular Necrosis of Bone)

Bone infarcts may be FDG photopenic, demonstrate increased FDG avidity, or demonstrate FDG avidity similar to background bone, depending upon the individual lesion. During the acute bone infarction, there is lack of blood flow to the involved bone, and thus the lesion will appear FDG photopenic. Remember that in addition to uptake of FDG through glucose transport proteins, FDG avidity is also dependent upon blood

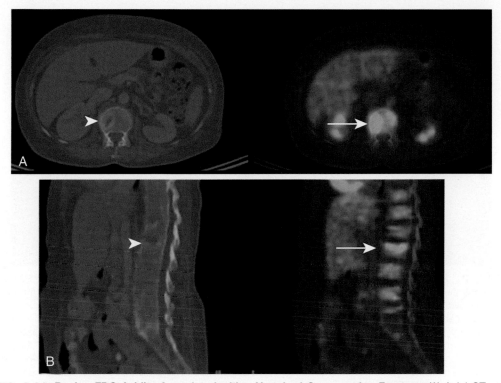

FIG. 3.20 Benign FDG Avidity Associated with a Vertebral Compression Fracture. (A) Axial CT and fused PET/CT demonstrate an FDG-avid focus corresponding to a vertebral body *(arrow)*. The axial CT image demonstrates a mixed sclerotic/lucent lesion at the site of FDG avidity *(arrowhead)*. (B) Sagittal CT and fused FDG PET/CT better evaluate this lesion than axial imaging. Sagittal CT demonstrates the typical appearance of a superior end plate compression fracture *(arrowhead)*. Sagittal PET demonstrates linear morphology to the FDG avidity in the superior end plate *(arrow)*, more consistent with a benign compression fracture rather than a malignant pathologic fracture.

flow. An area with no current blood flow will lack a mechanism to deliver FDG to this site, and thus the lesion will appear FDG photopenic. After the acute bone infarction, blood flow may return. During this phase, repairing bone may demonstrate increased FDG avidity compared with background bone. Clues to diagnosing bone infarcts on FDG PET/CT include the serpentine morphology of FDG avidity in the lesion, as well as corresponding serpentine sclerosis seen on CT images (Fig. 3.22). Bone infarcts may be idiopathic and are also associated with alcohol use, pregnancy, and pancreatitis. They are also commonly associated with exogenous steroids, which may be part of cancer therapy.

Paget Disease
Paget disease (also known as osteitis deformans) is a disorder of bone remodeling, with both early-phase excessive bone reabsorption and later abnormal bone deposition. This may affect the single bone or be multifocal. Pagetoid bone is weaker than normal bone, despite often being larger and more sclerotic than normal bone. Paget disease is common in people older than 50 years. The majority of patients with Paget disease are asymptomatic, and imaging may be the first time manifestations of the disease are encountered. On FDG PET, Paget disease may be FDG photopenic, demonstrate increased FDG avidity, or demonstrate FDG avidity similar to background bone, depending upon the individual lesion. Active Paget disease may be FDG avid and could easily be confused with osseous malignancy. Often, it is the corresponding CT characteristics of the FDG-avid bone which demonstrate benign Paget disease rather than osseous malignancy (Fig. 3.23). These CT characteristics include expansion of the bone, thickening of the cortex, and coarsening of the trabeculae.

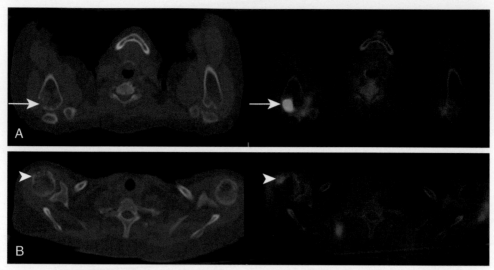

FIG. 3.21 **Benign FDG Avidity Associated with a Hill-Sachs Fracture.** (A) Axial CT and fused PET/CT demonstrate an FDG-avid focus corresponding to a lytic lesion in the superolateral right humerus *(arrows)*. An FDG-avid lytic lesion would initially raise suspicion for an osseous metastasis. However, this patient has colon cancer, without evidence of other metastatic disease. It would be highly unusual for colon cancer to first distantly metastasize to bone, thus an alternative explanation was sought. (B) Axial CT and fused FDG PET/CT of the patient 1 year previously demonstrate that the osseous lesion was present on CT but not FDG avid *(arrowheads)*. (Different rotation of the arm results in a different apparent position of the lesion on CT but was consistently in the superolateral aspect of the humerus.) This patient had recurrent right shoulder dislocations, and the FDG-avid humerus lesion represented an acutely inflamed Hill-Sachs fracture, rather than an osseous metastasis. This case demonstrates how correlation of the FDG PET images, CT images, and clinical scenario allows for the best interpretation of imaging findings.

Transient Osteoporosis of the Hip

Transient osteoporosis of the hip (TOH) is characterized by bone pain, osteopenia, and bone marrow edema in the absence of trauma. Usually it is transient, requires no treatment, and resolves spontaneously. When sufficient bone loss occurs, TOH may be visualized on radiographs or CT. TOH has been shown to be FDG avid and may be confused with osseous malignancy (Fig. 3.24). MR demonstrates a characteristic pattern of bone marrow edema, often with preservation of high T1-signal fat within the marrow, which can distinguish benign TOH and prevent misdiagnosis as a more aggressive process.

Benign Neoplasms

As we have seen, FDG avidity is not specific for malignancy. Benign neoplasms represent an additional category of pathology which may be FDG avid and must be distinguish from malignancy. Characteristic imaging findings on the CT component of an FDG PET/CT may be critical for distinguishing benign neoplasms from osseous malignancy. For example, the ring and arc

appearance of chondroid neoplasms on CT will greatly assist in the diagnosis of these lesions (Fig. 3.25). If necessary, plain radiographs could be obtained to further evaluate the ring and arc morphology of chondroid calcifications, which may be more easily characterized on radiograph than on FDG PET/CT.

Nonossifying Fibromas

Nonossifying fibromas are the most common nonneoplastic fibrous bone lesion. They are common in children and adolescents, and extremely uncommon over the age of 30. The term "nonossifying" may be a misnomer because during adolescence these lesions spontaneously heal and ossify. The majority of nonossifying fibromas are asymptomatic, although larger lesions may be painful and lead to pathologic fracture. These lesions usually occur in the metaphysis of long bones, most commonly the metaphysis of the distal femur or proximal tibia. Although the majority of nonossifying fibromas are not of clinical concern, and if it has been labeled a "touch" lesion, their incidental detection on radiologic examinations may lead to

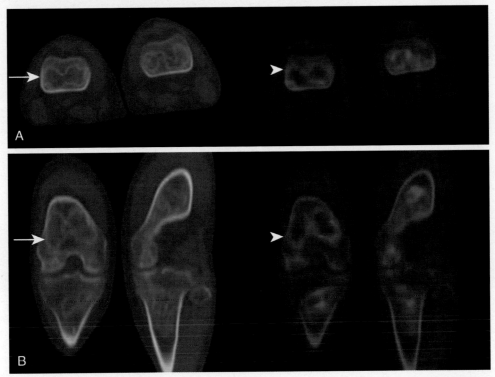

FIG. 3.22 **Benign FDG Avidity Associated with Bone Infarcts.** (A) Axial CT and fused PET/CT through the distal femur in a patient with long-term steroid use demonstrate FDG-avid bilateral osseous sclerotic lesions. (B) Coronal CT and fused FDG PET/CT demonstrate the lesions are apparent in the distal femur as well as the proximal tibia. Both the CT lesions *(arrows)* and the FDG avidity *(arrowheads)* are serpentine in morphology. The serpentine morphology, as well as the location in the distal femur and proximal tibias, strongly favors benign avascular necrosis.

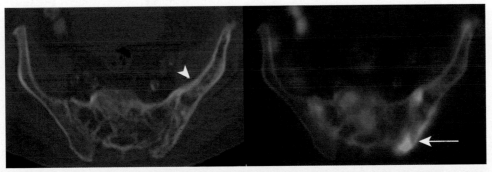

FIG. 3.23 **Benign FDG Avidity Associated with Paget Disease.** Axial CT and fused PET/CT through the pelvis in a patient with Merkle cell carcinoma demonstrate an FDG-avid osseous lesion in the left ilium *(arrow)*. An FDG-avid osseous lesion initially raises suspicion or malignancy. However, corresponding CT images demonstrate expansion of the bone compared with the contralateral normal side *(arrowhead)*, cortical thickening, and coarsening of the trabeculae. These findings would be unusual in an osseous metastasis. This patient has benign osseous Paget disease, which needs to be distinguished from osseous malignancy.

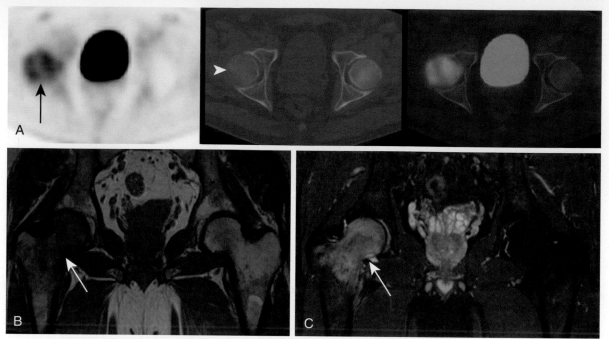

FIG. 3.24 **Benign FDG Avidity Associated with Transient Osteoporosis of the Hip (TOH).** (A) Axial PET, CT, and fused PET/CT through the pelvis in a patient with leukemia, currently on observation, demonstrate FDG avidity in the right femoral head *(arrow)*. The corresponding CT image demonstrates subtle lucency in the region of FDG avidity *(arrowhead)*, compared with the contralateral normal left femoral head. The presence of FDG-avid osseous leukemia could alter patient management and induce more aggressive therapy. (B) Coronal T1-weighted magnetic resonance (MR) demonstrates areas of preserved high T1 signal fat within the area of abnormality *(arrow)*. The preservation of the marrow fat demonstrates that the low signal abnormality is not a mass lesion which would focally replace marrow fat. (C) Coronal T2-weighted MR demonstrates high T2 signal edema *(arrow)*. This MR appearance is characteristic of the bone marrow edema seen in TOH and helps to prevent a misdiagnosis of osseous malignancy.

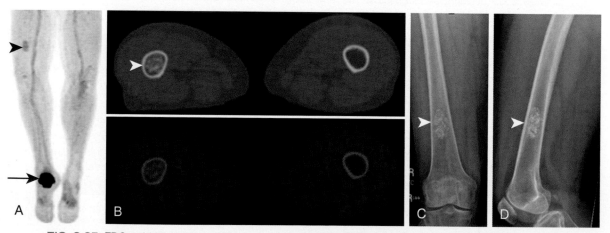

FIG. 3.25 **FDG-avid Malignant Angiosarcoma but Benign FDG-avid Enchondroma.** (A) PET maximum intensity projection (MIP) demonstrates an FDG-avid lesion in the right foot *(arrow)*, which corresponds with a lytic destructive mass on axial images (images not show). There is also a mildly FDG-avid focus in the right thigh *(arrowhead)*. (B) Axial CT-infused PET/CT images demonstrate the right thigh focus represents a moderately FDG-avid lesion localizing to the right femur *(arrowhead)*. If this were a metastasis, it could dramatically change patient management and prognosis. However, CT images demonstrate benign-appearing patchy sclerosis. (C) Anteroposterior and (D) lateral radiographs were obtained for further characterization. Radiographs more definitively demonstrate the ring and arc calcifications of a low-grade chondroid neoplasm *(arrowheads)*, probably an enchondroma.

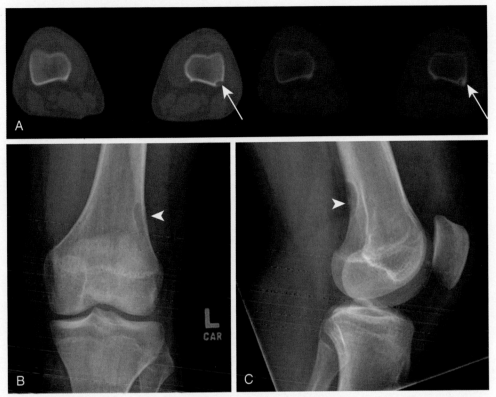

FIG. 3.26 Benign FDG-avid Nonossifying Fibroma in a 16-Year-Old Boy with Treated Left Shoulder Soft Tissue Sarcoma. (A) Axial CT and fused PET/CT demonstrate an FDG-avid lytic lesion in the distal left femur *(arrows)*. An FDG-avid lytic lesion at first raises suspicion of an osseous metastasis. However, the age of the patient (16 years) and the location of the lesion (distal femoral metaphysis) would be typical of a benign nonossifying fibroma. (B) Anteroposterior and (C) lateral radiographs demonstrate the well-circumscribed lucency and sclerotic rim of a benign nonossifying fibroma *(arrowheads)*. The radiograph confirms this is a "don't touch me" lesion, and biopsy is not necessary.

an appropriate intervention such as biopsy. The age of the patient and the location of the lesion within the bone are critical for recognize this benign entity. For example, a well-circumscribed distal metaphyseal lesion in a teenager would have the age and location typical of a benign nonossifying fibroma (Fig. 3.26). If necessary, plain radiographs could be obtained for further evaluation to demonstrate the well-circumscribed lucency with sclerotic border characteristic of this benign lesion.

Biopsy Tracts

Bone biopsies are commonly performed for diagnosis of osseous lesions and evaluation of the bone marrow in patients with lymphoid malignancy. Often, the history of a recent bone marrow biopsy is unknown to radiologists evaluating imaging studies including FDG PET/CT.

Recent bone marrow biopsies may be FDG avid and mistaken for osseous malignancy. Consider the case of a patient with lymphoma in a single biopsied lymph node. This patient will likely undergo bone marrow biopsy for marrow stage, as well as a staging FDG PET/CT. Because the presence of FDG-avid osseous lesions on PET/CT will often be considered evidence of osseous lymphoma, even given benign findings on the bone marrow biopsy, the accurate evaluation of the skeleton on the FDG PET/CT is critical. The misdiagnosis of osseous lymphoma on FDG PET/CT will upstage the patient's lymphoma and have an effect on the patient management. Fig. 3.27 demonstrates an early-stage lymphoma patient who underwent bone marrow biopsy in the left pelvis prior to the staging FDG PET/CT. The extension of linear FDG avidity into the soft tissues overlying the osseous FDG avidity demonstrates that

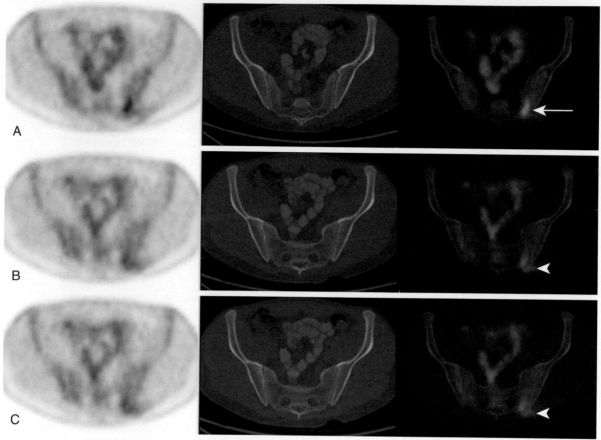

FIG. 3.27 **Benign FDG-avid Biopsy Tract in a Patient with Early-Stage Notable Lymphoma and a Recent Bone Marrow Biopsy.** (A) Axial PET, CT, and fused PET/CT demonstrate an FDG-avid focus in the left sacrum *(arrow)*. If this is interpreted as osseous lymphoma, this would have had a substantial impact on the patient's staging and treatment. (B and C) However, axial PET, CT, and fused PET/CT images from adjacent imaging sections demonstrate the linear morphology of the biopsy tract and extension to the overlying soft tissues *(arrowheads)*. This is recognized as benign FDG-avid inflammation from a recent bone marrow biopsy, rather than osseous lymphoma.

this is benign inflammation from a recent biopsy tract, rather than an FDG-avid osseous lymphoma.

Radiation-Induced Osteoradionecrosis

Radiotherapy is a component of the treatment of many malignancies. Osteoradionecrosis is a benign complication of bone within external beam radiation ports. Often, the radiation port is unknown to the interpreting radiologist; however, imaging findings may suggest prior radiation therapy. Finding an FDG-avid destructive osseous lesion in a prior radiation port is a conundrum for the interpreting radiologist because benign osteoradionecrosis, as well as malignant etiologies including metastases and primary radiation-associated

sarcoma, may have very similar CT and FDG PET appearance. In fact, it may be difficult to distinguish benign osteoradionecrosis from malignancy on all current imaging modalities. The identification of an FDG-avid destructive lesion in a known radiation port should prompt consideration of a biopsy to distinguish between benign and malignant potential lesions. Fig. 3.28 demonstrates an FDG-avid destructive sternal lesion within a prior radiation port for breast cancer therapy. This was benign osteoradionecrosis; however, malignancy would have similar imaging characteristics and biopsy is needed for diagnosis. Fig. 3.29 demonstrates an FDG-avid destructive clavicular lesion within a prior radiation port for thyroid cancer therapy. This was a biopsy-proven

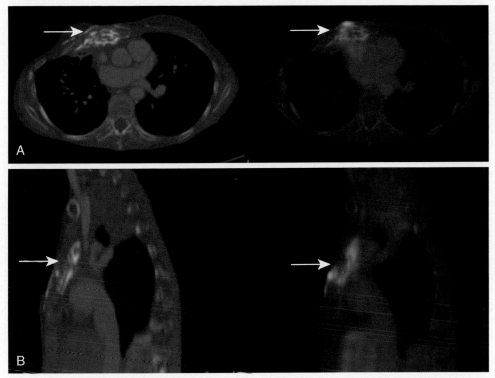

FIG. 3.28 **Benign FDG-avid Osteoradionecrosis of the Sternum in a Patient Previously Treated with External Beam Radiation for Breast Cancer.** (A) Axial CT and fused PET/CT, as well as (B) sagittal CT and fused PET/CT demonstrate an FDG-avid destructive osseous lesion in the sternum *(arrows)*. Differential diagnosis for this lesion includes benign osteoradionecrosis as well as breast cancer osseous metastasis and primary radiation-associated sarcoma. Biopsy was needed to make the diagnosis of benign osteoradionecrosis.

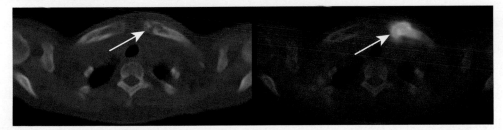

FIG. 3.29 **Primary Radiation-Associated Sarcoma of the Clavicle in a Patient Previously Treated with External Beam Radiation for Thyroid Cancer.** Axial CT and fused PET/CT demonstrate an FDG-avid destructive osseous lesion in the left clavicle *(arrows)*. Differential diagnosis for this finding includes benign osteoradionecrosis, as well as osseous metastasis and primary radiation-associated sarcoma. Biopsy was needed to make the diagnosis of primary radiation-associated sarcoma.

radiation-associated sarcoma; however, again, biopsy was needed for diagnosis.

CONCLUSION

FDG PET/CT provides substantial value for detecting osseous malignancy that may be overlooked with anatomic imaging. However, it is important to remember that not all malignancy is FDG avid and not everything that is FDG avid is malignant.

In this chapter on the skeleton, as well as all organ systems, **correlate FDG PET findings with corresponding CT findings, as well as the clinical scenario, to optimally diagnose findings on FDG PET/CT**. For example, a round FDG-avid focus in a bone, without a CT correlate, and in a patient with a malignancy predisposed to osseous metastases is highly suspicious for an osseous metastasis. However, joint-centered FDG avidity with corresponding joint space narrowing and osteophytes on CT is probably a result of benign degenerative changes, and FDG avidity in the posterior ilium or sacrum of a patient with lymphoma may represent a recent bone marrow biopsy tract.

Here are a few suggestions to help optimize your interpretation of FDG PET/CT of the osseous structures:

1. Evaluate lesions of the spine and sternum on multiple planar projections. Often, spinal and sternal lesions are better characterized on sagittal images than on axial images.

2. Use corresponding CT images to localize skeletal FDG avidity into bone-centered and joint-centered lesions. Bone-centered FDG avidity, even without a CT correlate, is often malignant. Joint-centered FDG avidity is usually benign, and consider benign etiologies such as degenerative changes and inflammatory arthropathies.

3. Treatment response is often better evaluated by FDG PET than by anatomic imaging. This is true for response to systemic therapies, radiation therapy, and ablations.

4. Adjust the PET window level to "see" through benign FDG avidity such as bone marrow repopulation from colony-stimulating factors. Adjusting the PET window level may allow you to visualize FDG-avid malignancy as separate from benign FDG-avid bone marrow repopulation.

5. Consider radiographs or MR for further evaluation of unclear osseous lesions on FDG PET/CT. Do not hesitate to obtain plain radiographs to work to unclear osseous lesions on FDG PET/CT. Radiographs are often helpful in characterizing osseous lesions in ways that are not apparent on FDG PET/CT or even MR.

6. FDG-avid destructive osseous lesions within a radiation port have a differential of benign osteoradionecrosis, as well as malignancy, including metastases and primary radiation-associated sarcoma. Biopsy is needed to determine the diagnosis.

SUGGESTED READINGS

Cavo M, et al: Role of 18F-FDG PET/CT in the diagnosis and management of multiple myeloma and other plasma cell disorders: a consensus statement by the International Myeloma Working Group, *Lancet Oncol* 18:e206–e217, 2017.

Cheson BD, et al: Recommendations for initial evaluation, staging, and response assessment of Hodgkin and non-Hodgkin lymphoma: the Lugano classification, *J Clin Oncol* 32:3059–3068, 2014.

Choi YY, et al: PET/CT in benign and malignant musculoskeletal tumors and tumor-like conditions, *Semin Musculoskelet Radiol* 18:133–148, 2014.

Costelloe CM, et al: FDG PET for the detection of bone metastases sensitivity, specificity and comparison with other imaging modalities, *PET Clin* 5:281–295, 2010.

Dashevsky BZ, et al: Appearance of untreated bone metastases from breast cancer on FDG PET/CT: importance of histologic subtype, *Eur J Nucl Med Mol Imaging* 42:1666–1673, 2015.

Morris PG, et al: Integrated positron emission tomography/ computed tomography may render bone scintigraphy unnecessary to investigate suspected metastatic breast cancer, *J Clin Oncol* 28:3154–3159, 2010.

Rajkumar, et al: International Myeloma Working Group updated criteria for the diagnosis of multiple myeloma, *Lancet Oncol* 15:e538–e548, 2014.

Tateishi U, et al: Bone metastases in patients with metastatic breast cancer: morphologic and metabolic monitoring of response to systemic therapy with integrated PET/CT, *Radiology* 247(1):189–196, 2008.

Ulaner GA, et al: Identifying and distinguishing treatment effects and complications from malignancy at FDG PET/CT, *Radiographics* 33:1817–1834, 2013.

White ML, et al: Spectrum of benign articular and periarticular findings at FDG PET/CT, *Radiographics* 36:824–839, 2016.

CHAPTER 4

Muscle and Nerve on FDG PET/CT

Muscles are a less common site of malignancy, yet are very important to the proper interpretation of 18F-flourodeoxyglucose (FDG) positron emission tomography/computed tomography (PET/CT) in their own right. Benign skeletal muscle may demonstrate substantial FDG uptake, and this should not be confused with malignancy. Physiologic FDG avidity in skeletal muscle is often related with muscular exertion, which is why at most FDG PET facilities patients are asked to refrain from exercise the day before and the day of a PET/CT scan. Linear FDG avidity corresponding to normal appearing muscles on CT is usually physiologic (Fig. 4.1).

Extensive physiologic FDG avidity could initially be alarming on PET/CT examinations. For example, large segments of FDG-avid back musculature are uncommon and could mimic an aggressive process. However, correlation with the corresponding CT images usually allows for the proper identification of physiologic muscular FDG avidity. Note the patient in Fig. 4.2. This patient has extensive FDG avidity in the region of back musculature. The corresponding CT images demonstrate normal fat planes within the FDG-avid muscle, consistent with benign muscle, despite the extensive FDG avidity. FDG-avid masses would be expected to displace or obliterate the normal fat planes within musculature (Fig. 4.3). While areas of FDG-avid malignancy underlying the physiologic muscular FDG avidity cannot be entirely excluded, the presence of normal fat planes within musculature is a very reassuring sign that FDG avidity is probably physiologic.

As with the skeleton, FDG PET helps visualize metastases that may be occult or overlooked on anatomic imaging. Muscle is an uncommon site for metastasis; therefore it is an organ that may not be scrutinized by the radiologist on every scan. FDG avidity highlights potentially important findings for additional scrutiny (Fig. 4.4).

Unfortunately, as with other organ systems, FDG avidity could lead to the misinterpretation of benign findings. Focal areas of physiologic muscular FDG avidity could be mistaken for FDG-avid lymph nodes or other suspicious FDG-avid lesions. One area of muscle for which mistakes may occur is the crura of the diaphragm. The diaphragmatic crura may appear to have focal FDG avidity on individual axial slices, and this may be confused with retrocrural or upper abdominal lymph nodes (Fig. 4.5). Similarly, not all histologies of malignancy will be readily apparent on FDG PET, and the corresponding CT images may demonstrate an abnormality within the muscle better than the FDG PET images. For example, myxoid tumors will demonstrate low attenuation compared to skeletal muscle, and muscular metastases from myxoid tumors may be more readily apparent on the CT component of the PET/CT (Fig. 4.6).

Another important issue is that muscles have a high potential for glucose uptake, and when glucose moves into muscles, FDG follows. If the patient recently consumed a meal, then endogenous secretion of insulin by the pancreas will drive glucose and FDG into the muscles (Fig. 4.7). The propensity for insulin-induced FDG uptake in muscles is the reason why patients must fast for at least 4 to 6 hours prior to FDG administration. Fasting lowers endogenous insulin levels, helping prevent physiologic FDG uptake within musculature.

Greater than expected physiologic FDG uptake within musculature may compromise interpretation of FDG PET/CT in multiple ways. First, there is a finite supply of FDG within the body following FDG injection. Substantial uptake of FDG within musculature reduces the amount of FDG available for uptake within malignancy, and may reduce standard uptake value (SUV) measurements taken on malignant masses (Fig. 4.8). If follow-up examinations have a greater or lesser extent of muscular FDG uptake, then comparison of the SUV values taken from masses at different time points may not be directly comparable. Under most conditions, it takes a very substantial amount of physiologic muscular FDG uptake to cause an effect on SUV values of masses; however, at its extreme, markedly excessive physiologic muscular FDG uptake could have a substantial impact on measured SUV values and even cause an FDG-avid mass to fail to be visualized on FDG PET. Uptake of FDG avidity in body musculature is just one of many factors that may affect the SUV measurement of masses, and thus direct comparison of SUV values of masses

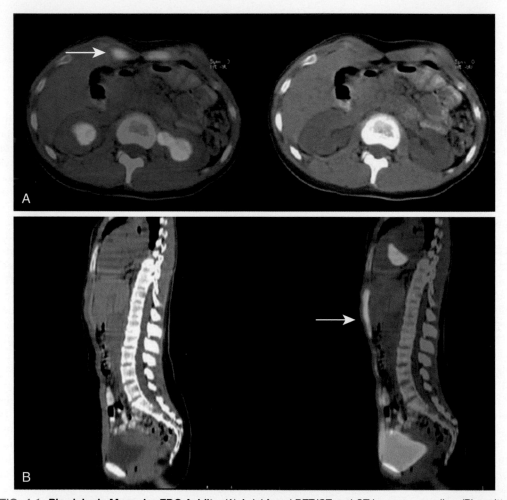

FIG. 4.1 **Physiologic Muscular FDG Avidity.** (A) Axial fused PET/CT and CT images, as well as (B) sagittal CT and fused PET/CT images, demonstrate physiologic FDG avidity within the bilateral rectus abdominus muscles *(arrows)*, in a patient who performed sit-ups the morning of FDG PET/CT scan, despite instructions not to exercise before the examination.

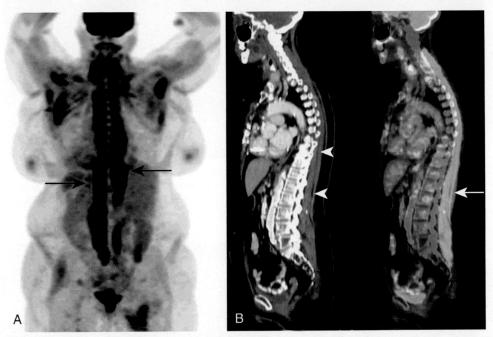

FIG. 4.2 Extensive Physiologic Muscular FDG Avidity. (A) Maximum intensity projection (MIP) PET demonstrates extensive FDG-avid musculature, including bilateral FDG avid paraspinal musculature *(arrows)*. (B) Sagittal CT and fused PET/CT images demonstrate the FDG avidity in paraspinal musculature *(arrow)*. The CT image demonstrates normal fat planes *(arrowheads)* traversing the FDG-avid muscles, a reassuring sign that the FDG avidity is probably physiologic.

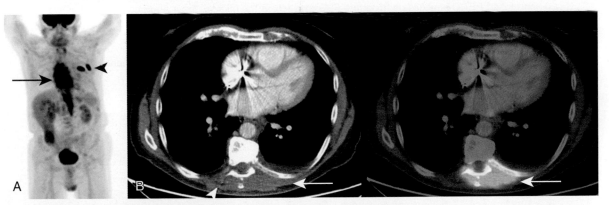

FIG. 4.3 FDG-avid Muscular Lymphoma. (A) MIP PET demonstrates midline FDG avidity overlying the chest and upper abdomen *(arrow)*, as well as additional lesions osseous foci *(arrowhead)*. (B) Axial CT and fused PET/CT images demonstrate the midline FDG avidity localizes to paraspinal musculature *(arrow)*. The CT image demonstrates obliteration of normal fat planes in the region of the FDG avidity *(arrow)*, as compared with the preservation of fat planes in the contralateral muscle *(arrowhead)*. The obliteration of fat planes is worrisome for a pathologic process, and biopsy demonstrated lymphomatosis infiltration of the muscle.

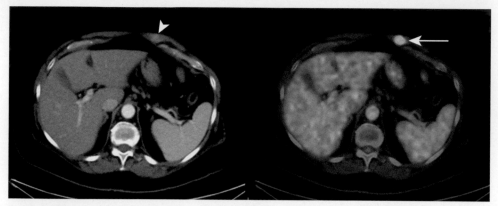

FIG. 4.4 **FDG-avid Muscular Metastasis.** Axial CT and fused PET/CT images demonstrate an FDG-avid focus in the left rectus muscle *(arrow)*. Corresponding CT image demonstrates a subtle enhancing lesion at this location *(arrowhead)*, suspicious for metastasis, which could easily have been overlooked without FDG guidance. Biopsy confirmed a muscular metastasis.

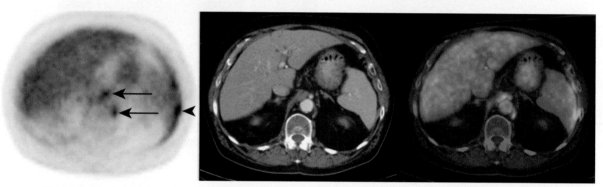

FIG. 4.5 **Benign FDG Avidity in the Diaphragm, Which Could be Mistaken for Malignancy.** Axial PET, CT, and fused PET/CT images demonstrate FDG-avid foci in the midline upper abdomen *(arrows)* as well as in the region of the left costodiaphragmatic recess *(arrowhead)*. The midline foci could be confused with retrocrural or upper abdominal lymph nodes, while the left costodiaphragmatic foci could be confused with pleural metastases. The CT and fused images demonstrate that the midline foci localize to normal-appearing diaphragmatic crura, while the left costodiaphragmatic foci localize to the lateral pleura, without any nodal or pleural masses.

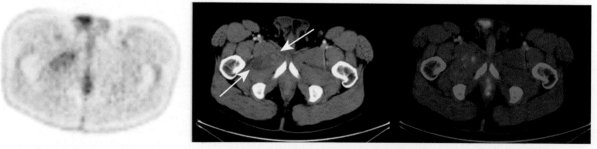

FIG. 4.6 **Muscular Metastasis from Myxoid Liposarcoma More Readily Apparent on CT Than FDG PET Images.** Axial PET, CT, and fused PET/CT images demonstrate minimal FDG avidity in right thigh musculature. The CT image demonstrates a low-attenuation mass in the musculature with faint areas of enhancement *(arrows)*. The mild FDG avidity was not mentioned in the FDG PET/CT report, probably overlooked as physiologic muscular FDG avidity. The abnormality was mentioned in a separate contrast-enhanced CT report. Biopsy confirmed muscular metastasis. This case highlights the importance of evaluating CT images to detect non- or mildly FDG-avid malignancy. This case also highlights the importance of knowing the tumor histology. Myxoid tumors often produce low-attenuation masses, leading the radiologist to carefully evaluate for low-attenuation lesions.

from different time points is predicated on the knowledge of multiple factors, including muscular FDG uptake, blood glucose levels, time between tracer injection and imaging acquisition, lesion size, sensitivity of the PET camera, method of processing acquired data, and others. Second, as with any physiologic FDG avidity, FDG uptake within musculature could obscure visualization of FDG-avid muscular metastases.

The head and neck is a particularly challenging area to determine if FDG avidity in the region of muscles is physiologic or malignant in etiology. The four paired muscles of mastication (temporalis, masseter, and medial and lateral pterygoids) least often demonstrate benign physiologic FDG avidity on FDG PET/CT scans, as they are exercised at every meal (Fig. 4.9). Benign physiologic FDG avidity in the muscles of mastication could be mistaken for suspicious findings, or malignancy may be mistaken for benign avidity in muscles of mastication. For example, when muscular FDG avidity is asymmetric, which is not uncommon, this could be suspicious for an underlying lesion (Fig. 4.10). Direct physical examination or contrast-enhanced imaging such as CT or magnetic resonance (MR) could be used to exclude an underlying lesion. Potentially more worrisome, an FDG-avid mass could be mistaken for physiologic muscular FDG avidity (Fig. 4.11). Determining how sensitive you wish to be for calling suspicious FDG avidity in the region of the muscles of mastication is often more of an art than a science. Setting a low bar for suspicious findings will lead to workups that are benign, while setting a high bar will eventually lead to a missed area of malignancy.

Nerves are an uncommon site of malignancy. They are often better evaluated on MR imaging than by FDG PET/CT. (Malignancy involving nerve structures is certainly a potential area of exploration for PET/MR scanners.) Like osseous and muscular FDG avidity, FDG avidity within nerve structures may be physiologic, inflammatory, or malignant. Knowledge of common areas of physiologic nerve FDG avidity and correlation with anatomic imaging will help optimize the interpretation of nerve FDG avidity.

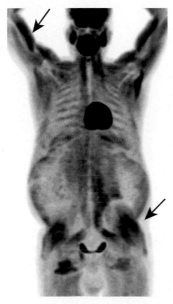

FIG. 4.7 Significant glucose uptake in body musculature *(arrows)* in a patient who ate lunch prior to and FDG PET/CT and "forgot" to inform the PET facility staff.

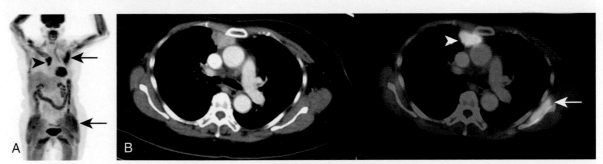

FIG. 4.8 **Uptake of FDG Within Body Musculature May Reduce SUV Measurements of Malignancy.** (A) PET MIP demonstrating substantial FDG uptake within body musculature *(arrows)*. Another focus of FDG avidity overlies the central chest *(arrowhead)*. (B) Axial contrast-enhanced CT and fused FDG PET/CT demonstrate FDG avidity in physiologic muscle *(arrow)*. The FDG focus overlying the central chest localizes to an anterior mediastinal soft tissue mass *(arrowhead)*. A PET/CT report will often provide an SUV value for the anterior mediastinal soft tissue mass. Care must be taken to remember that the SUV of the mass may be artificially reduced by excessive FDG uptake within skeletal muscle.

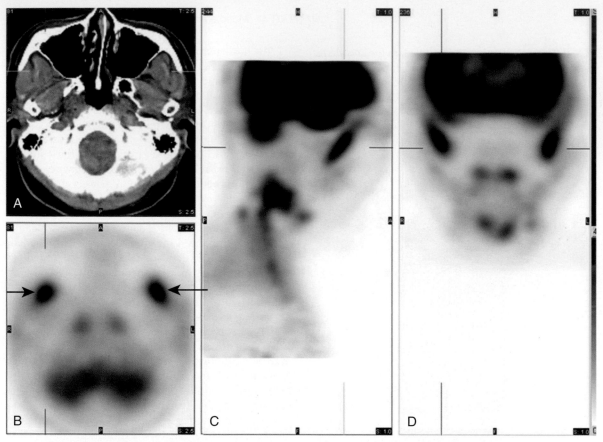

FIG. 4.9 **Physiologic FDG Avidity in the Bilateral Temporalis Muscles.** (A) Axial CT through the temporalis muscles. (B) Axial, (C) sagittal, and (C) coronal PET images through the temporalis muscles demonstrate physiologic FDG avidity in these muscles of mastication *(arrows)*. No abnormality is visualized within the musculature on the corresponding CT images.

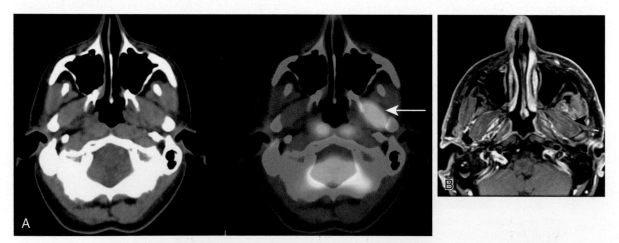

FIG. 4.10 **Physiologic FDG Avidity in the Left Lateral Pterygoid Muscle.** (A) Axial CT and fused PET/CT images through the pterygoid musculature demonstrate focal FDG avidity in the left lateral pterygoid *(arrow)* without correlate on noncontrast CT. Unilateral physiologic FDG avidity in a muscle of mastication is not uncommon; however due to clinical concern a magnetic resonance image (MRI) was obtained for further evaluation. (B) Axial T1 postgadolinium MRI demonstrates a normal lateral pterygoid, including preservation of high T1 signal fat planes *(arrowhead)*. This was physiologic FDG avidity in a unilateral muscle of mastication.

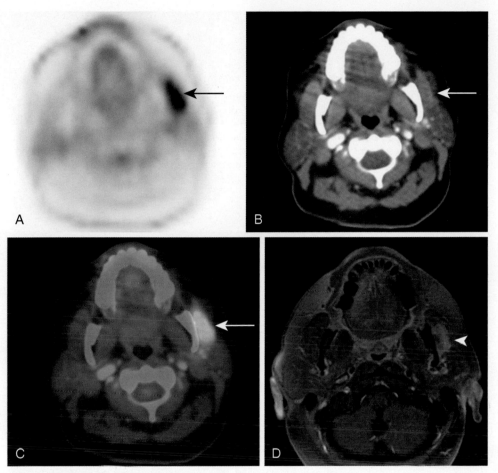

FIG. 4.11 **Metastasis in the Left Masseter Muscle.** (A) Axial PET, (B) axial CT, and (C) axial fused PET/CT through the level of the masseter muscles demonstrate an FDG-avid focus correlating to only normal muscle on contrast-enhanced CT *(arrows)*. Unilateral physiologic FDG avidity in a muscle of mastication is not uncommon; however, due to left facial numbness, an MRI was obtained for further evaluation. (D) Axial T1 fat-sat postgadolinium MRI demonstrates an enhancing mass in the left masseter muscle *(arrowhead)*. This was biopsy-proven to represent a muscle metastasis. This demonstrates the difficulty sometimes encountered in distinguishing benign muscular FDG avidity from clinically significant lesions.

The spinal cord may demonstrate physiologic FDG avidity. This is usually greatest at the levels of the brachial (C5-T1) and lumbosacral (T12-S4) plexi. Physiologic FDG avidity of the spinal cord is normally well centered within the cord, and without corresponding abnormality on CT or MR (Fig. 4.12). In contrast, asymmetric FDG avidity within the spinal canal is more suspicious for pathology. Of course, FDG PET and CT images should be compared to evaluate for misregistration before deciding upon asymmetric FDG avidity on a fused image. Asymmetric FDG avidity within the spinal canal may represent a benign process such as

inflammation from a disc herniation (Fig. 4.13) or an abscess (Fig. 4.14), or a malignant process such as a primary malignancy, metastasis (Fig. 4.15), or neural lymphoma.

FDG PET/CT may play a particular level evaluation of patients with neurofibromatosis type I (NF1). Neurofibromas often appear as mildly FDG-avid soft tissue masses on FDG PET/CT. Periodic FDG PET/CT evaluation may help identify areas of transformation to higher grade malignancy, such as malignant peripheral nerve sheath tumors, which commonly demonstrate interval increases in FDG avidity and/or size (Fig. 4.16).

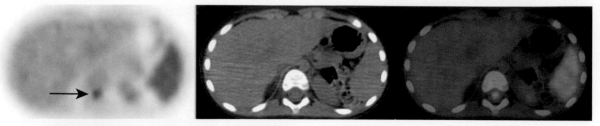

FIG. 4.12 **Physiologic FDG Avidity in the Spinal Cord.** Axial PET, CT, and fused PET/CT images through the level of T12, at the superior margin of the lumbosacral plexus. Focal FDG avidity can be seen centered within the spinal cord *(arrow)*, probably a benign finding at this level.

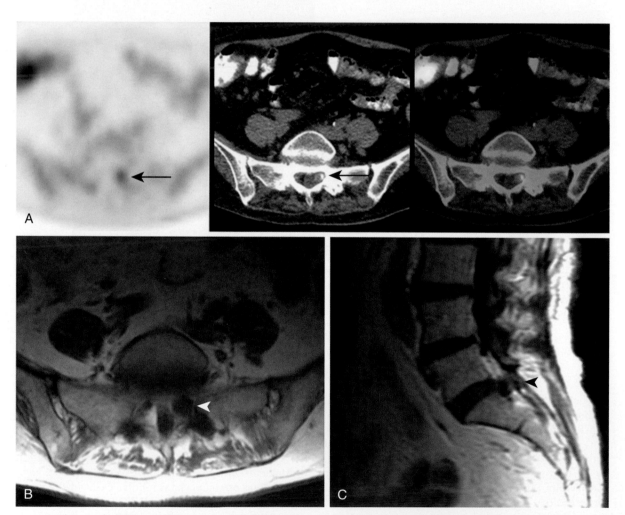

FIG. 4.13 **FDG-avid Disc L5-S1 Herniation.** (A) Axial PET, CT and fused PET/CT images through the level of the lumbosacral junction demonstrate mild FDG avidity asymmetrically in the left aspect of the spinal canal, corresponding with a calcified lesion on CT *(arrows)*. (B) Axial T1 and (C) sagittal T1 images demonstrate a low T1 disc herniation is the cause of the FDG-avid finding on FDG PET/CT *(arrowheads)*.

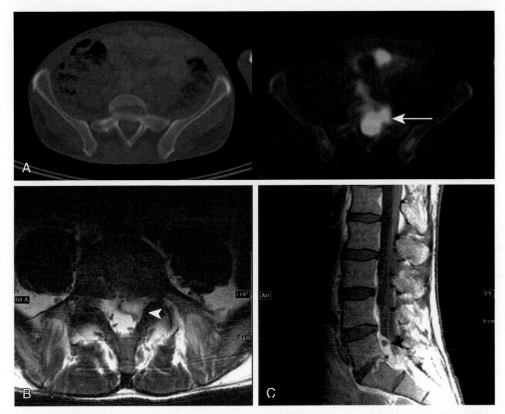

FIG. 4.14 **FDG-avid Spinal Abscess In a Patient With History of Humerus Angiosarcoma and Recent Back Pain, Fever, and Elevated White Blood Cell Count.** (A) Axial CT and fused PET/CT images through the level of the lumbosacral junction demonstrate asymmetric FDG avidity in the left aspect of the spinal canal, probably extending out of a neural foramen *(arrows)*. (B) Axial T2 and (C) sagittal T1 postgadolinium images demonstrate a peripherally enhancing abscess in the spinal canal *(arrowheads)*.

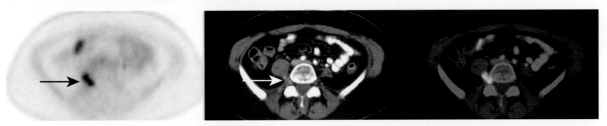

FIG. 4.15 **FDG-avid Neural Metastasis in a Patient With Ductal Breast Cancer.** Axial PET, CT, and fused PET/CT images through the level of the lumbar spine demonstrate asymmetric FDG extending out of a neural foramen *(arrows)*. Follow-up imaging demonstrated this was a growing neural metastasis.

CONCLUSION

Similar to the interpretation of skeletal FDG PET/CT findings in Chapter 3, consider the following issues for the interpretation of muscle/nerve lesions in this chapter, as well as lesions in the subsequent organ systems. First, PET findings, CT findings, and clinical scenarios should be integrated to arrive at an optimal differential or diagnosis. Second, it should be realized that FDG avidity in any organ system may be physiologic, inflammatory, or malignant. Correlation with CT findings and the

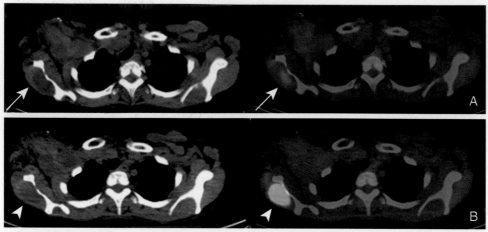

FIG. 4.16 **Transformation of a Neurofibroma to a Malignant Peripheral Nerve Sheath Tumor in a Patient With Neurofibromatosis Type I (NF1).** (A) Axial CT and fused PET/CT images through the level of the lumbar spine demonstrate a dominant mildly FDG-avid low-attenuation mass within the right shoulder musculature *(arrows)*, as well as additional low-attenuation lesions in the right shoulder and axilla, all representing neurofibromas in a patient with NF1. (B) Follow-up imaging demonstrates an interval increase in size and FDG avidity *(arrowheads)* of the dominant mass. Biopsy confirmed transformation to a malignant peripheral nerve sheath tumor.

clinical scenario often help distinguish between these possibilities. Third, familiarity with common sites of physiologic or inflammatory FDG avidity will help increase accuracy in the identification of malignant lesions.

Here are a few suggestions to help optimize your interpretation of FDG PET/CT of the muscles and nerves:

1. Physiologic muscular FDG avidity may mask FDG-avid malignancy. Likewise, physiologic muscular FDG avidity could be mistaken for FDG-avid malignancy.

2. Preservation of normal fat planes within muscle is a valuable finding on CT or MR. FDG-avid masses would be expected to displace or obliterate the normal fat planes within musculature. While FDG-avid malignancy underlying the physiologic muscular FDG avidity cannot be entirely excluded, the presence of normal fat planes within musculature is a very reassuring sign that FDG avidity is probably physiologic.

3. Compare FDG uptake within musculature of sequential scans. Endogenous or exogenous insulin can result in substantial muscular FDG uptake, reducing FDG available for tumor uptake. Substantial muscular FDG uptake could artificially alter SUV measurements of masses, making comparison of SUV values difficult.

4. The spinal cord may have physiologic FDG avidity, greatest at the brachial and lumbosacral plexi. Physiologic FDG avidity in the spinal cord is usually symmetric, and asymmetric FDG avidity in the spinal canal should prompt further evaluation.

5. Consider MR for further evaluation of unclear muscle or nerve lesions on FDG PET/CT.

SUGGESTED READINGS

Emmering J, et al: Intramuscular metastases on FDG PET-CT: a review of the literature, *Nucl Med Commun* 33:117–120, 2012.

Grant FD, et al: Normal variations and benign findings in pediatric 18F-FDG-PET/CT, *PET Clin* 9:195–208, 2014.

Karunanithi S, et al: Spectrum of physiologic and pathologic skeletal muscle (18)F-FDG uptake on PET/CT, *AJR Am J Roentgenol* 205:W141–W149, 2015.

Parida GK, et al: FDG PET/CT in skeletal muscle: pitfalls and pathologies, *Semin Nucl Med* 47:362–372, 2017.

Tovmassian D, et al: The role of 18F-FDG PET/CT in predicting malignant transformation of plexiform neurofibromas in neurofibromatosis-1, *Int J Surg Oncol* 2016:6162182, 2016.

CHAPTER 5

Skin and Breast on FDG PET/CT

The skin and subcutaneous tissues are common sites of inflammatory lesions such as acne, sebaceous cysts, warts, and pilonidal cysts (Fig. 5.1). These benign etiologies may produce abnormalities on 18F-fluorodeoxyglucose positron emission tomography/computed tomography (FDG PET/CT), or both. However, the skin is also the site of primary malignancies such as melanoma, squamous cell carcinoma, and Kaposi sarcoma (Fig. 5.2), as well as lymphoma (Fig. 5.3) or metastases (Fig. 5.4). It is usually not possible to distinguish these benign and malignant lesions on whole-body FDG PET/CT. Fortunately, the skin allows for direct inspection of abnormalities. Thus often the best method for further evaluation of abnormality seen on FDG PET/CT is the suggestion to perform a physical examination to correlate with imaging findings. Usually the patient is no longer available to the radiologist when a skin or subcutaneous lesion is identified on PET/CT images. In clinics where the patient is available to the interpreting radiologist, this is one abnormality where the radiologist can perform their own physical examination. A PET/CT report which describes the radiologist's physical examination findings is sure to raise eyebrows in your institution.

In patients with known breast cancer, the FDG-avid soft tissue lesions within the breast probably represent the primary breast malignancy (Fig. 5.5). However, in patients without known breast malignancy, FDG PET/CT is not sensitive for the detection or diagnosis of breast lesions. Due to physical examination and mammographic screening, many breast cancers are small, early stage lesions at diagnosis, which are often not visualized by either whole-body FDG PET or CT, even though they are readily apparent on dedicated breast imaging such as mammography, ultrasound, or breast magnetic resonance (MR) (Fig. 5.6).

In addition to the low sensitivity of whole-body FDG PET/CT for primary breast cancers, FDG PET/CT also has low specificity. Breast parenchyma may demonstrate normal FDG avidity, heightened by physiologic activity such as breast-feeding (Fig. 5.7). Benign processes within the breast may also demonstrate FDG avidity, such as fibroadenomas (Fig. 5.8) or fat necrosis (Fig. 5.9). Benign or inflammatory processes may be more FDG avid than many primary breast malignancies. For example, following lumpectomy, mastectomy, and/or axillary lymph node dissections, the resulting postsurgical inflammation may be more FDG avid than the original primary malignancy, but should be able to be recognized as benign given the corresponding CT findings and clinical scenario (Fig. 5.10). Recognizing benign FDG-avid postsurgical inflammation will prevent misdiagnosis of malignancy in surgical beds. In general, surgeons are loathe to be told they have left large FDG-avid tumors in their surgical beds.

Although whole-body FDG PET/CT demonstrates both low sensitivity and specificity for primary breast malignancy, this does not mean that incidentally visualized FDG-avid lesions within the breasts can be ignored. Approximately one-third of incidentally visualized FDG-avid lesions within the breasts end up being diagnosed as malignancy, including incidental primary breast cancers (Fig. 5.11), breast lymphoma, or metastases to the breast (Fig. 5.12).

A reasonable approach to FDG-avid lesions within the breasts would be as follows: (1) In a patient with a known primary breast malignancy, the FDG-avid breast lesion is probably the primary breast malignancy. (2) Incidental FDG-avid lesions within the breast in a patient without known primary breast malignancy should be further evaluated with dedicated breast imaging, starting with mammogram if over the age of 30, and breast ultrasound if under the age of 30. Dedicated breast imaging may be able to definitively diagnose the lesion as benign. If the lesion is suspicious (Breast Imaging Reporting and Data System [BIRADS] 4 or 5) on dedicated breast imaging, then biopsy could be performed for tissue diagnosis.

Text continued on p. 50

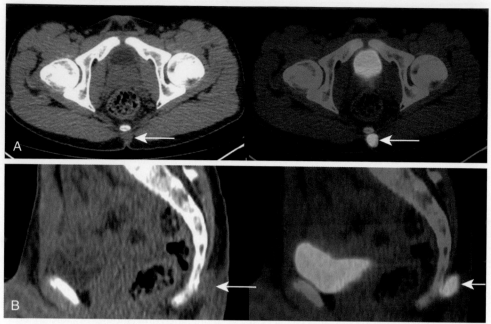

FIG. 5.1 **FDG-avid Benign Pilonidal Cyst.** (A) Axial CT and fused PET/CT images, as well as (B) sagittal CT and fused PET/CT images demonstrate an FDG-avid soft tissue lesion posterior to the inferior coccyx *(arrows)*. This patient had treated lymphoma, and the differential would include a benign skin/subcutaneous lesion and recurrent lymphoma. Physical examination and tissue sampling diagnosed a benign pilonidal cyst.

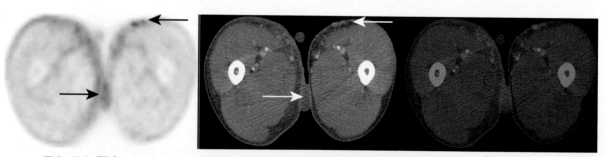

FIG. 5.2 **FDG-avid Kaposi Sarcoma.** Axial PET, CT, and fused PET/CT images demonstrate multiple FDG-avid soft tissue lesions in the skin and subcutaneous tissues *(arrows)*. This patient had human immunodeficiency virus (HIV), and the findings were suspicious for HIV-associated lymphoma or Kaposi sarcoma. Physical examination and tissue sampling diagnosed Kaposi sarcoma.

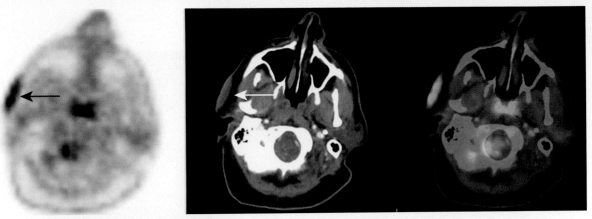

FIG. 5.3 **FDG-avid Lymphoma of the Skin.** Axial PET, CT, and fused PET/CT images demonstrate FDG-avid soft tissue in the right facial skin *(arrows)*. This patient was treated for lymphoma, and the differential would include a benign skin/subcutaneous lesion and recurrent lymphoma. Physical examination and tissue sampling diagnosed recurrent lymphoma.

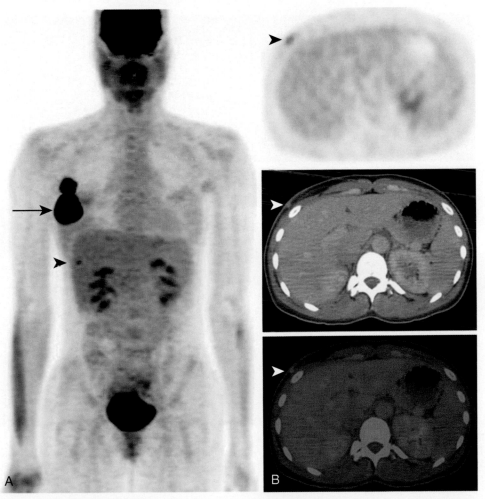

FIG. 5.4 **FDG-avid Skin Metastasis.** (A) PET maximum intensity projection (MIP) in a patient with ductal breast cancer demonstrates FDG-avid right breast malignancy and right axillary nodal metastasis *(arrow)*. There is also a small abnormal FDG-avid focus overlying the right liver *(arrowhead)*. (B) Axial PET, CT, and fused PET/CT images demonstrate this focus localizes to a small skin/subcutaneous nodule in the inferior right chest wall *(arrow heads)*. Physical examination and tissue sampling diagnosed a breast cancer metastasis of the skin.

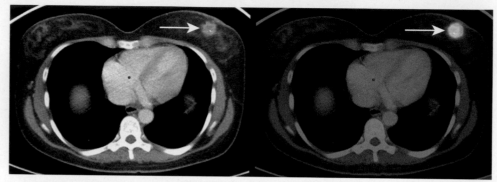

FIG. 5.5 **FDG-avid Primary Breast Malignancy.** Axial CT and fused PET/CT images in a patient with newly diagnosed ductal breast cancer demonstrates an FDG avid soft tissue mass in the left breast *(arrows)*. In a patient with known breast malignancy, these findings represent the primary breast malignancy.

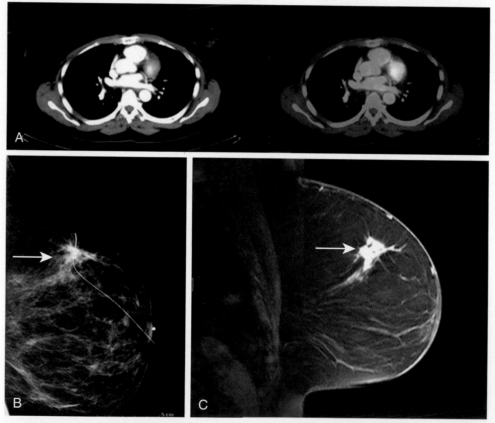

FIG. 5.6 **Primary Breast Malignancy, Which is Occult on Both Whole-Body FDG PET and CT.** (A) Axial CT and fused PET/CT images in a patient with newly diagnosed ductal breast cancer fail to visualize the primary breast malignancy. (B) Mammographic image from a needle localization of the primary breast cancer and (C) sagittal image from contrast enhanced breast MR, both readily visualize the primary malignancy *(arrows)*, which is occult on FDG PET/CT.

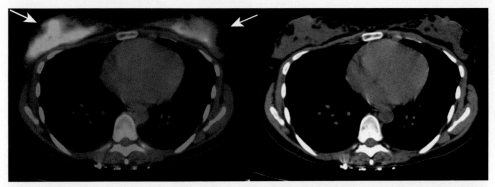

FIG. 5.7 Physiologic FDG Avidity in the Breasts due to Breast-feeding. Axial fused PET/CT and CT images demonstrate substantial FDG avidity within the bilateral breast parenchyma *(arrows)*. This patient was currently breast-feeding. Breast-feeding induces increased FDG avidity within the breast parenchyma, which should not be confused with malignancy or infection.

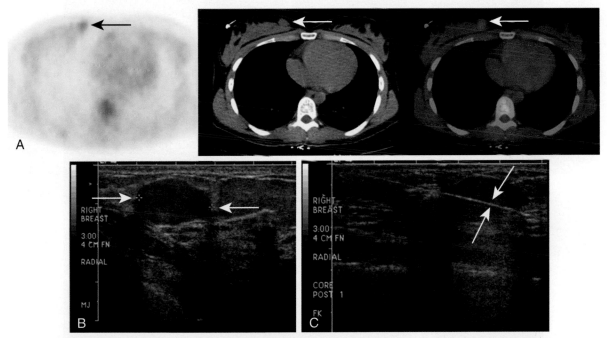

FIG. 5.8 FDG Avidity in a Benign Breast Fibroadenoma. (A) Axial PET, CT, and fused PET/CT demonstrate an FDG-avid soft tissue nodule in the medial right breast *(arrows)*. (B) Ultrasound, performed for further evaluation, demonstrates a well-circumscribed hypoechoic nodule *(arrows)*. (C) Ultrasound-guided biopsy was performed, an image acquired at the biopsy needle within the nodule *(arrows)*. Pathology demonstrated a benign fibroadenoma.

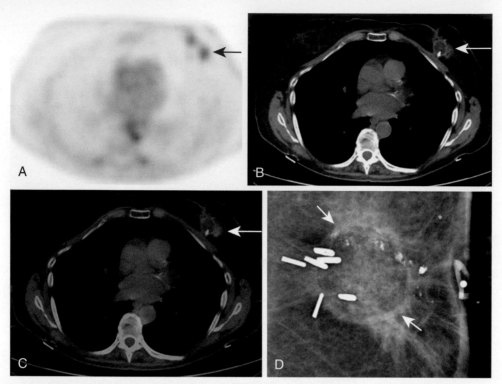

FIG. 5.9 **FDG Avidity Benign Fat Necrosis.** (A) Axial PET, (B) axial CT, and (C) axial fused PET/CT demonstrate FDG-avid soft tissue in the left breast, following lumpectomy *(arrows)*. (D) Mammogram was performed for further evaluation and demonstrated fat within the lesion (outlined by *arrowheads*), diagnostic of benign fat necrosis. No further workup was needed.

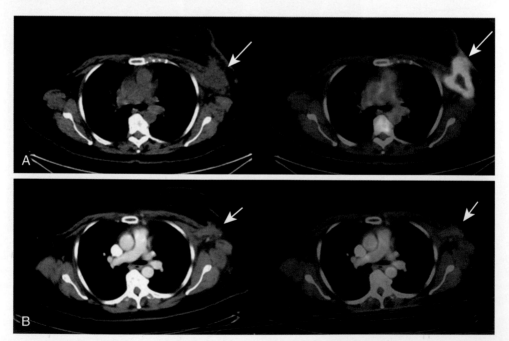

FIG. 5.10 **Benign FDG-avid Postsurgical Inflammation, Which Resolves on Follow-up.** (A) Axial CT and fused PET/CT the patient 1 month after left mastectomy and left axillary lymph node dissection for breast cancer demonstrates FDG-avid soft tissue in the surgical bed *(arrows)*. (B) Axial CT and fused PET/ CT 5 months postsurgery demonstrate resolution of FDG avidity and decreased size of the soft tissue lesion *(arrows)*. These findings represent benign FDG-avid postsurgical inflammation which resolves on follow-up.

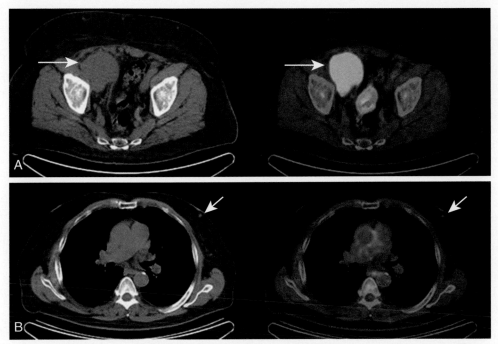

FIG. 5.11 **Incidental FDG-avid Primary Breast Malignancy Detected in a Patient With Lymphoma.** (A) Axial CT and fused PET/CT through the pelvis demonstrate an FDG-avid soft tissue mass *(arrows)* representing nodal lymphoma in a patient with lymphoma. (B) Axial CT and fused PET/CT through the chest of the same patient demonstrate a small FDG-avid nodule in the left breast *(arrowheads)*. Mammogram and ultrasound were performed for further evaluation. Ultrasound-guided biopsy led to the diagnosis of a synchronous primary breast malignancy.

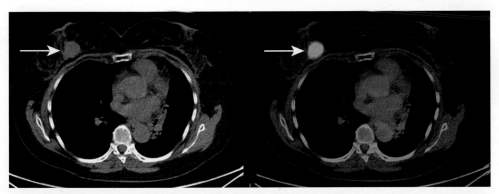

FIG. 5.12 **FDG-avid Metastasis to the Breast.** Axial CT and fused PET/CT through the chest demonstrate an FDG-avid soft tissue mass *(arrows)* in a patient with atypical carcinoid of the lung. Mammogram and ultrasound were performed for further evaluation. Ultrasound-guided biopsy led to the diagnosis of a metastasis to the breast.

Here are a few suggestions to help optimize your interpretation of FDG PET/CT of the skin and breast parenchyma:

1. The skin and subcutaneous tissues are common sites of benign lesions; however, they may be involved by primary malignancies, lymphoma, or metastasis. In a patient with a known skin malignancy, FDG-avid skin lesions probably represent the known malignancy. Incidentally visualized FDG-avid skin lesions in patients without known skin malignancy can be further evaluated by direct physical examination, which will dictate whether biopsy is necessary.

2. Breast tissue is also a common site of benign lesions; however, it is also the site of primary breast malignancy, lymphoma, and metastases. In a patient with a known breast malignancy, FDG-avid breast lesions probably represent the known malignancy. Incidentally visualized FDG-avid breast lesions in patients without known breast malignancy can be further evaluated by dedicated breast imaging, starting with mammogram if over the age of 30, and breast ultrasound if under the age of 30. Results of dedicated breast imaging will dictate whether biopsy is necessary.

SUGGESTED READINGS

Adejolu et al: False-positive lesions mimicking breast cancer on FDGPET and PET/CT, *AJR Am J Roentgenol* 198: W304–W314, 2012.

Benveniste et al: Incidental primary breast cancer detected on PET-CT, *Breast Cancer Res Treat* 151:261–268, 2015.

Bertagna et al: Prevalence and clinical significance of incidental F18-FDG breast uptake: a systematic review and meta-analysis, *Jpn J Radiol*. 32(2):59–68, 2014.

Duncan et al: The utility of positron emission tomography with and without computed tomography in patients with nonmelanoma skin cancer, *J Am Acad Dermatol* 75:186–196, 2016.

Groheux et al: Performance of FDG PET/CT in the clinical management of breast cancer, *Radiology* 266:388–405, 2013.

Juan et al: Malignant skin and subcutaneous neoplasms in adults: multimodality imaging with CT, MRI, and 18F-FDG PET/CT, *AJR Am J Roentgenol* 202:W422–W438, 2014.

Kang, et al: Clinical significance of incidental finding of local activity in the breast at 18F-FDG PET/CT, *AJR Am J Roentgenol* 197:341–347, 2011.

Korn, et al: Unexpected focal hypermetabolic activity in the breast: significance in patients undergoing 18F-FDG PET/CT, *AJR Am J Roentgenol* 187:81–85, 2006.

Kumar, et al: Clinicopathologic factors associated with false negative FDG-PET in primary breast cancer, *Breast Cancer Res Treat* 98:267–274, 2006.

Qiu et al: The role of 18F-FDG PET and PET/CT in the evaluation of primary cutaneous lymphoma, *Nucl Med Commun* 38:106–116, 2017.

Rohren et al: PET/computed tomography and patient outcomes in melanoma, *PET Clin* 10:243–254, 2015.

CHAPTER 6

Brain on FDG PET/CT

NORMAL BRAIN

18F-Fluorodeoxyglucose (FDG) was initially designed to be a brain metabolism tracer and today has multiple applications in neurologic disorders, such as dementias and seizures. The demonstration of the value of FDG in metabolically active tumors has led to a vast majority of clinical FDG positron emission tomography/computed tomography (PET/CT) studies being performed for evaluation of malignancy, and this chapter will focus on FDG PET/CT for oncologic findings in the brain.

The brain accounts for about 20% of the body's glucose consumption; thus the brain demonstrates very high physiologic uptake on FDG PET. To view the brain appropriately, it will be necessary to optimize the PET window settings. For example, when the PET window is set at a maximum standardized uptake value (SUV) display of 5, all voxels with an SUV of 5 or above will appear identically black on a gray-scale display. This is a common setting for evaluating most of the body, but the brain will appear nearly uniformly black and provide little information. By changing the PET window to a maximum SUV display of 15, 20, or more, the details of the brain will become visible (Fig. 6.1). Each brain you examine may have a different PET window for optimal evaluation.

Once the display is properly windowed for the brain, the metabolism of the brain becomes evident (Fig. 6.2). Brain FDG avidity is normally symmetric, higher in the gray matter than white matter. Gray matter gyri will be apparent. There may be slightly lower uptake in the temporal lobes than the frontal, parietal, and occipital lobes. The basal ganglia often have the highest intracranial physiologic uptake. There may also be slightly higher uptake in the midline cerebellum. Extracranially, the optic muscle may be highly FDG avid.

INITIAL DETECTION OF BRAIN MALIGNANCY

Malignancy involving the brain includes metastases, lymphoma, and primary brain gliomas. Due to the high physiologic FDG uptake in normal brain, visualization of FDG-avid intracranial malignancies may be obscured. High-grade metastases may exhibit FDG avidity even greater than brain background and be identified as foci of high FDG avidity (Fig. 6.3). The corresponding anatomic mass may not be visualized on noncontrast CT, or even contrast-enhanced CT. Contrast-enhanced multiparametric magnetic resonance (MR) is the most sensitive method for the initial detection of brain metastases (see Fig. 6.3B). However, not all brain metastases will have FDG avidity greater than the normal brain. In cases where FDG avidity is less than normal brain, metastases may be visualized as photopenic defects in normal brain avidity (Fig. 6.4). In some cases, the avidity of metastases may not be discernible from normal brain avidity. In these cases, evaluation of the corresponding CT images may reveal metastases that are not apparent on FDG PET (Fig. 6.5). In all cases, inconclusive findings can be further evaluated by contrast-enhanced multiparametric MR.

High-grade lymphomas, particularly primary central nervous system (PCNS) lymphomas, will usually be more FDG avid than normal brain and discernible as FDG-avid foci (Fig. 6.6). Lower-grade lymphomas may not be apparent on FDG PET. Again, MR will be the most sensitive method for initial detection of disease extent in the brain. A specific indication for brain FDG PET/CT is in acquired immunodeficiency syndrome (AIDS) patients with a new enhancing lesion on MR. The most common differential diagnoses for this scenario are toxoplasmosis and AIDS-related lymphoma. An FDG PET/CT may assist in making this distinction, as AIDS-related lymphoma is normally more FDG avid than background brain, while toxoplasmosis is relatively photopenic (Fig. 6.7).

Primary brain gliomas run a spectrum of low to high grade. Low-grade gliomas, such as astrocytomas, often have FDG avidity lower than normal brain and may appear as a photopenic defect (Fig. 6.8). High-grade gliomas, such as glioblastoma multiforme, have variable extent of FDG avidity, ranging from above normal gray matter to below white matter. And again, MR will be the most sensitive method for initial detection of disease extent in the brain.

Text continued on p. 57

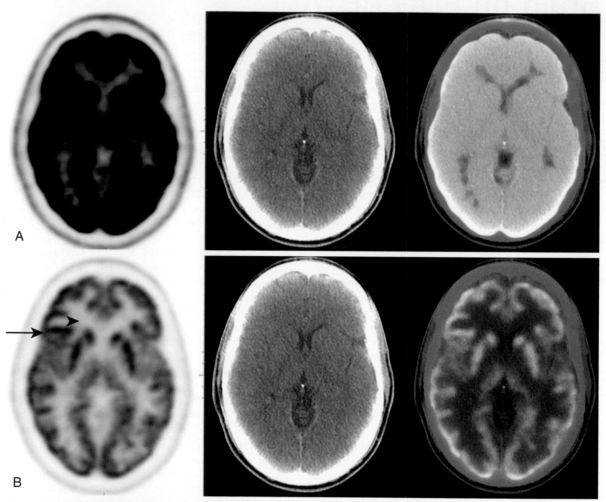

FIG. 6.1 **Optimal Windowing of the Brain on FDG PET.** (A) Axial PET, CT, and fused PET/CT images on a window display where all standard uptake values (SUVs) greater than 5 have maximal darkness. The metabolic features of the brain are indiscernible. (B) Axial PET, CT, and fused PET/CT images after the window display has been changed to a setting where SUVs greater than 15 have maximal darkness. The metabolic features of the brain are now much more apparent, demonstrating the gray matter gyri *(arrow)* in gray scale and the less metabolically active white matter *(arrowhead)* closer to white.

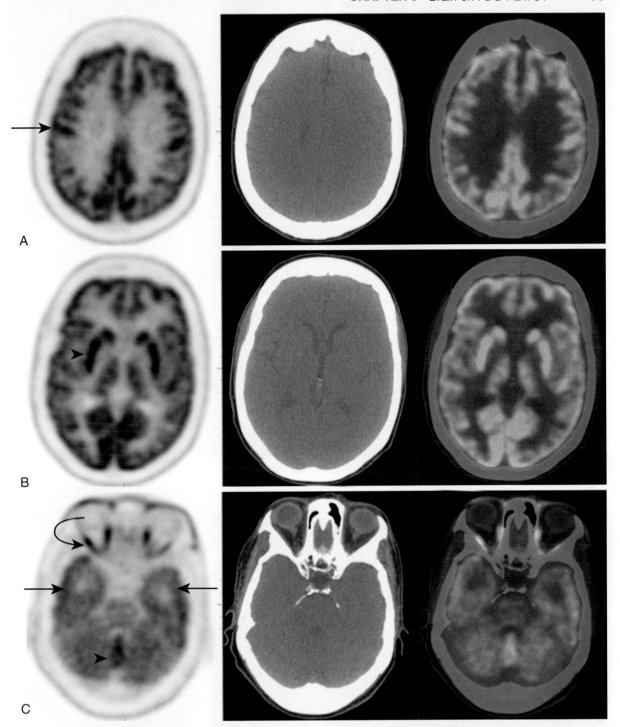

FIG. 6.2 **Normal Brain on FDG PET/CT.** Axial PET, CT, and fused PET/CT images through three levels of the brain. (A) Superior brain demonstrates symmetric FDG avidity in the gray matter gyri of the frontal *(arrow)* and parietal lobes. (B) More inferior slice demonstrates that the basal ganglia *(arrowhead)* are often the most FDG-avid normal structure in the brain. (C) Most inferior slice demonstrates that the avidity in the temporal lobes *(arrows)* is often slightly lower than the frontal, parietal, and occipital lobes more superiorly. There is often an area of linear FDG avidity between the cerebellar hemispheres *(arrowhead)*. The extraocular muscles may be normally FDG avid *(curved arrow)*.

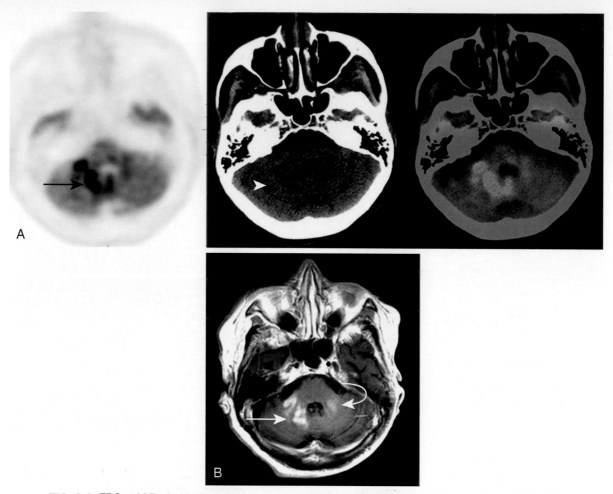

FIG. 6.3 **FDG-avid Brain Metastases in a Patient with Non-Small Cell Lung Cancer.** (A) Axial PET, CT, and fused PET/CT images through the cerebellum demonstrate FDG-avid cerebellar foci *(arrow)* without a correlate on noncontrast CT *(arrowhead)*, consistent with brain metastases. (B) T1 postgadolinium MR demonstrates the enhancing lesions corresponding to the FDG-avid foci *(arrow)*, as well as additional enhancing metastases *(curved arrow)*.

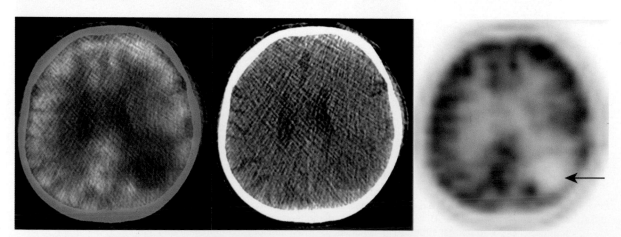

FIG. 6.4 **FDG-Photopenic Brain Metastases in a Patient with Melanoma.** Axial PET, CT, and fused PET/CT images through the cerebrum demonstrate a round FDG-photopenic defect in the left parietal lobe *(arrow)*, consistent with a brain metastasis.

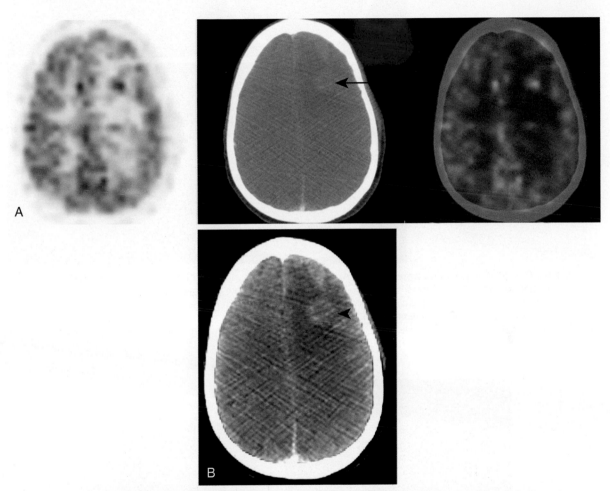

FIG. 6.5 Brain Metastases Detected on CT Component of FDG PET/CT in a Patient with Ductal Breast Cancer. (A) Axial PET, CT, and fused PET/CT images through the cerebellum are without clear FDG abnormality, but a high-attenuation lesion is visible on CT at the soft tissue window *(arrow)*. (B) Adjusting the CT to a brain window allows better visualization of the high-attenuation brain metastasis *(arrowhead)* and surrounding low-attenuation edema.

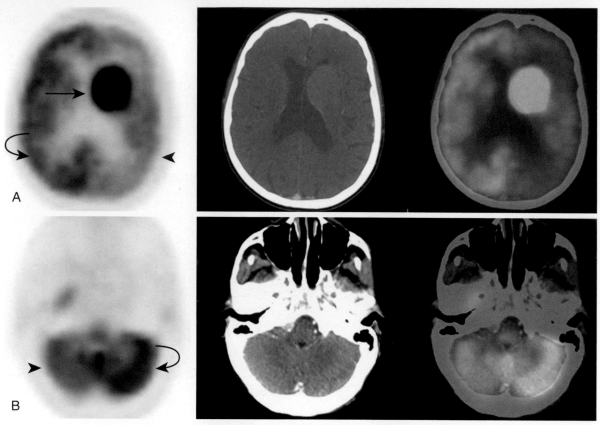

FIG. 6.6 **FDG-avid Brain Lymphoma.** (A) Axial PET, CT, and fused PET/CT images through the cerebrum demonstrate an FDG-avid mass representing lymphoma *(arrow)*. Note the lower avidity in the ipsilateral left cerebrum *(arrowhead)* compared with the contralateral right cerebrum *(curved arrow)*, probably due to the lymphoma. (B) Axial PET, CT, and fused PET/CT images through the cerebrum demonstrate crossed cerebellar diaschisis. The cerebellum contralateral to the depressed cerebrum (right cerebellum, *arrowhead*) has lower avidity compared with the left cerebellum *(curved arrow)*.

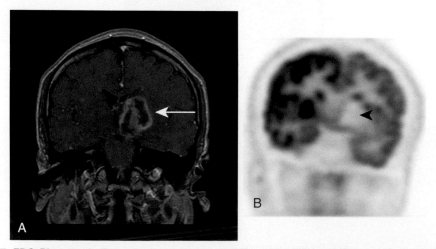

FIG. 6.7 **FDG-Photopenic Toxoplasmosis.** (A) Coronal T1 postgadolinium MR in a patient with acquired immunodeficiency syndrome (AIDS) demonstrates a ring-enhancing lesion *(arrow)*. A new ring-enhancing lesion in a patient with AIDS is most commonly toxoplasmosis or AIDS-related lymphoma. (B) Coronal PET demonstrates the lesion is photopenic *(arrowhead)*, consistent with toxoplasmosis. AIDS-related lymphoma would be expected to be avid.

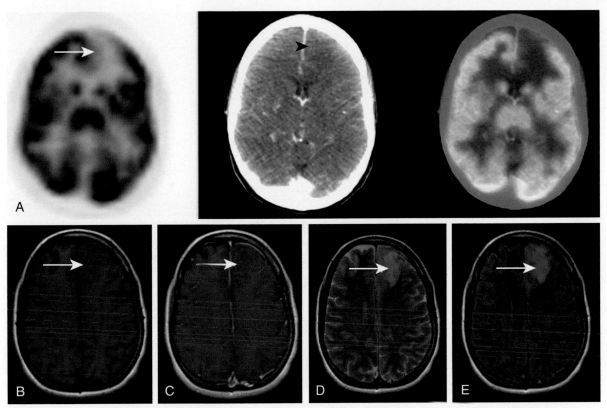

FIG. 6.8 FDG-Photopenic Glioma. (A) Axial PET, CT, and fused PET/CT images in a patient with ductal breast cancer demonstrate focal photopenia in the medial left frontal lobe *(arrow)*, without corresponding abnormality on CT *(arrowhead)*. MR was performed for further evaluation. (B) T1 MR shows no abnormality *(arrow)*. (C) T1 postgadolinium also shows no abnormality *(arrow)*. However, (D) T2 and (E) T2 fluid-attenuated inversion recovery images demonstrate a high signal abnormality *(arrows)* that was subsequently proven to be a low-grade glioma. This represents incidental detection of an FDG-photopenic low-grade glioma by FDG PET/CT.

An interesting metabolic phenomenon is the decrease in cerebellar metabolism contralateral to a large cerebral abnormality. This is known as crossed-cerebellar diaschisis (see Fig. 6.6B), and this probably occurs because the cerebellum receives neurons through the cerebropontine-cerebellar pathway, which decussates in the pons. Interruption of this pathway results in relatively lower innervation of the cerebellum contralateral to a cerebral injury.

TREATMENT RESPONSE OF BRAIN MALIGNANCY

The most commonly used criteria for treatment response of brain malignancies is based on MR imaging, the Response Assessment in Neuro-Oncology criteria. However, MR has some limitations, including

pseudoprogression (disruption of the blood-brain barrier leading to increased enhancement and presumed progression, when the lesion is truly responding) and pseudoresponse (reduction of blood-brain barrier disruption leading to decreased enhancement and presumed response, when the lesion is truly progressing). FDG uptake is independent from blood-brain barrier disruption and may help evaluate treatment response (Fig. 6.9), although inflammatory causes of FDG avidity must still be distinguished from malignancy.

TUMOR RECURRENCE VERSUS RADIATION NECROSIS

This is an area of tumor evaluation where FDG PET has demonstrated superiority over traditional MR methods (although newer MR measurements such as blood

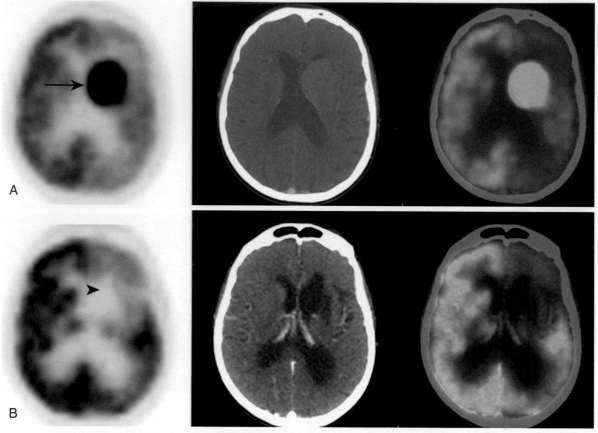

FIG. 6.9 **Treatment Response on FDG PET/CT.** (A) Axial PET, CT, and fused PET/CT images following therapy demonstrate resolution of the FDG-avid lesion *(arrowhead)*, representing treatment response.

volume are showing considerable promise). Following radiation therapy, new enhancing lesions on contrast-enhanced MR may represent high-grade tumor recurrence or radiation necrosis. While less perfect, there is about 80% accuracy for FDG PET/CT to distinguish these two very different options. If the postradiation therapy MR-enhancing lesion corresponds with FDG avidity, then it is probably high-grade tumor recurrence (Fig. 6.10). If the postradiation therapy MR-enhancing lesion lacks FDG avidity, then it is probably radiation necrosis (Fig. 6.11). The descriptor "probably" is apt in this scenario, as there are many examples where this paradigm is incorrect, and clinically imaging follow up is needed in most cases. This can be applied to multiple enhancing lesions in a single patient to determine the lesion that is most suspicious for tumor recurrence or to a single lesion to determine the most suspicious area of the lesion (Fig. 6.12), when biopsy is planned.

BENIGN INTRACRANIAL LESIONS

As is true for other organ systems, not all FDG-avid intracranial foci are malignant. A common benign FDG-avid intracranial lesion is a pituitary adenoma (Fig. 6.13). Often the FDG-avid focus in the sella will not have a corresponding abnormality on CT. MR could be used to visualize the pituitary adenoma.

Meningiomas are benign extra-axial growths from the meninges. They are typically not FDG avid, but may appear as photopenic areas on FDG PET if large enough to displace normal brain parenchyma. The meningioma will be visualized on contrast-enhanced CT or MR (Fig. 6.14).

INFARCTS AND SEIZURES

It is beyond the scope of this oncology textbook to describe the many uses of FDG PET/CT in neurology.

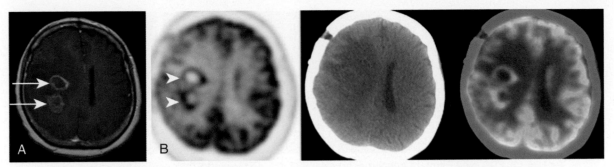

FIG. 6.10 FDG-avid postradiation tumor recurrence. (A) T1 postgadolinium MR in a patient with glioblastoma postradiation therapy demonstrates new ring-enhancing lesions in the radiation field *(arrows)*. The differential is recurrent tumor versus radiation necrosis. (B) Axial PET, CT, and fused PET/CT images demonstrate corresponding rings of FDG avidity *(arrowheads)*, probably recurrent tumor.

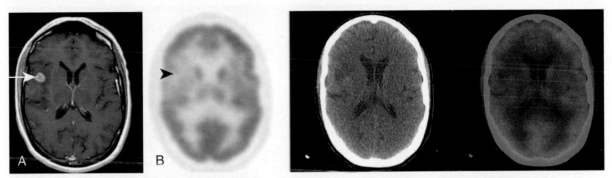

FIG. 6.11 **Non-FDG-avid Postradiation Necrosis.** (A) T1 postgadolinium MR in a patient with glioblastoma postradiation therapy demonstrates a new ring-enhancing lesion in the radiation field *(arrow)*. The differential is recurrent tumor versus radiation necrosis. (B) Axial PET, CT, and fused PET/CT images demonstrate corresponding FDG photopenia *(arrowhead)*, probably radiation necrosis.

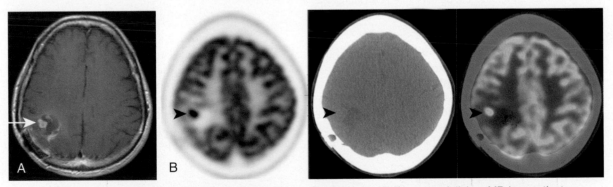

FIG. 6.12 **Focally FDG-avid Postradiation Tumor Recurrence.** (A) T1 postgadolinium MR in a patient with glioblastoma postradiation therapy demonstrates a new ring-enhancing lesion in the radiation field *(arrow)*. The differential is recurrent tumor versus radiation necrosis. (B) Axial PET, CT, and fused PET/CT images demonstrate corresponding focal FDG avidity in the lateral aspect of the lesion *(arrowheads)*, probably tumor recurrence. This helps localize the most suspicious portion on the lesion.

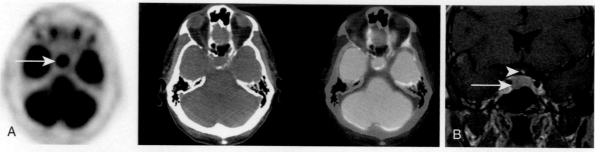

FIG. 6.13 **FDG-avid Pituitary Adenoma.** (A) Axial PET, CT, and fused PET/CT images demonstrate and FDG-avid focus in the pituitary fossa *(arrow)*. (B) Coronal T1 postgadolinium MR demonstrates the adenoma in the right sella *(arrow)* with relatively less enhancement than the normal pituitary. Note the normally enhancing pituitary stalk is deviating to the left *(arrowhead)*.

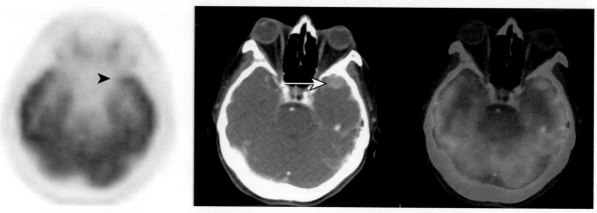

FIG. 6.14 **Non-FDG-avid Meningioma.** Axial PET, CT, and fused PET/CT images demonstrate an extra-axial enhancing lesion in the left middle cranial fossa *(arrow)*, without associated FDG avidity *(arrowhead)*. This is a common incidental finding on contrast CT or MR of the head, a benign meningioma. Meningiomas may appear as photopenic defects if large enough.

However, some manifestations of malignant pathology should be recognized to prevent overcalling malignancy. Wedge-shaped photopenic defects may represent infarcts (Fig. 6.15). When chronic, these will be accompanied by encephalomalacia on CT. Infarcts may also be rounded in the basal ganglia or thalamus. If there is uncertainty, MR could be obtained for further evaluation.

During an active seizure (ictal phase), the seizure focus demonstrates greater than normal FDG avidity. The avidity may be gyriform, rather than mass-like, in morphology (Fig. 6.16). It is uncommon to scan during the ictal phase. It is more common to scan between seizure episodes (inter-ictal) when the seizure focus is photopenic compared with normal brain.

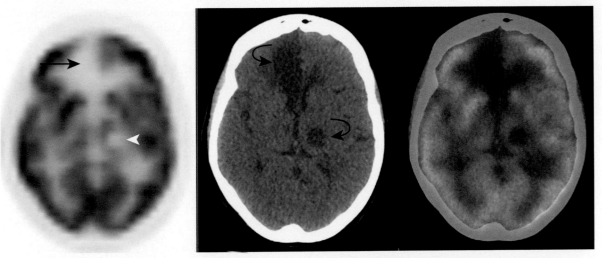

FIG. 6.15 FDG-photopenic infarcts. Axial PET, CT, and fused PET/CT images demonstrate wedge shaped FDG photopenia in the medial right frontal lobe *(arrow)* and round photopenia in the left thalamus *(arrowhead)*. CT image demonstrates corresponding encephalomalacia from chronic infarcts *(curved arrows)*.

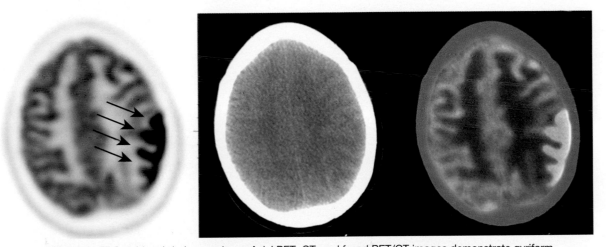

FIG. 6.16 FDG-avid gyri during a seizure. Axial PET, CT, and fused PET/CT images demonstrate gyriform FDG avidity in a patient with glioma *(arrows)*. The morphology is not consistent with tumor. Upon questioning, the patient has been experiencing repeated seizures and may have had a seizure during the PET/CT scan. This FDG avidity resolved on follow-up. The low-grade glioma was not FDG-avid.

Here are a few suggestions to help optimize your interpretation of FDG PET/CT of the brain:

1. Contrast-enhanced multiparametric MR is the most sensitive modality for initial detection intracranial malignancy. Always compare FDG PET/CT images with any available contrast-enhanced MR images for optimal characterization of lesions.

2. Intracranial malignancy may be visualized on FDG PET/CT as FDG avidity above normal brain, FDG photopenia, or lesions on the corresponding CT images. When there is any indecision on FDG PET/CT, consider MR for further evaluation.

3. FDG PET/CT adds value in distinguishing recurrent malignancy (probably avid) from postradiation necrosis (probably nonavid). These two very different lesions are often indistinguishable on contrast-enhanced MR.

4. In AIDS patients with a new enhanced brain lesion, FDG PET/CT has added value in distinguishing AIDS-related lymphoma (avid) from toxoplasmosis (nonavid), the two leading differentials in this scenario.

SUGGESTED READINGS

Berti, et al: Brain: normal variations in benign findings and FDG PET/CT imaging, *PET Clin* 9:129–140, 2014.

Fink, et al: Multimodality brain tumor imaging: MR imaging, PET, and PET/MR imaging, *J Nucl Med* 56:1554–1561, 2015.

Herholz: Brain tumors: an update on clinical PET research in gliomas, *Semin Nucl Med* 47:5–17, 2017.

Kawai, et al: 18F-FDG PET in the diagnosis and treatment of primary central nervous system lymphoma, *Biomed Res Int* 2013:247152, 2013.

Segtnan, et al: ^{18}F-fluorodeoxyglucose PET/computed tomography for primary brain tumors, *PET Clin* 10(1):59–73, 2015.

Wray, et al: 18F-flourodeoxy-glucose PET/computed tomography in brain tumors: value to patient management and survival outcomes, *PET Clin* 10:423–430, 2015.

CHAPTER 7

Head and Neck on FDG PET/CT

HEAD AND NECK ANATOMY

The head and neck has complex anatomy. Proper identification of benign and malignant lesions depends on an understanding of this anatomy and how it may be altered by surgery, chemotherapy, and radiation.

The suprahyoid neck is divided by fascial planes into spaces. While the fascia is not visible on imaging studies, the spaces created by the fascia contain specific structures and the differential diagnosis of a lesion depends on which space the lesion is found in. Thus it is important to be able to localize a mass into one of the spaces. This can often be accomplished by concentrating on the parapharyngeal space (PPS; Fig. 7.1). The PPS contains mostly fat and is an uncommon site for abnormalities, but the fat in the PPS is displaced by masses in other spaces in characteristic directions (Fig. 7.2).

When the PPS fat is displaced posterolaterally, the mass originates in the pharyngeal mucosal space. The pharyngeal mucosal space contains the naso- and oropharyngeal mucosa. Masses in the pharyngeal mucosal space are often malignant and most commonly include squamous cell carcinoma (SCC) of the naso- and oropharynx. Other differentials in the pharyngeal mucosal space include minor salivary gland tumors, lymphoma, and abscess.

When the PPS fat is displaced posteromedially, the mass originates in the masticator space. Masses in the masticator space are usually benign, most commonly dental infections. Other differentials in the masticator space include accessory parotid tissue and muscle hypertrophy. Malignancy in the masticator space is less common, but does occur.

When the PPS fat is displaced anteromedially, the mass originates in the parotid space. Masses in the parotid space are most commonly salivary gland tumors, both benign and malignant. Of course, lymphoma, metastases, and benign lesions from parotitis and sialolithiasis also occur.

And when the PPS fat is displaced anterolaterally, the mass originates in the carotid space. Carotid space masses are usually benign, most commonly paraganglioma and nerve sheath tumors. Of course, malignant lesions, such as nodal metastases, occur here.

Knowing the differential diagnoses based on neck spaces will help interpret imaging findings. While benign and malignant lesions are found in all spaces, a pharyngeal mucosal space mass should first raise concern for SCC, while masticator and carotid space masses should be recognized as most commonly benign. 18F-fluorodeoxyglucose (FDG)-avid foci along the mandible are examples of masticator space lesions which are usually benign dental inflammation.

Lymph nodes in the neck are commonly involved in head and neck malignancy. To help localize nodes and understand nodal drainage pathways in the head and neck, there is a commonly utilized system of nodal levels (Fig. 7.3). Above the hyoid bone are found nodal levels I, II, and the superior portion of V. Level I is anterior to the posterior edge of the submandibular gland. Level V is posterior to the sternocleidomastoid muscle. Level II is between levels I and V, along the internal jugular vein, above the hyoid bone. Below the hyoid bone are found levels III, IV, VI, and the inferior portion of V. Level VI is medial to carotid arteries. Again, level V is posterior to the sternocleidomastoid muscle. Levels III and IV are between levels VI and V, with level III between the hyoid bone and the cricoid cartilage and level IV between the cricoid cartilage and the clavicle. Is takes some practice to properly classify nodes in this system, but it is worth it. Head and neck surgeons use the nodal levels to classify neck nodes; thus using this system will help you communicate with surgeons. Furthermore, primary head and neck SCCs drain to predictable nodal levels. For instance, pharynx cancers and supraglottic larynx usually drain to levels II to V, while infraglottic and thyroid cancers usually drain to level VI. Oral cavity cancers drain first to level I. Thus understanding the nodal levels will help you determine where to expect nodal metastases from head and neck squamous cell cancers.

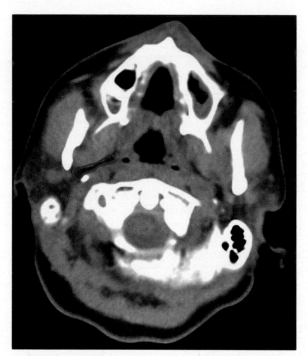

FIG. 7.1 **The Parapharyngeal Space (PPS) on Axial CT.** The fat in the parapharyngeal space *(red outline)* can be identified on CT. This fat is displaced by masses in the spaces around it. You can identify the space a mass is located in by determining which direction the fat in the PPS is displaced. Masses in the different neck spaces have different differential diagnoses.

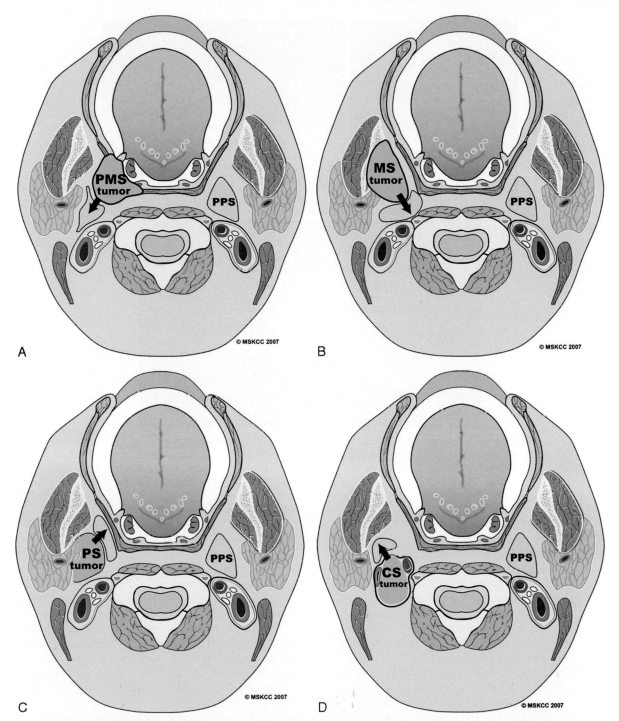

FIG. 7.2 Determining the Space a Head and Neck Mass Originates From. (A) When the parapharyngeal space (PPS) fat is displaced posterolaterally, the mass originates in the pharyngeal mucosal space (PMS). (B) When the PPS fat is displaced posteromedially, the mass originates in the masticator space (MS). (C) When the PPS fat is displaced anteromedially, the mass originates in the parotid space (PS). (D) When the PPS fat is displaced anterolaterally, the mass originates in the carotid space (CS). (Reprinted from Stambuk HE, Patel SG: Imaging of parapharyngeal space, *Otolaryngol Clin North Am* 41(1):77–101, 2008. Courtesy of Memorial Sloan-Kettering Cancer Center, New York, NY; with permission. Copyright 2007 MSKCC.)

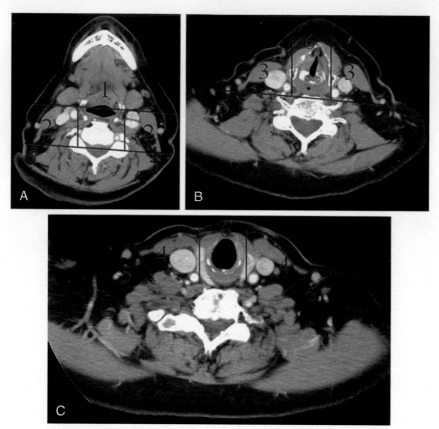

FIG. 7.3 **The Nodal Levels in the Neck.** Axial CT images of the neck (A) above the hyoid, (B) between the hyoid and cricoid, and (C) below the cricoid. Note that nodal levels 1 and 2 are above the hyoid bone. Levels 3, 4, and 6 are below the hyoid bone. Level 5 is posterior to the sternocleidomastoid muscle, both above and below the hyoid.

PHYSIOLOGY FDG AVIDITY IN THE HEAD AND NECK

There are multiple organs in the head and neck with physiologic FDG avidity. This makes comparison of FDG positron emission tomography (PET) images with the corresponding computed tomography (CT) images particularly useful in the head and neck. Localization of FDG avidity to an organ known to have physiologic FDG avidity, without a corresponding CT abnormality, is almost always benign.

Organs in the head and neck with physiologic FDG avidity include the salivary glands (parotid, submandibular, and sublingual glands) and the lymphoid tissue of Waldeyer ring (Fig. 7.4). Waldeyer ring extends from the adenoids superiorly, and extends posterolaterally through the palatine tonsils to converge in the midline again at the base of tongue. The intensity of FDG avidity in these tissues varies among patients and may also vary

between scans of a single patient. The intensity of avidity in any of these organs may range from background avidity to the most avid structure on the image, and any level of avidity may still be physiologic and benign. There may be left-right asymmetry in the level of FDG avidity in any of these organs from physiologic variation or caused by resection or radiation in one side of the neck.

Muscles of the head and neck may be avid (see Chapter 4). These include the muscles of mastication, the ocular muscles, and neck musculature. Curvilinear FDG avidity in muscles, without corresponding CT abnormality, is usually benign. More focal FDG avidity may require further evaluation with contrast-enhanced CT or magnetic resonance (MR) to exclude an underlying mass.

Brown fat may be FDG avid. It is called "brown" because of the more numerous pigmented mitochondria compared with typical "white" fat. These two types of

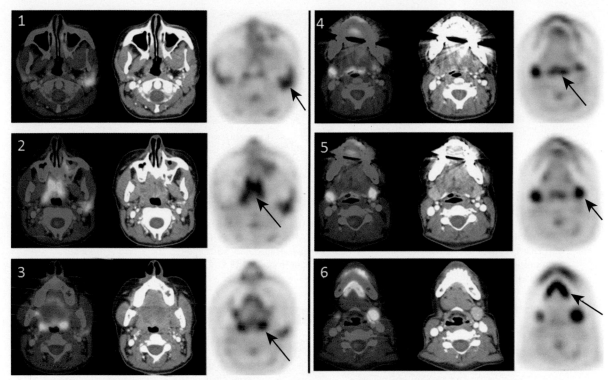

FIG. 7.4 Physiologic FDG Avidity in the Salivary Tissues and Lymphoid Tissues of Waldeyer Ring.
Six axial levels of the head and neck are demonstrated from superior to inferior. (1) Parotid glands *(arrow)*.
(2) Palate and adenoids *(arrow)*. (3) Palatine tonsils *(arrow)*. (4) Base of tongue *(arrow)*. (5) Submandibular
glands *(arrow)*. (6) Sublingual glands *(arrow)*.

fat have the same attenuation and are indistinguishable on CT. The CT component of the PET/CT is crucial for distinguishing brown fat from more ominous findings (see Chapter 21). Unless the patient has a very rare liposarcoma or malignant teratoma, the presence of fat can be a reliable sign that something is benign. FDG avidity in the neck that corresponds to fat on the CT is almost certainly benign brown fat. If the FDG avidity corresponds to soft tissue on CT, then brown fat can be excluded.

The tremendous variability in physiologic FDG avidity in the head and neck may make distinguishing FDG-avid malignancy from benign physiologic FDG avidity difficult.

ANATOMIC AND METABOLIC ALTERATIONS BY SURGERY AND CHEMORADIATION

Surgery and chemoradiation may alter the physiologic FDG-avid structures in the head and neck. Identifying the surgical and chemoradiation changes in a scan will help prevent missing malignancy or misinterpreting a remaining physiologic structure as malignant.

Neck dissections are a common surgical procedure in patients with SCCs of the head and neck. In addition to nodes, neck dissections may or may not include resection of additional structures, including the submandibular gland, sternocleidomastoid muscle, accessory nerve (cranial nerve XI), and/or internal jugular vein. Having an unpaired submandibular gland, due to resection of one in a neck dissection, could easily be mistaken for an FDG-avid node (Fig. 7.5). Resection of a sternocleidomastoid muscle could lead to confusion in the contour of the neck (Fig. 7.6) or if the remaining sternocleidomastoid muscle is FDG avid. The accessory nerve cannot be seen on CT; however, the effects of accessory nerve resection may still be identified. The accessory nerve innervates the trapezius and the sternocleidomastoid muscles. Atrophy of these muscles often helps identify an accessory nerve resection (Fig. 7.7).

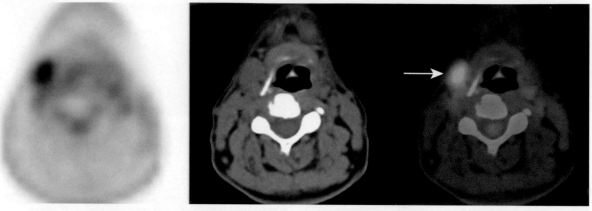

FIG. 7.5 **Unilateral Benign Submandibular Gland in a Patient with Squamous Cell Carcinoma of the Left Tonsil Postresection and Left Neck Dissection.** Axial PET, CT, and fused PET/CT images demonstrate an FDG-avid soft tissue lesion in the right neck *(arrow)*. This could be mistaken for a nodal metastasis. Recognizing that the left submandibular gland has been resected is key to recognizing this as a benign FDG-avid right submandibular gland.

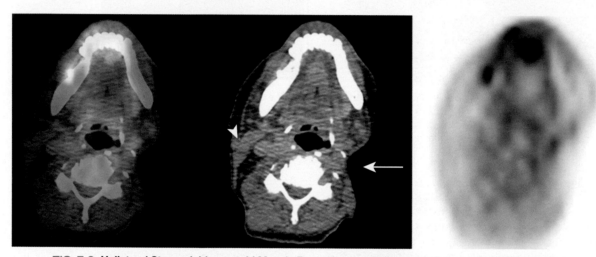

FIG. 7.6 **Unilateral Sternocleidomastoid Muscle Resection in a Patient with Squamous Cell Carcinoma of the Left Tonsil Postresection and Left Neck Dissection.** Fused PET/CT, CT, PET, axial PET images demonstrate absence of the left sternocleidomastoid muscle *(arrow)* creating an abnormality in neck morphology. Compare with the normal sternocleidomastoid muscle on the right *(arrowhead)*.

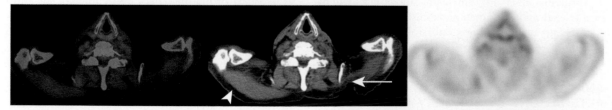

FIG. 7.7 **Unilateral Accessory Nerve Resection as Evidence by Atrophy of the Trapezius Muscle.** Fused PET/CT, CT, PET, axial PET images demonstrate atrophy of the left trapezius muscle *(arrow)* in a patient who has undergone a left neck dissection. Compare with the normal trapezius muscle on the right *(arrowhead)*.

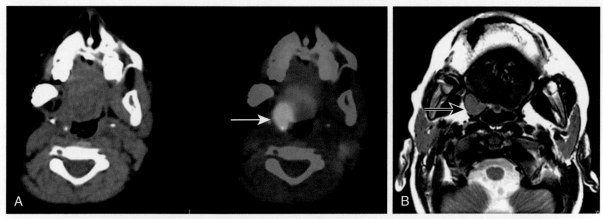

FIG. 7.8 **Unilateral Right Palatine Tonsil in a Patient Following Resection of a Left Oval Cavity Sarcoma.** (A) CT and fused PET/CT images demonstrate FDG-avid soft tissue in the right neck *(arrow)*. (B) Magnetic resonance image demonstrates the unilateral right palatine tonsil *(arrow)* in this patient who has had the left tonsil resected. This prevents misinterpreting the FDG avidity as a nodal metastasis.

In addition to neck dissections, surgical resection of a primary malignancy may alter the appearance of normally FDG-avid structures in the head and neck (Fig. 7.8). Resection of a salivary gland or tonsil may leave an unpaired FDG-avid structure that could be mistaken for a nodal metastasis. Following resection of a head and neck malignancy, the area may be reconstructed. Reconstructions with myocutaneous flaps may contain fatty elements, as well as muscle. The muscular component of flaps may have FDG avidity, which must be recognized as benign (Fig. 7.9).

Chemotherapy and other systemic therapies may have side effects that may be FDG avid. One notable example is bisphosphonate therapy. Bisphosphonates help prevent bone resorption and may be used in patients with osseous metastases. Osteonecrosis of the mandible is a well-recognized side effect of bisphosphonate therapy (Fig. 7.10). Radiotherapy may cause FDG-avid postradiation inflammation or may alternatively injure structures and decrease physiology FDG avidity. Salivary glands or lymphoid tissue in a radiation port may demonstrate reduced FDG avidity, and this may cause asymmetry in pair structures. Radiation may injure nerves, and this may lead to asymmetric FDG avidity in muscular structures. A known example is radiation injury to the hypoglossal nerve causing unilateral tongue FDG avidity (Fig. 7.11).

SALIVARY GLANDS

The parotid, submandibular, and sublingual glands may all demonstrate physiologic FDG avidity (see Fig. 7.4). This avidity may vary from scan to scan and may be asymmetric. Focal areas of FDG avidity in a salivary gland should be correlated with the corresponding CT images for an anatomic correlate. An FDG-avid mass within a salivary gland may be benign or malignant. The most common benign salivary tumors include pleomorphic adenomas and Warthin tumors. The most common malignant salivary tumors are mucoepidermoid carcinoma, adenoid cystic carcinoma, and adenocarcinoma. Benign and malignant salivary tumors cannot be distinguished by the intensity of FDG avidity (Fig. 7.12). Both benign and malignant salivary tumors may have low standardized uptake value (SUV) values or very high SUV values. Invasion of adjacent structures on CT, nodal, and distant metastases are good predictors of malignancy. If these features are not present, then the FDG-avid salivary lesion should either be tissue sampled or followed up by imaging to determine stability or growth. Growth should prompt tissue sampling.

It is interesting that the larger the salivary gland, the more likely a neoplasm is to be benign. In the largest salivary glands, the parotids, neoplasms are more likely to be benign than malignant. Neoplasms in the submandibular glands and sublingual glands have a higher chance of being malignant. Salivary neoplasms of the small accessory salivary glands, which are found throughout the oral cavity, are almost always malignant.

THYROID GLAND

FDG avidity in the thyroid gland should be determined to be diffuse or focal. Diffuse FDG avidity without a CT correlate is almost always inflammatory (Fig. 7.13).

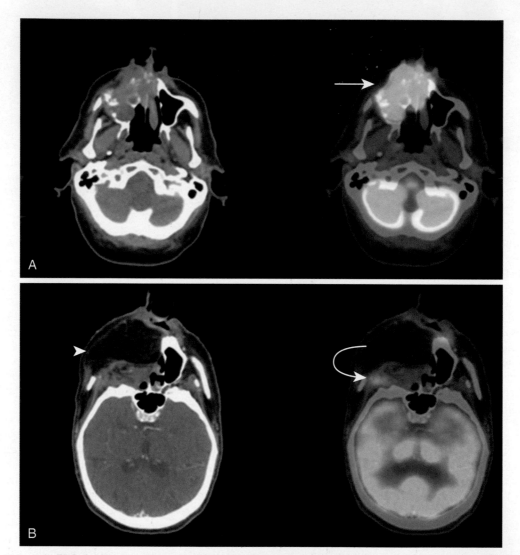

FIG. 7.9 **FDG Avidity in a Myocutaneous Flap Reconstruction.** (A) Axial CT and fused FDG PET/CT demonstrate and FDG-avid adenoid cystic carcinoma *(arrow)*, a salivary malignancy of a minor salivary gland in this patient. (B) Following resection of the malignancy and myocutaneous flap reconstruction, there is fatty *(arrowhead)* and muscle *(curved arrow)* components of the flap reconstruction. Mild FDG avidity in the muscular components, with a focal mass on CT, should be recognized as benign.

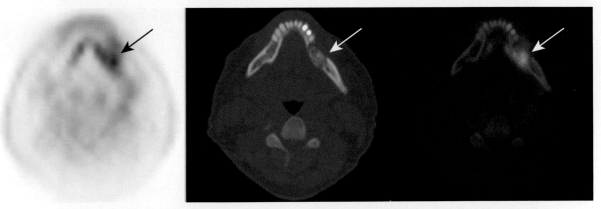

FIG. 7.10 **FDG-avid Osteonecrosis of the Jaw in a Patient on Bisphosphonate Therapy.** Axial PET, CT, and fused PET/CT images demonstrate an FDG-avid lytic lesion in the mandible *(arrows)*. This patient had multiple osseous metastases which were all responding to therapy when this mandibular lesion appeared. Given the response in other metastases, a benign etiology was suspected. Biopsy diagnosed osteonecrosis.

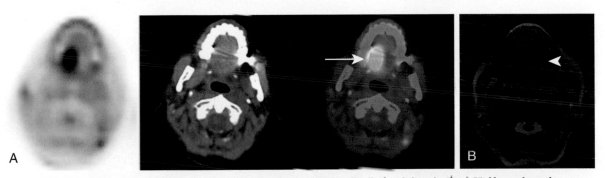

FIG. 7.11 **Asymmetric FDG Avidity in the Tongue Following Radiation Injury to the Left Hypoglossal.** Asymmetric FDG avidity in the tongue following radiation injury to the left hypoglossal nerve. (A) Axial PET, CT, and fused PET/CT images demonstrate unilateral FDG avidity in the right tongue *(arrow)*. (B) T2 magnetic resonance image demonstrates high T2 signal in the left tongue representing edema *(arrowhead)*. This patient had radiation injury to the left hypoglossal nerve, resulting in left tongue paralysis. The paralyzed left tongue is FDG photopenic, while the compensating right tongue is FDG avid.

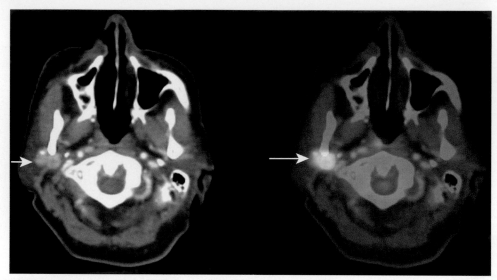

FIG. 7.12 **FDG-avid Parotid Nodule.** Axial CT and fused FDG PET/CT in a patient with ductal breast cancer demonstrate an FDG-avid parotid nodule *(arrows)*. Differential for this lesion includes benign and malignant salivary tumor and breast cancer metastasis. The standard uptake value (SUV) of this nodule cannot distinguish whether it is benign or malignant. Tissue sampling or follow-up imaging is needed. This nodule was biopsied and proven to be a benign Warthin tumor.

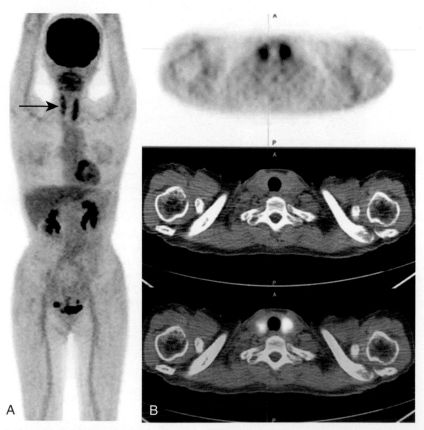

FIG. 7.13 **Inflammatory FDG Avidity in the Thyroid.** (A) FDG maximum intensity projection (MIP) demonstrates linear FDG avidity on both sides of the neck *(arrow)*. (B) Axial PET, CT, and fused PET/CT images demonstrate the avidity corresponds with the two lobes of the thyroid gland, without corresponding CT abnormality. Diffuse thyroid avidity such as this is almost always benign.

Consider describing this as inflammatory or benign in dictations, rather than as "thyroiditis." Thyroiditis is a diagnosis of clinical symptoms and laboratory values. While diffuse FDG avidity in the thyroid will be found in many patients with thyroiditis, not all patients with diffuse thyroid FDG avidity will have clinical and laboratory findings of thyroiditis. Depending on the amount of thyroid tissue in the thyroid isthmus, diffuse thyroid FDG avidity may appear as one continuous avid thyroid or two separate FDG-avid thyroid lobes. If one thyroid lobe has been resected or radiated, then there may only be unilateral FDG avidity.

Focal FDG avidity in the thyroid gland more often requires additional evaluation than diffuse thyroid avidity. The differential for focal thyroid FDG avidity includes benign and malignant thyroid tumors, lymphoma, and metastases to the thyroid. SUV values cannot distinguish benign from malignant thyroid foci. Both benign and malignant thyroid nodules may have low SUV values or very high SUV values. Invasion of adjacent structures on CT, nodal, and distant metastases is a good predictor of malignancy. If these features are not present, then the FDG-avid thyroid nodule should be either subsequently evaluated by ultrasound or followed up by PET/CT to determine stability or growth (Figs. 7.14–7.16). Suspicious features on ultrasound or growth should prompt tissue sampling.

Developmental anomalies may result in thyroid tissue in uncommon anatomic locations. The thyroid gland forms at the base on the tongue and then descends along the thyroglossal duct in the midline anterior to the hyoid bone until it reaches its usual location anterior to the thyroid cartilage. In cases where there is incomplete migration of the thyroid tissue during development, residual thyroid tissue may be found anywhere along the thyroglossal duct. This includes an ectopic lingual thyroid gland, which never migrated from the base of the tongue, and residual thyroid tissue along the thyroid glossal duct (Fig. 7.17).

Both nuclear iodine imaging with iodine-123 or iodine-131 and metabolic imaging with FDG may be valuable for the imaging of thyroid malignancy. The choice between utilizing nuclear iodine imaging and FDG PET/CT may be influenced by the thyroid tumor histology. For papillary thyroid cancer, there may be reciprocal uptake of iodine and FDG, depending on the differentiation of the papillary malignancy. Well-differentiated papillary thyroid cancer may maintain iodine uptake but have low metabolism, and thus be better visualized by iodine imaging than FDG PET/CT. If the tumor dedifferentiates, it may lose iodine uptake, but increase in metabolism and become better visualized by FDG. If recurrent papillary thyroid cancer is suspected due to elevated thyroglobulin but is not

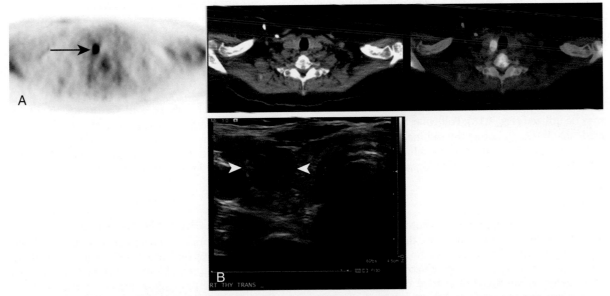

FIG. 7.14 **Focal FDG Avidity in the Thyroid.** (A) Axial PET, CT, and fused PET/CT images in a patient with lymphoma demonstrate focal FDG avidity in the right thyroid gland *(arrow)*. Differential for this lesion includes benign and malignant thyroid neoplasms and lymphoma. (B) Ultrasound demonstrated a solid thyroid nodule *(arrowheads)* prompting tissue sampling. Pathology diagnosed an incidental papillary thyroid carcinoma.

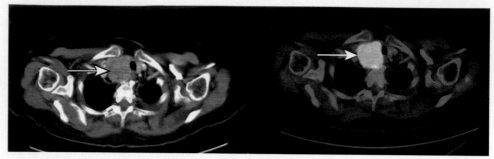

FIG. 7.15 **Focal FDG Avidity in the Thyroid.** Axial CT and fused PET/CT images in a patient with lymphoma demonstrate an FDG-avid soft tissue lesion in the right thyroid gland *(arrows)*. Differential for this lesion includes benign and malignant thyroid neoplasms and lymphoma. Tissue sampling diagnosed a benign thyroid adenoma.

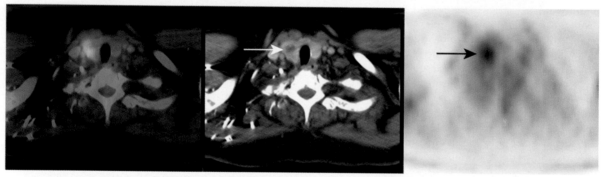

FIG. 7.16 **Focal FDG Avidity in the Thyroid.** Axial CT and fused PET/CT images in a patient with ductal breast cancer demonstrate an FDG-avid soft tissue lesion in the right thyroid gland *(arrows)*. Differential for this lesion includes benign and malignant thyroid neoplasms and breast cancer metastasis. Ultrasound was performed demonstrating a solid nodule and prompted tissue sampling. Tissue sampling diagnosed a breast cancer metastasis.

detected on nuclear iodine imaging, then FDG PET/CT may be utilized (Fig. 7.18). Follicular, poorly differentiated, anaplastic, and other thyroid malignancies, where iodine imaging is less likely to be valuable, may benefit from FDG PET/CT if recurrent malignancy is suspected.

VOCAL CORDS

The muscular portion of the vocal cords is the thyroarytenoid muscles. Like other muscles, these may demonstrate physiologic FDG avidity. In the case of unilateral vocal cord paralysis, the paralyzed cord is FDG photopenic, while the contralateral cord, overworked by compensating for the paralyzed cord, is often FDG avid (Fig. 7.19). This should not be mistaken for FDG-avid malignancy of the vocal cord. CT findings that help make the diagnosis of vocal cord paralysis are a keyhole appearance of the paralyzed cord, due to atrophy of the muscle, and expansion of the ipsilateral pyriform sinus. Primary malignancies of the vocal cord will be best characterized by contrast-enhanced CT or MR. FDG PET/CT provides value in the evaluation of nodal and distant metastases.

SQUAMOUS CELL CARCINOMAS

By far the most common malignancies in the head and neck are SCCs. SCCs may arise from the mucosal surfaces of the oral cavity, nasal cavity, nasopharynx, larynx, and pharynx. The pharynx includes the nasopharynx, oropharynx, and hypopharynx. As for all malignancies, initial staging requires evaluation of the primary tumor (T), local nodal metastases (N), and distant metastases (M).

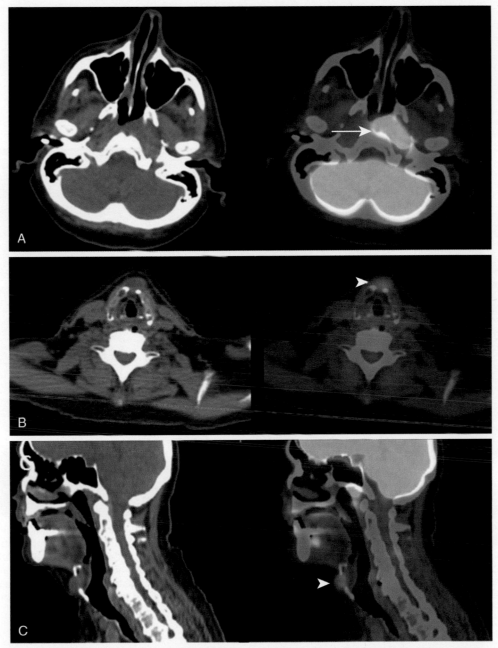

FIG. 7.17 **FDG Avidity in a Nasopharyngeal Carcinoma and a Thyroid Glossal Duct Cyst.** (A) Axial CT and fused FDG PET/CT images in a patient with a known nasopharyngeal carcinoma demonstrate FDG-avid soft tissue in the left nasopharynx which is the nasopharyngeal carcinoma *(arrow)*. (B) Axial and (C) sagittal CT and fused PET/CT images demonstrate FDG-avid soft tissue anterior to the thyroid cartilage *(arrowheads)*. The midline location and distance from the carcinoma is typical of a benign thyroglossal duct lesion, rather than a nodal metastases. Tissue sampling demonstrated a benign thyroglossal duct cyst.

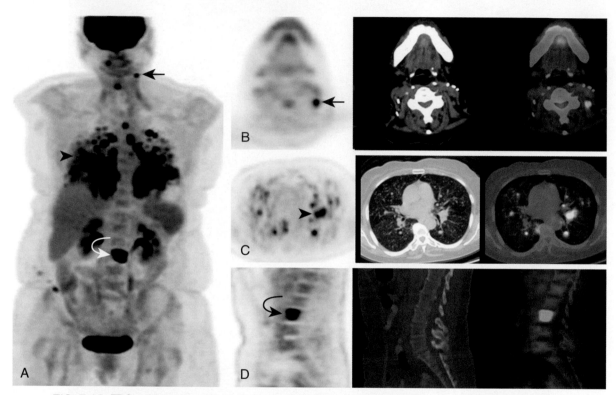

FIG. 7.18 **FDG-avid Papillary Thyroid Cancer Metastases.** (A) FDG maximum intensity projection (MIP) in a patient with papillary thyroid cancer and high thyroglobulin, but no uptake on iodine imaging, demonstrates multiple FDG-avid foci in the neck *(arrow)*, chest *(arrowhead)*, and abdomen *(curved arrow)*. Axial PET, CT, and fused PET/CT images through the (B) neck and (C) chest demonstrate FDG-avid nodal *(arrow)* and lung *(arrowhead)* metastases. (D) Sagittal PET, CT, and fused PET/CT images demonstrate an FDG-avid osseous metastasis *(curved arrow)*. This patient's malignancy may have dedifferentiated, losing avidity for iodine, but becoming more metabolically active and gaining avidity for FDG.

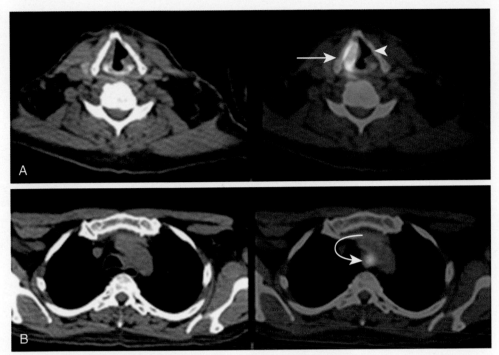

FIG. 7.19 **Vocal Cord Paralysis.** (A) Axial CT and fused PET/CT images through the vocal cords demonstrate unilateral vocal cord avidity *(arrow)*. The "keyhole" morphology of the contralateral vocal cord *(arrowhead)* suggests left vocal cord paralysis. Thus, the avidity in the right vocal cord is benign, related to excess work from compensating from the paralyzed cord. (B) Axial CT and fused PET/CT images through the aortic arch demonstrate and FDG-avid nodal metastasis *(curved arrow)* in this patient with esophageal cancer. The nodal metastasis is located where it could compromise the left recurrent laryngeal nerve as it passes under the aortic arch, leading to vocal cord paralysis.

T staging: In most cases, the primary SCC will be best characterized by contrast-enhanced CT or MR. Most primary malignancies will also be FDG avid on FDG PET/CT, although the local tumor extension will be better evaluated by contrast-enhanced examinations. On FDG PET/CT, superior and inferior extent of the primary malignancy may be appreciated on sagittal or coronal images (Fig. 7.20).

N staging: On CT and MR, evaluation of nodal metastases is based on morphologic and size criteria. Morphologic findings such as necrosis, extracapsular extension, rounding of the nodal shape, and loss of the fatty hilum are suspicious for metastases. For size criteria, different systems based on long-axis and short-axis measurements have been proposed. A commonly used system describes long-axis nodes greater than 15 mm in nodal levels I and II, and greater than 10 mm in nodal levels III to VI as abnormal and suspicious for metastases. However, even with evaluation of morphology and size, malignant nodes are often overlooked.

FDG PET/CT may help identify nodal metastases that are not recognized on contrast-enhanced CT or MR. In order to increase the sensitivity for detecting small neck nodal metastases on FDG PET/CT, a dedicated head and neck protocol is utilized by most centers. A dedicated head and neck protocol images the head and neck from the skull base to the clavicles with a small axial field of view with the arms down, in addition to the standard eyes-to-thighs scan with normal field of view (usually 70 cm) with the arms up. This is why you may see two files of PET/CT images for a patient with head and neck cancer.

In a patient with head and neck SCC, lymph nodes within the drainage system of the primary malignancy that have FDG avidity above local background raise suspicion for nodal malignancy (Fig. 7.21). The addition of FDG PET improves sensitivity for detection of small

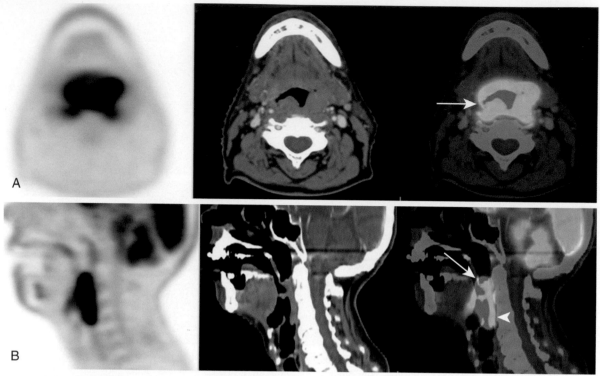

FIG. 7.20 Primary Squamous Cell Carcinoma of the Oropharynx. (A) Axial PET, CT, and fused FDG PET/CT images through the oropharynx demonstrate the FDG-avid primary malignancy *(arrow)*. (B) Sagittal PET, CT, and fused PET/CT images demonstrate the oropharynx primary *(arrow)*, as well as its extension into the hypopharynx *(arrowhead)*.

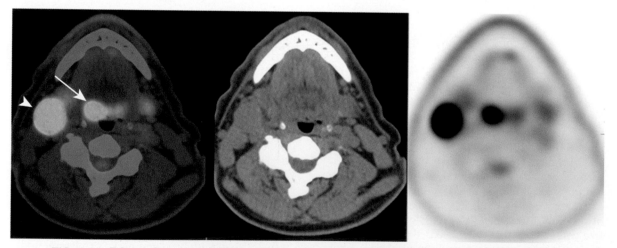

FIG. 7.21 Primary Squamous Cell Carcinoma of the Base of Tongue with Local Nodal Metastases. Fused FDG PET/CT, CT, and PET images through the base of tongue demonstrate the FDG-avid primary malignancy *(arrow)*, as well as an FDG-avid, enlarged right level II nodal metastasis *(arrowhead)*.

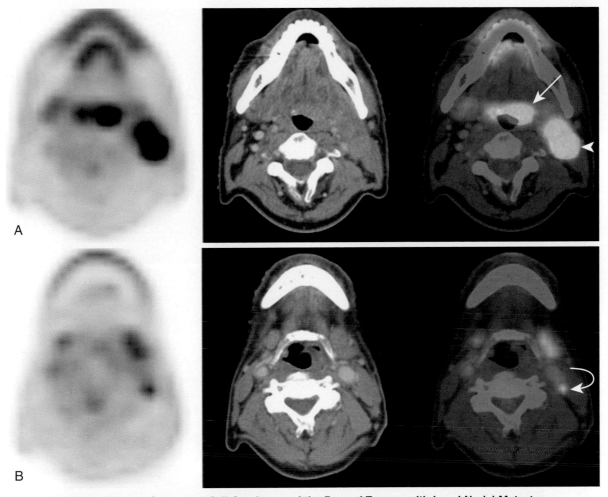

FIG. 7.22 Primary Squamous Cell Carcinoma of the Base of Tongue with Local Nodal Metastases.
(A) PET, CT, and fused FDG PET/CT images through the base of tongue demonstrate the FDG-avid primary malignancy *(arrow)*, as well as FDG-avid, enlarged left level II nodal metastases *(arrowhead)*. (B) More inferior PET, CT, and fused FDG PET/CT images demonstrate a small FDG-avid left level III node *(curved arrow)*, suspicious for an additional nodal metastasis. This node would likely be overlooked without FDG PET.

nodal metastases that would be overlooked by CT or MR (Fig. 7.22).

As inflammatory nodes may also be FDG avid, FDG-avid nodes may be false positive for malignancy. Tissue sampling should be used to confirm malignancy in FDG-avid nodes. False negatives on PET may be caused by necrosis, which may leave little volume of active malignancy in a node (Fig. 7.23).

M staging: The most common site of metastases from head and neck SCCs is the lung. Thus scrutiny of the lungs on CT is required in all patients with head and neck SCC. As discussed in Chapter 8, lung metastases

may be better appreciated on CT than on FDG PET. After lung, the next most common sites of metastases from head and neck SCCs are bone and liver. FDG PET/CT may identify malignancy in these organs, particularly the bone, which may not be appreciated without FDG PET.

FDG PET/CT plays an important role in the initial staging of patients with SCC found in a neck node, but with an unknown primary site. Identification of the primary malignancy is important for determining optimal treatment strategies. FDG PET/CT may identify the site of an unknown primary malignancy in a quarter to a third of cases (Fig. 7.24).

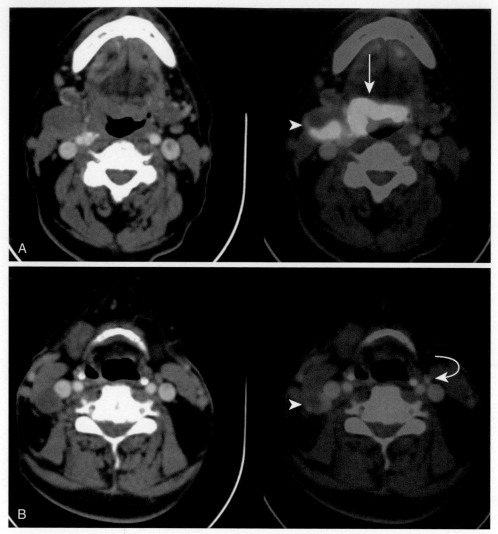

FIG. 7.23 **Primary Squamous Cell Carcinoma of the Base of Tongue with Necrotic Nodal Metastases.**
(A) Axial CT and fused FDG PET/CT images in a patient with a squamous cell carcinoma of the base of
tongue demonstrates the FDG-avid primary base of tongue malignancy *(arrow)*. In addition, a portion of a
right level II nodal metastases is FDG avid *(arrowhead)*. This node is necrotic; thus only part of the node is
avid. (B) Another necrotic node is seen in the right level III, with only mild peripheral FDG avidity *(arrowhead)*.
These necrotic nodes demonstrate how a necrotic node may be overlooked on FDG PET. In addition, there
is a small FDG-avid left level III node *(curved arrow)*, which is suspicious for metastases, but may be
overlooked if it were not for FDG PET.

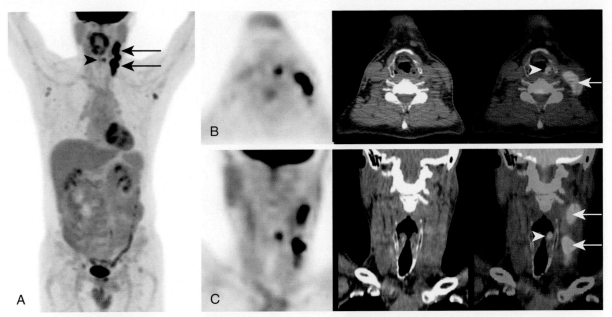

FIG. 7.24 Detection of the Primary Malignancy by FDG PET/CT in a Patient with Known Squamous Cell Carcinoma Left Neck Nodes But Unknown Primary. (A) FDG maximum intensity projection (MIP) demonstrates FDG avidity in the lateral left neck *(arrows)*, and a smaller focus in the more medial left neck *(arrowhead)*. (B) Axial and (C) coronal PET, CT, and fused FDG PET/CT images demonstrate the lateral FDG avidity localizes to FDG-avid nodal metastases *(arrows)*. The more medial focus corresponds to the left pyriform sinus *(arrowheads)*, without CT correlate. Endoscopy and biopsy confirmed the primary left pyriform sinus squamous cell carcinoma.

Given the impact FDG PET/CT has on staging head and neck SCCs, particularly with N and M staging, FDG PET/CT alters the management of a large percentage of patients who undergo FDG PET/CT. This includes changing surgical planning, particularly for nodal metastases, as well as altering radiotherapy planning.

Following therapy, FDG PET/CT again plays an important role in patients with head and neck SCCs. FDG PET is more accurate than CT or MR for measuring the response to chemoradiotherapy. A reduction in FDG avidity to background levels in the primary malignancy and local nodal metastases demonstrates a good tumor response, regardless of the size of the residual primary or neck nodes (Fig. 7.25). An FDG PET/CT without residual FDG-avid foci has a high negative predictive value. In these cases neck dissection may be avoided. The positive predictive value of a posttherapy FDG PET/CT (one with residual FDG-avid lesions) is not as high. This is because both residual malignancy and posttreatment inflammation may be FDG avid. In many cases, residual FDG-avid lesions require biopsy to prove residual active malignancy.

An important aspect of posttherapy FDG PET/CT is the timing of the study. FDG PET/CT is best performed at least 12 weeks following the end of treatment. FDG PET/CT performed earlier has a higher likelihood of false positives for malignancy.

FDG PET/CT is not recommended for routine follow-up of patients with treated SCC, although if recurrence is suspected due to clinical symptoms, then FDG PET/CT may have value in localizing the site of recurrence.

LYMPHOMA

Lymphoma in the head and neck on FDG PET/CT is similar to lymphoma elsewhere in the body. Lymphoma nodes are usually enlarged. Thus, while small mildly FDG-avid nodes in the drainage levels of a known head and neck SCC are suspicious for metastases, small mildly FDG-avid nodes without evidence of larger nodes are more likely to be reactive in patients with lymphoma. As lymphoma is not a primarily surgical disease, describing nodal levels in a patient with lymphoma is usually not important. They can just be called neck nodes. As Waldeyer ring contains lymphoid tissue, lymphoma may

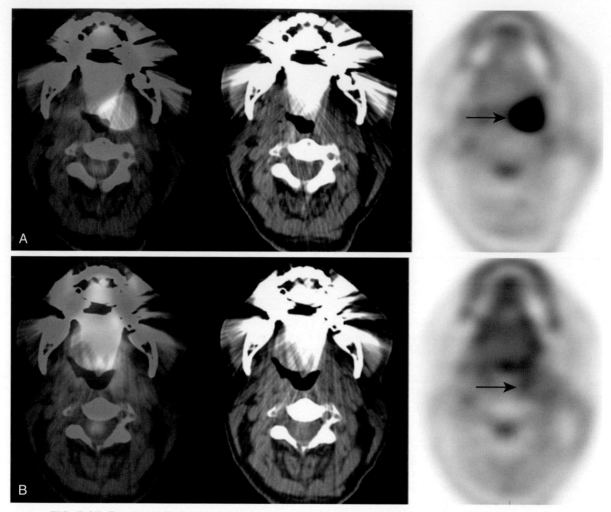

FIG. 7.25 Treatment Response in an Oropharyngeal Squamous Cell Carcinoma. (A) Axial fused FDG PET/CT, CT, and PET images in a patient with a squamous cell carcinoma of the oropharynx demonstrates the FDG-avid primary malignancy *(arrow)*. (B) Following chemoradiotherapy, there is reduction of FDG avidity to background *(arrow)*, indicative of a good tumor response.

be evidenced in the adenoids, palatine tonsils, or base of the tongue (Fig. 7.26). The presence of additional disease that is typical for lymphoma (nodes above and below the diaphragm, spleen, and other organ involvement) versus SCC (local nodal metastases and lung metastases) helps distinguish these malignancies, but Waldeyer ring lymphoma and SCC look identical on FDG PET/CT. Following therapy, the Lugano criteria are used, comparing the residual FDG avidity to the liver background to determine if residual active lymphoma is present.

ORBIT

The ocular muscles may demonstrate physiologic FDG avidity. This makes lesions near the ocular muscles more difficult to detect. The CT component of the FDG PET/CT should be scrutinized adjacent to the ocular muscles, to detect masses that may be obscured on FDG PET (Fig. 7.27). Primary malignancies of the lacrimal glands are similar to malignancies of salivary glands. Lymphoma and metastases may also be seen in the orbit.

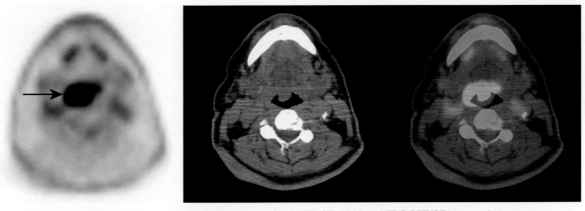

FIG. 7.26 **FDG-avid Base of Tongue Lymphoma.** Axial PET, CT, and fused FDG PET/CT images demonstrate FDG-avid soft tissue at the base of tongue *(arrow)*. Biopsy diagnosed lymphoma. A squamous cell carcinoma at this location may look identical on FDG PET/CT.

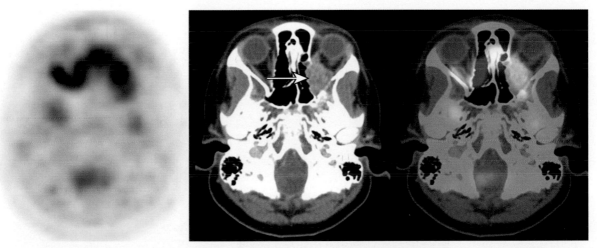

FIG. 7.27 **Orbital Lymphoma Obscured by FDG-avid Ocular Muscles.** Axial PET, CT, and fused FDG PET/CT images in a patient with lymphoma. The corresponding CT image better appreciates the retro-ocular mass *(arrow)* that represents the lymphoma, but it obscured on FDG PET by the FDG-avid ocular muscles.

PERINEURAL DISEASE

SCCs and adenoid cystic carcinomas have a propensity for growth along nerves, known as perineural spread. Other malignancies may demonstrate perineural spread as well. Anatomic findings of perineural malignancy include thickening and enhancement of the nerve, widening of osseous foramen, and loss of fat planes (Fig. 7.28). Perineural tumor may be FDG avid, although FDG PET/CT is less sensitive for perineural disease than contrast-enhanced MR or CT.

CONCURRENT PATHOLOGY

As with other areas of the body, the existence of two separate FDG-avid processes can be confusing. This may occur with two concurrent malignancies, one malignancy and one benign process, or two benign processes. Sometimes the processes can be individually identified because one is far more FDG avid than the other. Other times, the corresponding CT images can help distinguish the processes (Fig. 7.29). When the majority of malignant lesions respond to treatment but one is unaltered,

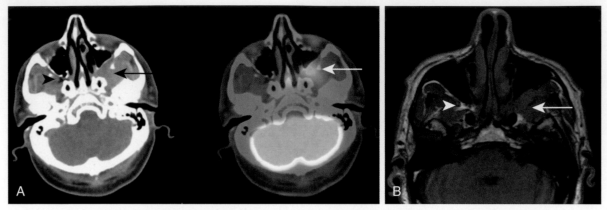

FIG. 7.28 **Perineural Lymphoma.** (A) Axial CT and fused FDG PET/CT images in a patient with lymphoma demonstrate FDG avidity in the region of the left pterygopalatine foramen (PPF) *(arrows)*. The corresponding CT image demonstrates the expansion of the PPF and loss of fat in the PPF, with more diagnostic of perineural malignancy. Compare with the normal right PPF on CT *(arrowhead)*. (B) T1 magnetic resonance demonstrates the loss of high T1 signal fat in the left PPF *(arrow)*, caused by perineural tumor. Compare with the normal right PPF *(arrowhead)*.

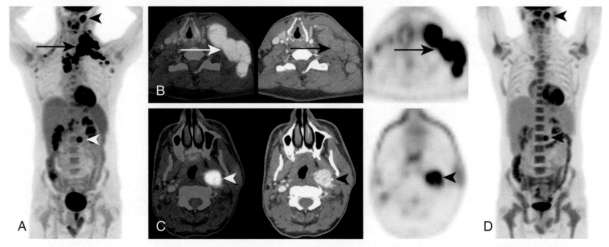

FIG. 7.29 **Concurrent FDG-avid Lymphoma and FDG-avid Benign Paragangliomas.** (A) FDG maximum intensity projection (MIP) demonstrating multiple FDG-avid foci in the neck, chest, and abdomen *(arrow and arrowheads)*. (B) Axial fused FDG PET/CT, CT, and PET images through the neck demonstrated multiple FDG-avid nodes *(arrows)*, with biopsy proven to represent lymphoma. (C) Axial-fused FDG PET/CT, CT, and PET images through the lower face demonstrate an FDG-avid soft tissue lesion with strong enhancement *(arrowheads)*, unlike the known lymphoma. This lesion splays the external and internal carotid arteries and represents a carotid space mass. An enhancing carotid space mass is consistent with a paraganglioma. (D) FDG MIP following lymphoma treatment demonstrates resolution of the vast majority of the FDG-avid lesions, representing the resolution of FDG-avid lymphoma. There are two remaining FDG-avid foci *(arrowheads)*, corresponding to the carotid space paraganglioma and another abdominal paraganglioma. These were distinguished from lymphoma by their strong contrast enhancement.

consider a second, independent process that may require further evaluation.

Here are a few suggestions to help optimize your interpretation of FDG PET/CT of the head and neck:

1. Neck anatomy is complex. The more you know, the better you can read FDG PET/CT.

2. Many structures in the head and neck have physiologic FDG avidity. Comparison with the corresponding CT images will help distinguish these from more ominous findings.

3. Surgery and chemoradiation may alter the physiologic FDG-avid structures in the head and neck. Identifying the surgical and chemoradiation changes in a scan will help prevent missing malignancy or misinterpreting a remaining physiologic structure as malignant.

4. FDG-avid salivary gland and thyroid nodules cannot be determined to be benign or malignant based on SUV. FDG-avid salivary nodules should be tissue sampled or followed up on imaging for stability/grow. FDG-avid thyroid nodules can be further evaluated by ultrasound to determine if tissue sampling is needed.

5. FDG PET/CT has multiple proven uses in patients with head and neck SCCs, including initial N and M staging, surgical and radiotherapy planning, detection of unknown primary tumor sites, and evaluating response to therapy.

6. Performing FDG PET/CT at least 12 weeks following radiotherapy of head and neck SCCs will help reduce false-positive FDG-avid findings. A post-therapy FDG PET/CT with no suspicious FDG-avid foci is highly valuable in demonstrating successful response to therapy and may prevent neck dissections. A post-therapy FDG PET/CT with suspicious FDG-avid foci often needs tissue sampling to prove residual malignancy, as both malignancy and posttherapy inflammation may be FDG avid.

SUGGESTED READINGS

Caetano, et al: Accuracy of positron emission tomography and positron emission tomography-CT in the detection of differentiated thyroid cancer recurrence with negative (131) I whole-body scan results: a meta-analysis, *Head Neck* 38:316–327, 2016.

Cheung, et al: Detecting residual/recurrent head neck squamous cell carcinomas using PET or PET /CT: systematic review and meta-analysis, *Otolaryngol Head Neck Surg* 154:421–432, 2016.

Evangelista, et al: Comparison between anatomical cross-sectional imaging and 18F-FDG PET/CT in the staging, restaging, treatment response, and long-term surveillance of squamous cell head and neck cancer: a systematic literature overview, *Nucl Med Commun* 35:123–134, 2014.

Goel, et al: Clinical practice in PET /CT for the management of head and neck squamous cell cancer, *AJR Am J Roentgenol* 209:289–303, 2017.

Højgaard, et al: Head and neck: normal variations and benign findings in FDG positron emission tomography/computed tomography imaging, *PET Clin* 9:141–145, 2014.

Lauridsen, et al: 18F-fluorodeoxyglucose-positron emission tomography/computed tomography in malignancies of the thyroid and in head and neck squamous cell carcinoma: a review of the literature, *PET Clin* 10:75–88, 2015.

Lonneux, et al: Positron emission tomography with [18F]fluorodeoxyglucose improves staging and patient management in patients with head and neck squamous cell carcinoma: a multicenter prospective study, *JCO* 28:1190–1195, 2010.

Paes, et al: Perineural spread in head and neck malignancies: clinical significance and evaluation with 18F-FDG PET/CT, *Radiographics* 33:1717–1736, 2013.

Park, et al: (18)F FDG PET/CT versus CT/MR imaging and the prognostic value of contralateral neck metastases in patients with head and neck squamous cell carcinoma, *Radiology* 279:481–491, 2016.

Plaxton, et al: Characteristics and limitations of FDG PET/CT for imaging of squamous cell carcinoma of the head and neck: a comprehensive review of anatomy, metastatic pathways, and image findings, *AJR Am J Roentgenol* 205:W519–W531, 2015.

Som, et al: An imaging-based classification for the cervical nodes designed as an adjunct to recent clinically based nodal classifications, *Arch Otolaryngol Head Neck Surg* 125:388–396, 1999.

Som, et al: Imaging-based nodal classification for evaluation of neck metastatic adenopathy, *AJR Am J Roentgenol* 174:837–844, 2000.

Stambuk, et al: Imaging of the parapharyngeal space, *Otolaryngol Clin North Am* 4:77–101, 2008.

Taghipour, et al: Use of 18F-fludeoxyglucose-positron emission tomography/computed tomography for patient management and outcome in oropharyngeal squamous cell carcinoma: a review, *JAMA Otolaryngol Head Neck Surg* 142:79–85, 2016.

Wassef, et al: PET/CT in head-neck malignancies: the implications for personalized clinical practice, *PET Clin* 11(3):219–232, 2016.

Zhu, et al: 18F-fluorodeoxyglucose positron emission tomography-computed tomography as a diagnostic tool in patients with cervical nodal metastases of unknown primary site: a meta-analysis, *Surg Oncol* 22:190–194, 2013.

CHAPTER 8

Lung on FDG PET/CT

The lung is an organ where the integration of findings on 18F-fluorodeoxyglucose positron emission tomography (FDG PET), findings on computed tomography (CT), and the clinical scenario is particularly important to arrive at the best conclusions. Many FDG-avid lung lesions will be determined to be malignant or benign only after correlation with CT findings and the clinical history. Non-FDG-avid lung lesions may also be malignant and need to be recognized on the CT component of the study.

It is useful to consider multiple differential diagnoses for pulmonary lesions. The lung is a common site of malignancy, including metastases, primary lung cancers, neuroendocrine tumors/carcinoid, and lymphoma. There are many benign etiologies of lung lesions: infectious (such as granulomas, pneumonia, abscesses), vascular (embolic, aterio-vascular malformations), autoimmune (rheumatoid nodules, Wegener/granulomatosis with polyangiitis), benign neoplasms (hamartomas), congenital (bronchogenic cysts), and traumatic (pneumatocele) lesions.

SOLITARY PULMONARY NODULES

A solitary pulmonary nodule (SPN) is a round intraparenchymal lung lesion less than 3 cm in greatest diameter, without adjacent atelectasis or local suspicious lymph nodes. I mention this definition, since many studies are ordered with a clinical indication of SPN, without actually being an SPN. FDG PET/CT has been estimated to have about 80% accuracy in defining an SPN greater than 8 mm as benign or malignant. This number will vary depending on where you live, as regions with endemic granulomatous diseases will have a greater prevalence of benign SPNs. This relatively high accuracy led to the evaluation of SPNs as one of the early approved applications for FDG PET (Fig. 8.1). However, an FDG-avid SPN is not always malignant (Fig. 8.2), and some primary lung malignancies such as adenocarcinoma in situ, minimally invasive adenocarcinoma (Fig. 8.3), well-differentiated adenocarcinoma (Fig. 8.4), and low-grade carcinoids

may not be FDG avid. All SPNs should be evaluated by tissue sampling or follow-up imaging. FDG PET/CT may help distinguish between these two choices, as a non-FDG-avid SPN may favor follow-up imaging, while FDG-avid SPN favors immediate tissue sampling.

MULTIPLE PULMONARY NODULES

Multiple pulmonary nodules also have a wide differential diagnosis, including malignant (metastases, primary lung cancers, lymphoma) and benign (embolic, autoimmune, infectious) etiologies. Both the CT and FDG PET characteristics, as well as the clinical scenarios, should be considered when characterizing multiple pulmonary nodules. In a patient with a malignancy with propensity to metastasize to the lung, multiple round pulmonary nodules should be considered suspicious for lung metastases, whether FDG avid (Fig. 8.5) or not (Fig. 8.6). Likewise, in a patient with lymphoma, multiple round nodules in the lungs should be considered lung lymphoma until proven otherwise (Fig. 8.7). Metastases are most commonly round nodules; thus the presence of multiple FDG-avid patchy nodules may suggest a different diagnosis (Fig. 8.8). As can be seen, both the CT and FDG PET characteristics of multiple pulmonary nodules are important for optimal diagnosis.

LUNG CANCER

Lung cancers are often divided into two main types: non-small cell lung cancer (NSCLC) and small cell lung cancer (SCLC). FDG PET/CT has demonstrated multiple valuable applications for patients with NSCLC, and almost all patients with NSCLC have an FDG PET/CT before initiating treatment. This is because FDG PET/CT has demonstrated substantial impact by detecting previously unknown nodal and distant metastases, which upstage the patient and may prevent a "futile" surgery (Fig. 8.9). FDG PET/CT may prevent from one-third to one-half of surgical resections by the demonstration of otherwise unknown extent of malignancy. FDG PET/CT

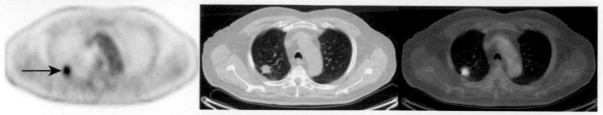

FIG. 8.1 **FDG-avid Solitary Pulmonary Nodule (SPN).** Patient was found to have a 2-cm nodule in the right upper lobe on a CT, prompting an FDG PET/CT scan. Axial FDG PET, axial CT, and fused FDG PET images demonstrated an FDG-avid SPN (standard uptake value (SUV) 6.5, *arrow*) without evidence of nodal or distant metastases. Subsequent biopsy diagnosed primary lung adenocarcinoma.

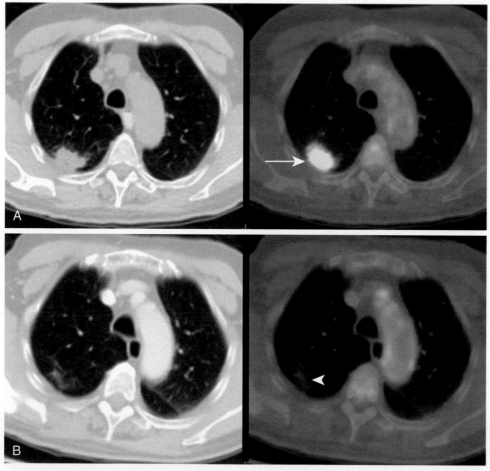

FIG. 8.2 **FDG-avid Solitary Pulmonary Nodule (SPN) That Was Nonmalignant.** Patient was found to have a 2.8-cm nodule in the right upper lobe on a CT, prompting an FDG PET/CT scan. (A) Axial CT and fused FDG PET/CT demonstrate the SPN is FDG avid (standard uptake value (SUV) 8.9, *arrow*). Subsequent biopsy diagnosed an abscess. (B) Four months later, axial CT and fused FDG PET/CT demonstrate resolution of FDG avidity and near resolution on the opacity *(arrowhead)*.

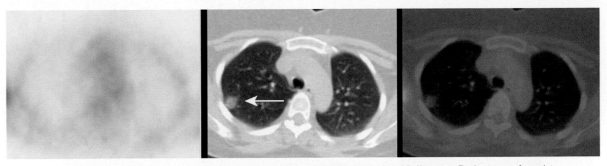

FIG. 8.3 **Non-FDG-avid Solitary Pulmonary Nodule (SPN) That Was Malignant.** Patient was found to have a 1.5-cm nodule in the right upper lobe on a CT, prompting an FDG PET/CT scan. Axial PET, CT, and fused FDG PET/CT demonstrate an SPN with FDG avidity less than mediastinal background (standard uptake value (SUV) 1.0, *arrow*). Biopsy was still performed and diagnosed a minimally invasive adenocarcinoma.

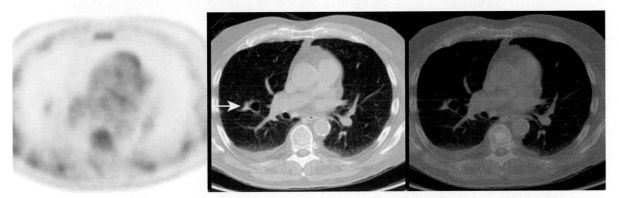

FIG. 8.4 **Non-FDG-avid Nodule That Was Malignant.** Patient with squamous cell carcinoma of the tonsil was found to have a mixed cystic and solid nodule in the right upper lobe on a CT, prompting an FDG PET/CT scan. Axial PET, CT, and fused FDG PET/CT demonstrate the nodule has FDG avidity less than mediastinal background (standard uptake value (SUV) 1.2, *arrow*). Biopsy was still performed and diagnosed a well-differentiated primary lung adenocarcinoma. Differential would have also included a cavitating metastases and benign cavitating lesions.

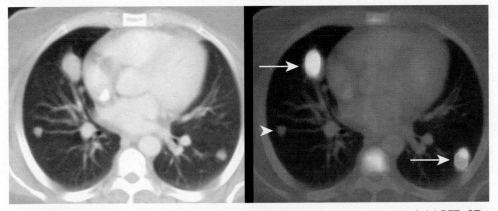

FIG. 8.5 **FDG-avid Lung Metastases in a Patient With Uterine Leiomyosarcoma.** Axial PET, CT, and fused FDG PET/CT demonstrate multiple rounded lung nodules, many of which are FDG avid *(arrows)*, although not all *(arrowhead)*. Biopsy diagnosed lung metastases.

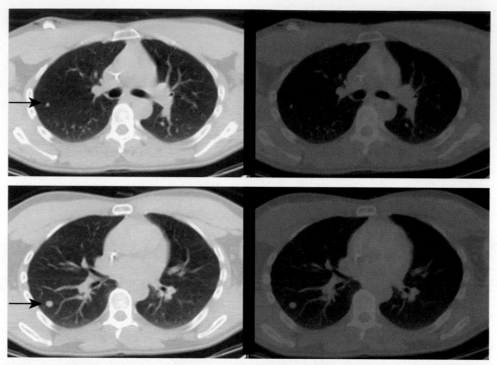

FIG. 8.6 **Non-FDG-avid Lung Metastases in a Patient With Synovial Sarcoma.** Axial CT and fused FDG PET/CT images at two levels demonstrate two of several rounded lung nodules with FDG avidity less than mediastinal background *(arrows)*. Despite the apparent lack of FDG avidity, the presence of multiple rounded lung nodules in a patient with a malignancy known to metastasize to the lung is suspicious for metastases. Biopsy confirmed lung metastases.

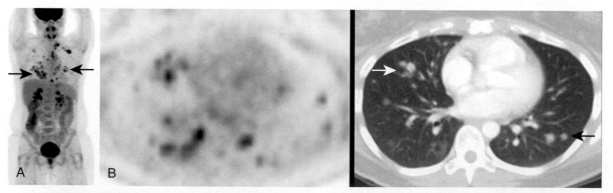

FIG. 8.7 **FDG-avid Lung Lymphoma.** (A) FDG maximum intensity projection (MIP) demonstrates multiple round foci of FDG avidity *(arrows)* in a patient with a history of lymphoma. (B) Axial FDG PET and CT images through the lungs demonstrate multiple FDG-avid rounded lung nodules *(arrows)*. Biopsy confirmed lung lymphoma.

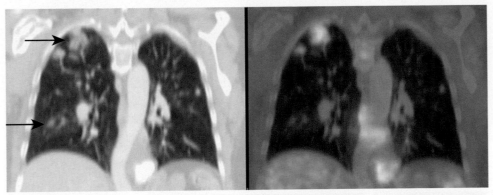

FIG. 8.8 FDG-avid Multiple Nodules That Were Benign in a Patient With Colon Cancer. Coronal CT and fused FDG PET/CT images through the lungs demonstrate multiple FDG-avid lung nodules *(arrows)*. However, the morphology on CT was patchy, rather than round, which is less characteristic of lung metastases. Biopsy confirmed infectious emboli.

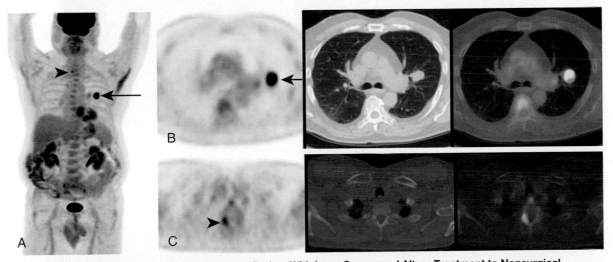

FIG. 8.9 FDG PET/CT Scan Upstages a Patient With Lung Cancer and Alters Treatment to Nonsurgical. (A) FDG maximum intensity projection (MIP) demonstrates an FDG-avid focus overlying the left lung *(arrow)*, but also an FDG-avid focus near the spine in the upper chest *(arrowhead)*. (B) Axial PET, CT, and fused FDG PET/CT images through the lungs demonstrate the known lung primary malignancy *(arrow)*. (C) Similar images through the upper chest demonstrate an FDG-avid focus in the spine *(arrowhead)*, without a CT correlate. Biopsy demonstrated osseous metastases, upstaging the patient to level IV (metastatic disease). The patient is no longer a surgical candidate.

has a high negative predictive value for mediastinal and hilar nodes, as well as distant metastases, and patients with an FDG PET/CT without evidence of nodal or distant disease may proceed to surgical resection of the primary lung malignancy. The positive predictive value of FDG PET is lower, and suspicious foci should be biopsied for confirmation of metastases. In the case of mediastinal/hilar nodes, this often requires mediastinoscopy and biopsy. In the cases of distant metastases, this often requires CT-guided biopsy. At some specialty centers, there is increased use of FDG PET/CT-guided biopsies to help pinpoint the most metabolically active portion of the lesion to biopsy or to allow biopsy of an FDG-avid lesion that may not be seen on CT.

SCLC is usually considered metastatic at diagnosis; thus FDG PET/CT has less proven value in initial staging

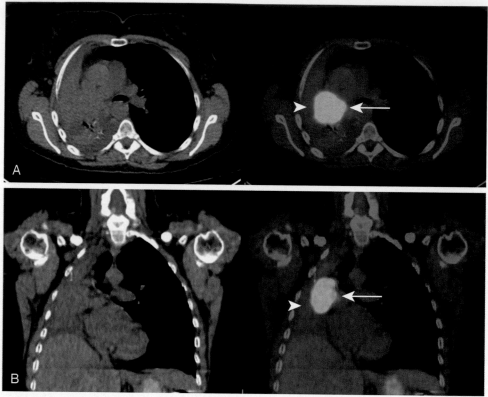

FIG. 8.10 **FDG PET/CT Scan Distinguishes Malignancy from Adjacent Postobstructive Atelectasis.** (A) Axial and (B) coronal CT and fused FDG PET/CT images through the lungs demonstrate the known lung metastasis *(arrows)* and distinguish it from the adjacent postobstructive atelectasis *(arrowheads)*. This confirms the malignancy does not extend to the pleural surface and may help localize the malignancy for radiotherapy contouring.

of SCLC. FDG PET/CT may still provide clinical value for radiotherapy contouring and detection of residual/recurrent malignancy following ablations.

FDG PET/CT can also distinguish malignancy from adjacent benign processes, such as postobstructive atelectasis, which can assist local staging and radiotherapy planning. It is often difficult on CT to distinguish the malignancy from postobstructive atelectasis, and FDG PET/CT improves the delineation of metabolically active tumor from adjacent atelectasis (Fig. 8.10).

There are currently no guidelines recommending the use of FDG PET/CT for evaluating lung cancer treatment response or detection of recurrent malignancy. The National Comprehensive Cancer Network (NCCN) suggests follow-up imaging of lung cancer with CT. That being said, there is potential for FDG PET/CT to be used in cases of suspected lung cancer recurrence following therapy, who are candidates for salvage therapies. There

is evidence that FDG PET/CT detects lung cancer recurrence earlier than CT. An example is the use of FDG PET/CT following the ablation of lung malignancies. Following an ablation, the ablation cavity is often larger than the initial malignancy, as a rim of normal tissue is sacrificed to ensure the entire malignant lesion was within the ablation cavity. This may make it difficult to distinguish postablation effects from residual or recurrent malignancy. In these instances, focal FDG avidity can help distinguish FDG-avid malignancy from nonavid postablation effects (Fig. 8.11). It is important to realize that the ablation may incite inflammation that may be avid days, weeks, or even months following the ablation. This FDG-avid postablation inflammation may even be more FDG avid than the ablated malignancy. Baseline postablation FDG PET/CT scans may demonstrate homogenous or peripheral FDG avidity which is inflammatory (Fig. 8.12). This is expected to

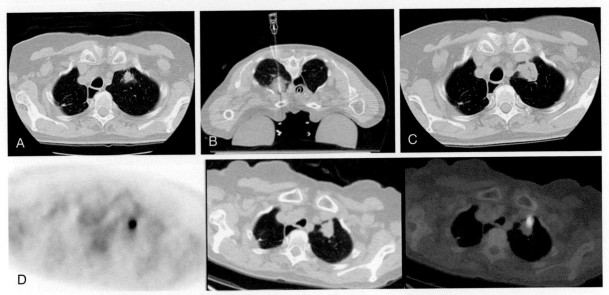

FIG. 8.11 **FDG-avid Lung Cancer Recurrence Following an Ablation.** (A) Axial CT demonstrating a known left upper lobe recurrent lung cancer. (B) Prone axial CT demonstrates interventional radiology ablation of the malignancy. (C) One month following ablation, the opacity on CT is larger, and it is difficult to distinguish postablation effects from residual malignancy. (D) Axial PET, CT, and fused FDG PET/CT images on the same day as (C) demonstrate a focus of FDG avidity in the superior aspect of the postablation opacity. PET/CT-guided biopsy helped localize the biopsy to the metabolically active portion of the lesion and diagnosed residual malignancy.

remain stable, decrease, or resolve on following imaging. It is the appearance of new focal FDG avidity within the ablation cavity that is most suspicious for recurrent malignancy.

There is some debate over the timing of FDG PET/CT if used following therapy. As radiation therapy often induces FDG-avid lung injury, which may last many months, most people recommend waiting 3 months after radiation therapy before undergoing FDG PET/CT. This will reduce but not eliminate the occurrence of FDG-avid postradiation lung damage, which could lead to false-positive interpretations. Chemotherapy and surgery induce relativity shorter lasting FDG-avid injury, and most people recommend waiting 3 to 4 weeks before undergoing FDG PET/CT. Of course, clinical need may override these recommendations in appropriate clinical situations.

BENIGN LUNG LESIONS WITH DISTINCT APPEARANCES

It is important to remember that not all FDG-avid lung lesions are malignant. There are several distinct appearances of FDG-avid lung lesions, which can help

distinguish them as benign. Dependent, patchy opacities in the lower lobes are not the typical appearance of malignancy, despite FDG avidity. This is the distribution of aspiration pneumonia, which may be highly FDG avid yet benign (Fig. 8.13). Tree-in-bud opacities are usually benign, but still display inflammatory FDG avidity (Fig. 8.14). A patchy opacity adjacent to a spinal osteophyte is usually benign and reactive to the osteophyte (Fig. 8.15). Of course, the opacity should remain stable or decrease over time. Radiation and systemic therapies may also induce FDG-avid but benign lung opacities. Following radiotherapy, FDG-avid patchy opacities within the radiation port are usually radiation-associated lung injury (Fig. 8.16). A number of systemic therapies, such as bleomycin, pralatrexate, and taxols, induce pneumonitis (Fig. 8.17). Often it is the patchy morphology of the lung opacities on CT that suggest the diagnosis of therapy-induced pneumonitis, rather than lung metastases. You may encounter an FDG-avid focus in the lung that has no CT correlate. First, scroll cranial and caudal on the CT images to see if the nodule on CT is misregistered from the FDG-avid focus on PET. If no corresponding CT abnormality is identified, this is usually an FDG tracer embolus (Fig. 8.18). When the FDG is administered

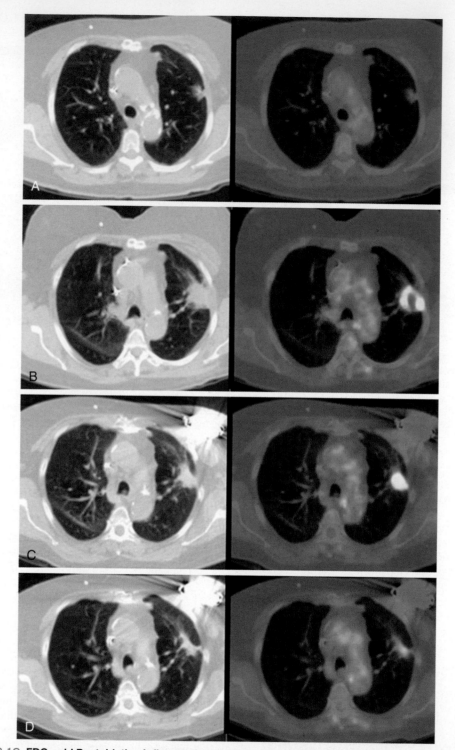

FIG. 8.12 **FDG-avid Postablation Inflammation.** (A) Axial CT and PET CT demonstrate a known recurrent left upper lobe lung cancer. Ablation was performed. (B) Three months following ablation, axial CT, and fused FDG PET/CT demonstrate a postablation opacity that is larger than the original malignancy and has periphery FDG avidity that is more intense than the original malignancy. (C) Seven months and (D) 11 months following ablation there is progressive decrease in size and FDG avidity of the opacity, consistent with resolving postablation inflammation.

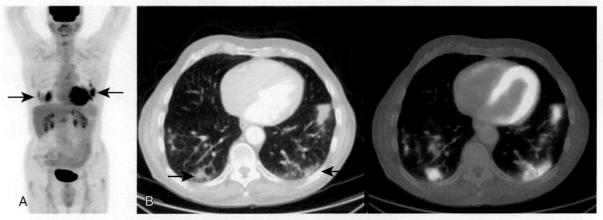

FIG. 8.13 **FDG-avid Aspiration Pneumonia.** (A) FDG maximum intensity projection (MIP) demonstrates multiple clustered FDG-avid foci overlying the lung bases *(arrows)*. (B) Axial CT and fused PET/CT demonstrate the FDG avidity corresponds to multiple patchy opacities in the lung bases *(arrows)*. This patient suffers from repeated aspirations.

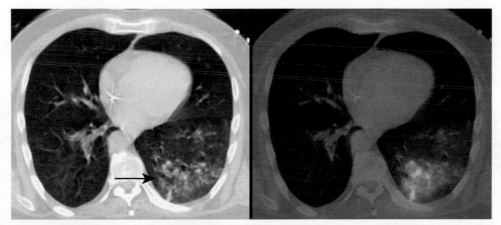

FIG. 8.14 **FDG-avid Inflammatory Opacities.** Axial CT and fused PET/CT demonstrate FDG-avid tree-in-bud lung opacities *(arrow)*. The CT morphology is consistent with a benign infectious process.

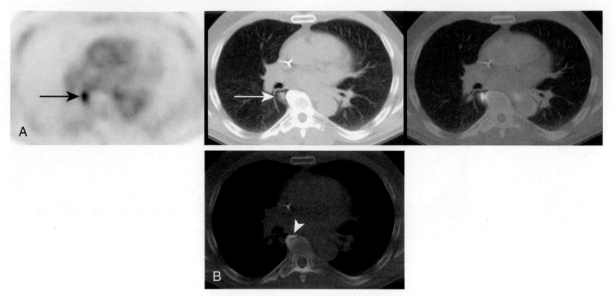

FIG. 8.15 **FDG-avid Inflammatory Opacity Adjacent to an Osteophyte.** (A) Axial PET, CT on lung window, and fused PET/CT demonstrate an FDG-avid opacity in the medial right lung *(arrows)*. (B) Changing the CT window to a bone window demonstrates the opacity is adjacent to a spinal osteophyte *(arrowhead)*. These opacities are usually benign and may be FDG avid.

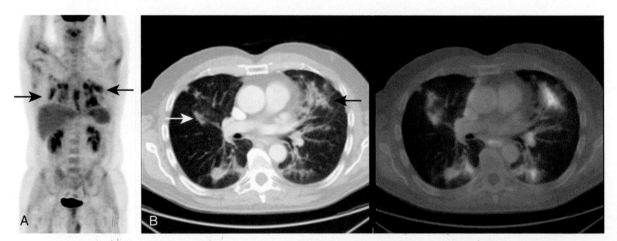

FIG. 8.16 **FDG-avid Postradiation Lung Injury.** (A) FDG maximum intensity projection (MIP) in a patient with esophageal cancer postradiation therapy demonstrates multiple FDG-avid foci overlying the medial lungs *(arrows)*. (B) Axial CT and fused PFDG PET/CT demonstrate the FDG-avid foci correspond with multiple patchy opacities within the radiation port *(arrows)* and represent benign radiation-induced lung injury.

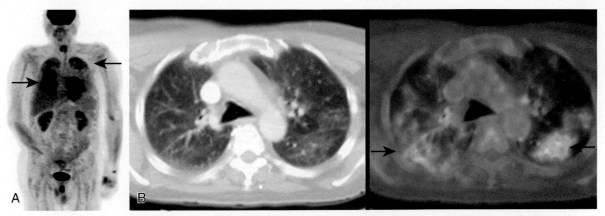

FIG. 8.17 **FDG-avid Bleomycin Pneumonitis.** (A) FDG maximum intensity projection (MIP) in a patient with lymphoma postchemotherapy therapy including bleomycin demonstrates multiple FDG-avid foci overlying the lungs *(arrows)*. (B) Axial CT and fused PFDG PET/CT demonstrate the FDG-avid foci correspond with multifocal patchy opacities on CT *(arrows)* and represent bleomycin-induced pneumonitis, rather than lung malignancy. These findings resolved on follow-up.

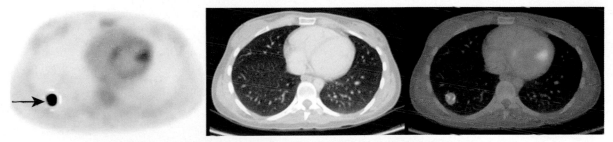

FIG. 8.18 **FDG Tracer Embolus.** Axial PET, CT, and fused FDG PET/CT in a patient with lymphoma demonstrate an FDG-avid focus without CT correlate *(arrow)*. This is a benign FDG tracer embolus, without clinical significance.

intravenously, a small clot may form at the administration site. This will travel through the veins into the right heart, through the pulmonary artery into the lungs, and lodge in a pulmonary capillary. The high concentration of FDG in the tracer embolus will appear as an FDG-avid focus in the lung without a CT correlate. This may be reported as a benign tracer embolus. It may be necessary to explain that this "embolus" is not the same as a central pulmonary embolism. A tiny capillary embolus like this has no clinical significance (your lungs trap and clear thousands, if not millions, of these tiny clots each day), and no treatment is needed. An FDG-avid tracer embolus should not occur in the same spot on a subsequent scan. If you find you have multiple FDG PET/CT scans containing tracer emboli, check if they are all associated with a single person administering the FDG. Training may be needed to optimize the tracer injection and prevent tracer emboli.

Compare the appearance of an FDG tracer embolus (a single FDG-avid focus in the lung without a CT correlate) with a similar FDG-avid focus in a bone. An FDG-avid focus in a bone without CT correlate is malignant until proven otherwise, since an osseous malignancy is often seen on FDG PET before the attenuation of the lesion changes enough to have a corresponding finding on CT. Contrarily, a single FDG-avid focus in the lung without a CT correlate is usually benign, since CT has excellent capacity to find small lung nodules, which are usually apparent on CT before demonstrating a correlating finding on FDG PET.

Here are a few suggestions to help optimize your interpretation of FDG PET/CT of the lung:

1. FDG PET/CT has value for the evaluation of SPNs. However, the presence or absence of FDG avidity does not prove benignity or malignancy. SPNs need either imaging follow-up or tissue sampling. Non-FDG-avid SPNs are often followed by serial imaging and tissue sampled if enlarging. FDG-avid SPNs are often tissue sampled due to the high rate of malignancy.

2. Multiple round pulmonary nodules in a patient with a malignancy with propensity to metastasize to the lungs should be considered suspicious for lung metastases, whether or not they are FDG avid.

3. Almost all patients with NSCLC undergo FDG PET/CT before initiating therapy. FDG PET/CT is currently the best modality to detect otherwise unsuspected nodal and distant metastases, which appropriately stages the patient and prevents futile surgeries.

4. FDG PET/CT can be used to distinguish metabolically active tumor from adjacent benign opacities such as postobstructive atelectasis or postablation opacities.

5. Not all FDG-avid lung lesions are malignant. There are many specific CT morphologic and lesion distributions which help distinguish benign FDG-avid lung opacities from malignancy.

SUGGESTED READINGS

Cronin, et al: Solitary pulmonary nodules: meta-analytic comparison of cross-sectional imaging modalities for diagnosis of malignancy, *Radiology* 246:772–782, 2008.

Fischer, et al: Preoperative staging of lung cancer with combined PET-CT, *N Engl J Med* 361:32–39, 2009.

Fischer, et al: Multimodality approach to mediastinal staging in non-small cell lung cancer. Faults and benefits of PET-CT: a randomised trial, *Thorax* 66:294–300, 2011.

Gould, et al: Accuracy of positron emission tomography for diagnosis of pulmonary nodules and mass lesions: a meta-analysis, *JAMA* 285:914–924, 2001.

Lardinois, et al: Staging of non-small-cell lung cancer with integrated positron-emission tomography and computed tomography, *N Engl J Med* 348:2500–2507, 2003.

Numan, et al: Peri- and postoperative management of stage I-III Non Small Cell Lung Cancer: which quality of care indicators are evidence-based?, *Lung Cancer* 101:129–136, 2016.

Ruilong, et al: Diagnostic value of 18F-FDG-PET/CT for the evaluation of solitary pulmonary nodules: a systematic review and meta-analysis, *Nucl Med Commun* 38:67–75, 2017.

Sheikhbahaei, et al: The value of FDG PET/CT in treatment response assessment, follow-up, and surveillance of lung cancer, *AJR Am J Roentgenol* 208:420–433, 2017.

van Tinteren, et al: Effectiveness of positron emission tomography in the preoperative assessment of patients with suspected non-small-cell lung cancer: the PLUS multicentre randomised trial, *Lancet* 359:1388–1393, 2002.

Zukotynski, et al: Molecular imaging and precision medicine in lung cancer, *PET Clin* 12:53–62, 2017.

CHAPTER 9

Pleura on FDG PET/CT

The pleura are the pair of membranous linings surrounding the lungs. The visceral pleura covers each lung surface, and the parietal pleura covers the inner surface of the thoracic cavity. Normally, the visceral and parietal pleura oppose each other, have negligible material between them, and are so thin as to be nearly imperceptible on computed tomography (CT). Thus, if you can see the pleura between lung and chest wall, it is abnormal. Pleural abnormalities are often associated with pleura effusions, which may obscure underlying solid pleural masses.

The differential for pleural abnormalities includes malignancies (metastases, lymphoma, mesothelioma) and benign (empyema, asbestos-related pleural disease, fibrous tumor, post-pleurodesis inflammation) etiologies.

POSTPLEURODESIS INFLAMMATION

Patients with large volume pleural effusions may undergo pleurodesis to help prevent future pleura fluid accumulation. The effectiveness of pleurodesis derives from the pleuritis produced by chemical irritation from talc which is introduced between the parietal and visceral pleural layers. The talc has high attenuation and persists indefinitely following the procedure. If a pleural lesion shows high attenuation on CT in a patient with a history of pleurodesis, this is consistent with postpleurodesis reactive inflammation because less than 10% of pleural malignancies develop calcifications. The chemical irritation from talc also may persist indefinitely, resulting in markedly 18F-fluorodeoxyglucose (FDG)-avid pleural thickening with areas of high attenuation. This may persist for years or decades and should not be confused with FDG-avid pleural metastases. Postpleurodesis inflammation is normally not associated with a pleural effusion. Thus FDG-avid pleural thickening with areas of high attenuation on CT, but without associated pleural effusion, is consistent with benign postpleurodesis inflammation and may persist indefinitely (Fig. 9.1). Follow-up imaging demonstrating new areas of pleural thickening or new pleural effusions is suspicious for recurrent malignancy.

PLEURAL METASTASES

Many primary malignancies (most commonly lung and breast cancers) metastasize to the pleura. This appears as pleural thickening or pleural-based masses on CT and is often avid on FDG positron emission tomography (PET). In contrast to postpleurodesis inflammation, pleural metastases are not usually calcified and are often associated with a pleural effusion (Fig. 9.2). In addition, unlike postpleurodesis inflammation, pleural metastases will increase or decrease during the course of treatment. Depending on the size and avidity of the pleural metastases, they may be visible on both the CT and FDG PET (see Fig. 9.2), the FDG PET but not CT (Fig. 9.3), or the CT but not the FDG PET. Pleural metastases may be occult on both CT and FDG PET but diagnosed through sampling of the pleural fluid. In patients with lung, breast, and ovarian cancers, the presence of a pleural effusion should raise suspicion for pleural metastases, even without pleural thickening/masses on CT or appreciable FDG avidity. Pleural fluid sampling may be needed to exclude the presence of pleural metastases.

PLEURAL MESOTHELIOMA

Mesothelioma is a rare, highly aggressive malignancy, most commonly originating from the pleura but may also arise from other membranous linings such as the peritoneum and pericardium. On CT, mesothelioma will be seen as pleural thickening or masses, often associated with a pleural effusion. Mesothelioma is usually markedly FDG avid, and the imaging findings are often indistinguishable from pleural metastases. FDG PET/CT may be valuable in mesothelioma by identifying the extent of disease outside of the pleura (Fig. 9.4).

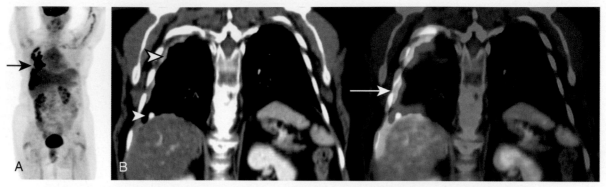

FIG. 9.1 **FDG-avid Postpleurodesis Inflammation.** (A) FDG maximum intensity projection (MIP) in a patient with history of ductal breast cancer demonstrates marked FDG avidity overlying the lateral right chest wall *(arrow)*. (B) Axial CT and fused FDG PET/CT demonstrate that the avidity corresponds with right pleura thickening *(arrow)*, which at first may be confused with pleural metastases. However, note the multiple high-attenuation foci in the thickened pleura *(arrowheads)* and the lack of a pleural effusion. These findings are consistent with benign post-pleurodesis inflammation, which may remain stable for many years.

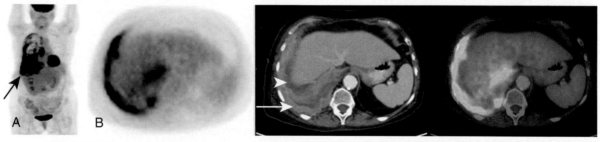

FIG. 9.2 **FDG-avid Pleural Metastases.** (A) FDG maximum intensity projection (MIP) in a patient with a history of ductal breast cancer demonstrates marked FDG avidity overlying the right chest wall *(arrow)*. (B) Axial PET, CT, and fused FDG PET/CT demonstrate that the avidity corresponds with right pleura thickening *(arrow)*. Note the lack of associated high-attenuation foci and the presence of a pleural effusion *(arrowhead)* in these FDG-avid pleural metastases. Compare with Fig. 9.1 demonstrating benign postpleurodesis inflammation.

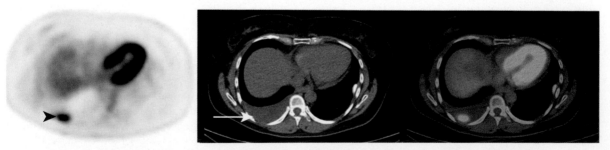

FIG. 9.3 **Pleural Metastases Seen on FDG PET but Not CT.** Axial PET, CT, and fused FDG PET/CT in a patient with non-small cell lung cancer demonstrate a pleural effusion *(arrow)*, which by itself in a patient with lung cancer raises suspicion for pleural metastases. There is a dependent FDG-avid focus within the pleural effusion *(arrowhead)*, which represents a pleural metastasis, despite no pleural mass on CT.

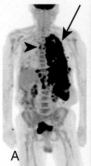
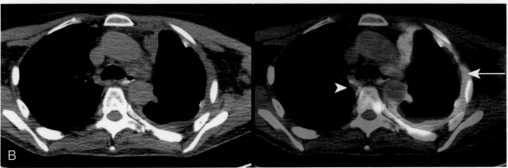

FIG. 9.4 **Pleural Mesothelioma.** (A) FDG maximum intensity projection (MIP) in a patient with mesothelioma demonstrates marked FDG avidity overlying the left chest wall *(arrow)*, as well as multiple additional FDG-avid foci *(arrowhead)*. (B) Axial CT and fused FDG PET/CT demonstrate that the avidity corresponds with left pleura thickening *(arrow)*. The imaging appearance of FDG-avid pleural mesothelioma is indistinguishable from FDG-avid pleural metastases. The FDG PET helps to visualize the extent of malignancy outside of the left pleura, in this case involving the right pleural *(arrowhead)* as well as peritoneal and nodal disease (not shown on axial images).

Here are a few suggestions to help optimize your interpretation of FDG PET/CT of the pleura:

1. Postpleurodesis inflammation appears as FDG-avid pleural thickening/masses with associated high attenuation (talc) foci and usually without a pleural effusion. This may remain stable over many years and should not be confused with malignancy.

2. Pleural malignancy (metastases, lymphoma, mesothelioma) appears as FDG-avid pleural thickening/masses but without high attenuation foci and often with a pleural effusion.

3. Pleural malignancy may be seen on both the FDG PET and CT, the FDG PET only, or the CT only or be occult on both the FDG PET and CT but diagnosed by pleural fluid sampling.

SUGGESTED READINGS

Ceresoli, et al: Early response evaluation in malignant pleural mesothelioma by positron emission tomography with [18F] fluorodeoxyglucose, *J Clin Oncol* 24:4587–4593, 2006.

Makis, et al: Spectrum of malignant pleural and pericardial disease on FDG PET/CT, *AJR Am J Roentgenol* 198:678–685, 2012.

Schaffler, et al: Non-small cell lung cancer: evaluation of pleural abnormalities on CT scans with 18F FDG PET, *Radiology* 231:858–865, 2004.

Truong, et al: Preoperative evaluation of patients with malignant pleural mesothelioma: role of integrated CT-PET imaging, *J Thorac Imaging* 21:146–153, 2006.

Wachsmann, et al: Thorax: normal and benign pathologic patterns in FDG-PET/CT imaging, *PET Clin* 9:147–168, 2014.

CHAPTER 10

Heart on FDG PET/CT

With a recent glucose load, the myocardium uses glucose as its primary energy source. When fasting, the myocardium switches to using fatty acids rather than glucose. The longer the fast, the more likely the myocardium will be using fatty acids. This is why for a cardiac 18F-fluorodeoxyglucose positron emission tomography/computed tomography (FDG PET/CT), when we want to evaluate cardiac ischemia and infarcts, the patient is given a glucose load prior to the PET/CT, to make the myocardium take up glucose and FDG. For an oncologic FDG PET/CT, the patient fasts at least 4 hours. This decreases glucose and FDG uptake in skeletal muscle. This also has the effect of decreasing glucose and FDG uptake in the myocardium. For most FDG PET/CT studies with a 4- to 6-hour fast, it is difficult to predict how much physiologic FDG uptake will be seen in the myocardium. This results in a highly variable appearance of the myocardium on oncologic FDG PET/CT. There may be no apparent FDG uptake, uptake in part or all of the left ventricle, even uptake in right ventricle or atria (Fig. 10.1). It is important not to mistake areas of no FDG uptake as infarctions on oncologic FDG PET/CT studies. Indeed, on an oncologic FDG PET/CT, focal areas of FDG photopenia are often physiologic, rather than infarcts or ischemia (see Fig. 10.1B).

Focal areas of FDG avidity in the heart may correspond with physiologic structures. One or more of the left ventricular papillary muscles may be focally FDG avid and are located in predictable locations (Fig. 10.2). The intraatrial septum may undergo lipomatous hypertrophy, and this may be focally FDG avid (Fig. 10.3).

Malignancy involving the myocardium is relatively infrequent but does occur. The differential of malignant myocardial lesions includes metastases (Fig. 10.4), lymphoma (Fig. 10.5), and primary cardiac sarcomas (Fig. 10.6). Given the relatively infrequent occurrence of cardiac malignancy and the highly variable appearance of physiologic myocardial FDG avidity, another imaging method such as echocardiography or cardiac magnetic resonance (MR) may be needed for more definite diagnosis of cardiac malignancy. These studies may not be needed because cardiac malignancy is often associated with widespread malignancy, obviating the need for definitive diagnosis of each site of malignancy. Myocardial involvement with malignancy may also already be suspected clinically due to an arrhythmia or another disturbance in cardiac physiology.

The myocardium may also be involved with a benign process such as sarcoidosis or amyloidosis. Inflammation associated with these benign processes may be FDG avid. If it is known that the heart or a lesion near the heart (such as the pericardium or a medial lung nodule) is the focus of an FDG PET/CT, consider increasing the length of the preexamination fast. The longer the fast, the more likely the myocardium will be using fatty acids. Some studies have found that a fast of 12 hours reduces physiologic FDG avidity in the heart and helps to visualize cardiac and pericardial lesions.

The pericardium may also be involved with malignant or benign processes. Pericardial lesions on FDG PET/CT are similar to pleural lesions (see Chapter 9). Pericardial masses may incite a pericardial effusion, which could obscure the underlying mass. Pericardial masses may be visualized on both CT and FDG PET/CT, on FDG PET only, on CT only, or on neither study but be diagnosed by fluid sampling. Pericardial FDG avidity may be further evaluated by cardiac MR or echocardiography, similar to myocardial lesions.

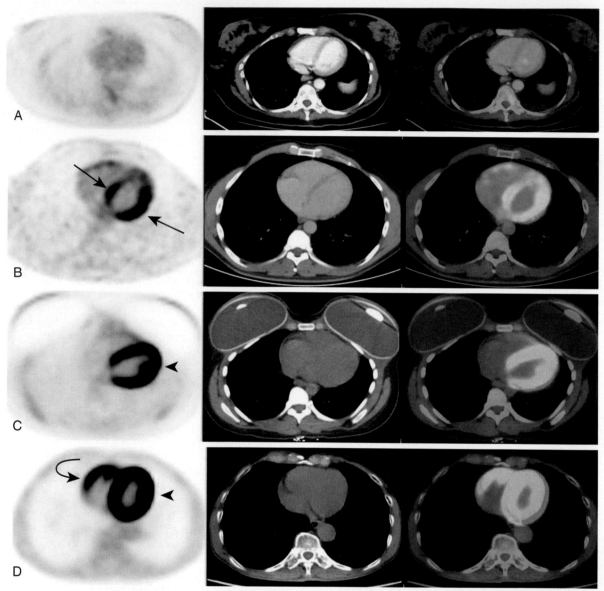

FIG. 10.1 **Axial PET, CT, and Fused FDG PET/CT Images in Four Different Patients Demonstrate Variations in the Extent of Physiologic FDG Avidity in Myocardium.** (A) Minimal myocardial FDG uptake. (B) Uptake in some of the left ventricle *(arrows)*. Do not confuse this with a left ventricular apical infarct. On a fasting oncologic FDG PET/CT scan, this appearance is often normal. (C) Uptake in the entire left ventricle *(arrowhead)*. (D) Uptake in the entire left ventricle *(arrowhead)* and in the right ventricle *(curved arrow)*.

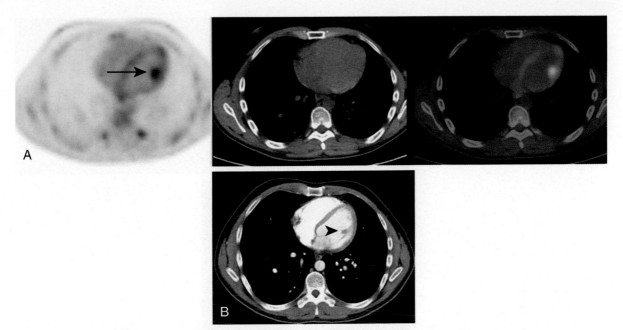

FIG. 10.2 **Focal FDG Avidity in a Papillary Muscle.** (A) Axial PET, CT, and fused FDG PET/CT images demonstrate an FDG-avid focus overlying the left ventricle *(arrow)*. (B) Corresponding contrast-enhanced CT image demonstrates that the FDG-avid focus localizes to a papillary muscle *(arrowhead)* and is physiologic.

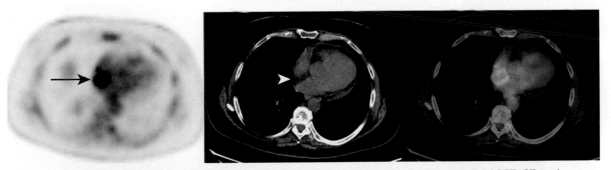

FIG. 10.3 **Focal FDG Avidity in Lipomatous Hypertrophy of the Intraaxial Septum.** Axial PET, CT, and fused FDG PET/CT images demonstrate an FDG-avid focus overlying the left atria *(arrow)*. Corresponding CT image demonstrates that the FDG-avid focus localizes to fat attenuation between the atria *(arrowhead)*, diagnostic of benign FDG-avid lipomatous hypertrophy of the intraaxial septum.

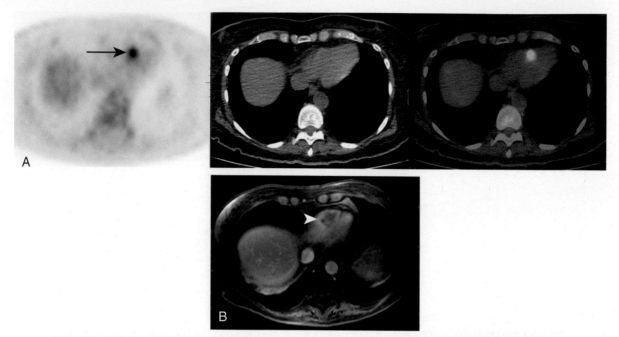

FIG. 10.4 **FDG-avid Cardiac Metastasis.** (A) Axial PET, CT, and fused FDG PET/CT images in a patient with history of squamous cell carcinoma demonstrate an FDG-avid focus overlying the left ventricle *(arrow)*. (B) Corresponding cardiac magnetic resonance demonstrated an enhancing mass at this location *(arrowhead),* and a cardiac metastasis was diagnosed.

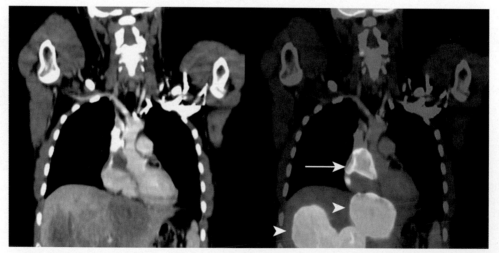

FIG. 10.5 **FDG-avid Cardiac Lymphoma.** Axial CT and fused FDG PET/CT images in a patient with lymphoma demonstrate FDG-avid thickening of the right atrial wall *(arrow)*. This represents cardiac lymphoma. The patient also has multifocal FDG-avid hepatic lymphoma *(arrowheads)*.

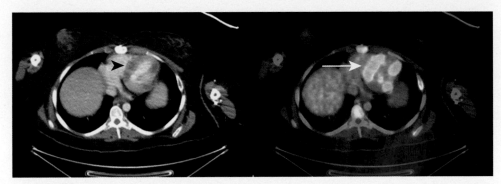

FIG. 10.6 **FDG-avid Primary Cardiac Sarcoma.** Axial CT and fused FDG PET/CT images in a patient with cardiac sarcoma demonstrate multiple FDG-avid cardiac foci *(arrow)*. The corresponding contrast-enhanced CT demonstrates that the FDG avidity localizes to low-attenuation cardiac masses *(arrowheads)*.

Here are a few suggestions to help optimize your interpretation of FDG PET/CT of the heart:

1. Physiologic FDG avidity in the myocardium is common and highly variable. It is often difficult to distinguish underlying FDG-avid lesions from physiologic myocardial FDG avidity.

2. If it is known that the heart or a lesion near the heart is the focus of an FDG PET/CT examination, consider increasing the length of the preexamination fast. The longer the fast, the less physiologic FDG avidity in the heart and the easier to see the pericardial lesion.

3. If an FDG-avid myocardial or pericardial finding needs further evaluation, consider cardiac MR or echocardiography.

SUGGESTED READINGS

Kaira, et al: The role of [^{18}F]fluorodeoxyglucose positron emission tomography in thymic epithelial tumors, *Cancer Imaging* 11:195–201, 2011.

Shammas, et al: Pediatric FDG PET/CT: physiologic uptake, normal variants, and benign conditions, *Radiographics* 29:1467–1486, 2009.

Sharma, et al: Evaluation of thymic tumors with 18F-FDG PET-CT: a pictorial review, *Acta Radiol* 54:14–21, 2013.

CHAPTER 11

Thymus Masses on FDG PET/CT

The thymus is a lymphoid organ located anterior to the heart in the anterior mediastinum. Thymic lesions include thymoma, thymic hyperplasia, invasive thymoma, thymic carcinoma, and carcinoid. 18F-fluorodeoxyglucose positron emission tomography/computed tomography (FDG PET/CT) may assist with the characterization of thymic lesions. Thymomas are usually non- to minimally FDG avid (Fig. 11.1), whereas invasive thymomas and thymic carcinomas typically demonstrate substantial FDG avidity (Fig. 11.2). A hallmark feature of invasive thymoma is unilateral pleural metastasis (see Fig. 11.2).

Following chemotherapy or other systemic therapies, it is common to have rebound thymic hyperplasia. This may be markedly FDG avid and needs to be distinguished from malignancy. The thymus is quite malleable, and the normal thymus is molded into a triangular morphology by the lungs (Figs. 11.3 and 11.4). Contrarily, anterior mediastinal masses are stiffer, form more rounded structures, and subsequently mold the lungs around them. Thus the morphology of an FDG-avid thymus provides substantial value in distinguishing benign from malignant lesions.

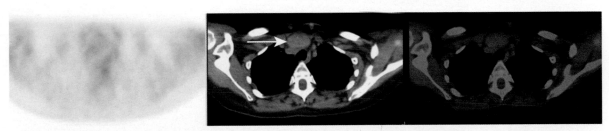

FIG. 11.1 **Thymoma.** Axial PET, CT, and fused FDG PET/CT in a patient with melanoma demonstrate an anterior mediastinal mass *(arrow)* with minimal, if any, FDG avidity. A single calcification can be seen within the mass. Given the lack of FDG avidity in the mass, it was followed conservatively and remained stable. Given the location, calcification, lack of FDG avidity, and stability, a benign thymoma is the preferred diagnosis.

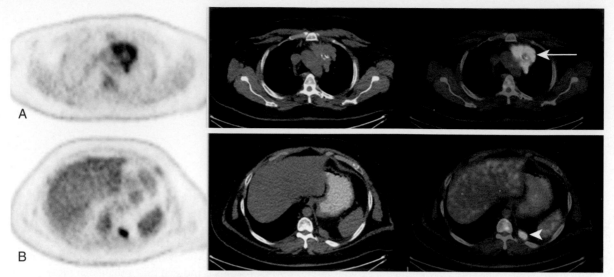

FIG. 11.2 **FDG-avid Invasive Thymoma.** (A) Axial PET, CT, and fused FDG PET/CT through the upper chest demonstrate an FDG-avid anterior mediastinal mass *(arrow)*. (B) Similar images through the lower chest demonstrate a unilateral FDG-avid pleural mass *(arrowhead)*. The presence of unilateral pleural spread raises suspicion for invasive thymoma, which was proven on histology.

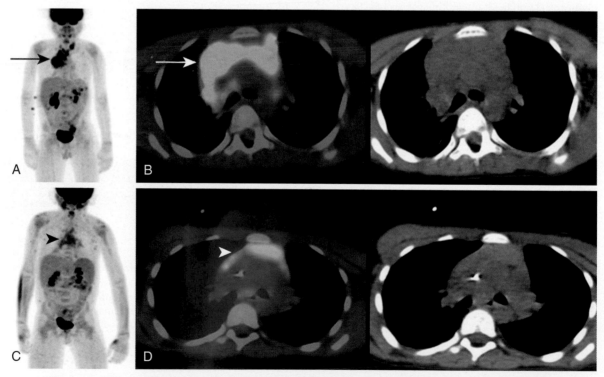

FIG. 11.3 **FDG-avid Benign Thymic Rebound.** (A) FDG maximum intensity projection (MIP) demonstrates FDG-avid anterior mediastinal masses *(arrow)* biopsy proven to be lymphoma. (B) Axial CT and fused FDG PET/CT demonstrate the FDG-avid anterior mediastinal lymphoma *(arrow)*. Note how the lymphoma mass pushes into and molds the adjacent lung. (C) FDG MIP following therapy demonstrates a change in morphology of the anterior mediastinal soft tissue. It is now triangular in shape *(arrowhead)*. (D) Axial CT and fused FDG PET/CT demonstrate the residual FDG-avid triangular structure *(arrowhead)*, which represents benign thymic rebound. Note how the residual soft tissue is molded into a triangular shape by the adjacent lungs. The triangular shape helps to distinguish this as benign, despite FDG avidity.

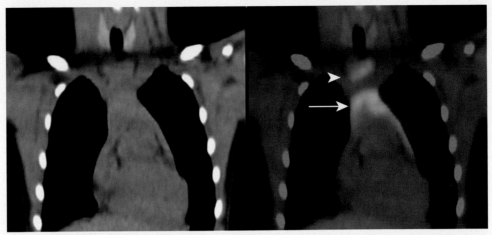

FIG. 11.4 FDG-avid Benign Thymic Rebound With Cervical Thymus. Coronal CT and fused FDG PET/CT in a 10-year-old boy with lymphoma following chemotherapy demonstrate FDG-avid triangular soft tissue consistent with benign thymic rebound *(arrow)*. There is separate linear FDG-avid soft tissue superior to the main thymus *(arrowhead)* representing cervical extension of the thymus. This is also benign FDG avidity related to thymic rebound.

Here are a few suggestions to help optimize your interpretation of FDG PET/CT of the thymus:

1. The thymus may demonstrate benign FDG-avid rebound following systemic therapies. The characteristic triangular shape will help to characterize this as benign thymic rebound and distinguish it from anterior mediastinal malignancy.

2. The thymus may have a cervical component which is separate from the main gland. This should not be mistaken for cervical nodal malignancy.

SUGGESTED READINGS

Kaira, et al: The role of [18F]fluorodeoxyglucose positron emission tomography in thymic epithelial tumors, *Cancer Imaging* 11:195–201, 2011.

Shammas, et al: Pediatric FDG PET/CT: physiologic uptake, normal variants, and benign conditions, *Radiographics* 29:1467–1486, 2009.

Sharma, et al: Evaluation of thymic tumors with 18F-FDG PET-CT: a pictorial review, *Acta Radiol* 54:14–21, 2013.

CHAPTER 12

Hepatobiliary FDG PET/CT

LIVER

The segmental anatomy of the liver is based on the hepatic veins, thus the segmental anatomy of the liver is more difficult to appreciate on contrast computed tomography (CT). The liver is divided into right and left lobes by the middle hepatic vein. The right lobe is divided into anterior and posterior segments by the right hepatic vein, and the left lobe is divided into medial and lateral segments by the left hepatic vein (Fig. 12.1). On a noncontrast CT, this may lead to confusion with defining the left and right hepatic lobes (Fig. 12.2). The falciform ligament may be confused as the structure that separates the left and right hepatic lobes, but this is actually the plane of the left hepatic vein, separating the medial and lateral segments of the left lobe. On a noncontrast CT scan, the intralobar fissure, separating the left and right hepatic lobes, is better approximated by the location of the gallbladder fossa.

When confronted with a focal liver lesion, knowledge of the differential diagnosis for solid and cystic liver masses is valuable. In the differential diagnosis, consider malignancies, including primary malignancies, metastases, and lymphoma, as well as benign etiologies including benign neoplasms and infections.

Let's start with solid liver lesions (Fig. 12.3). Solid liver lesions may be malignant or benign. Malignant solid liver lesions include metastases, lymphoma, and primary malignancies such as hepatocellular carcinoma (HCC) and cholangiocarcinoma (CC). Benign solid liver lesions are most commonly hemangiomas, focal nodular hyperplasia (FNH), or adenomas. With this differential diagnosis for solid liver lesions, clinical history and imaging characteristics can then be used to narrow the differential or determine diagnosis. Of course, biopsy may sometimes be required for the definitive diagnosis.

Now let's consider cystic liver lesions (Fig. 12.4). Cystic lesions may also be malignant or benign. For malignancies, metastases may be cystic, HCC and CC may be cystic, and we would add biliary cystadenocarcinomas. Lymphoma is less likely to be cystic. For benign cystic liver lesions, we would consider cysts, infections (pyogenic, amoebic, echinococcal), biliary hamartomas (von Meyenburg complexes), and biliary cystadenomas. This produces a differential diagnosis that is different from that of solid liver lesions.

With the knowledge of common differentials for solid and cystic liver lesions, we can now address specific scenarios of liver lesions on fluorodeoxyglucose positron emission tomography (FDG PET)/CT.

Hepatic Metastases

The liver is one of the most common organs for metastatic involvement. In a patient with a known malignancy with a propensity to metastasize to the liver, FDG-avid liver lesions are highly suspicious for liver metastases (Fig. 12.5). FDG-avid liver metastases may be visualized with corresponding low-attenuation lesions on CT; however, the lack of low-attenuation lesions on the corresponding CT does not prevent the diagnosis of metastasis. Several possible reasons may contribute to the lack of an apparent lesion on CT. First and foremost, most FDG PET/CT scans are performed without intravenous contrast, and scans without intravenous contrast will greatly limit the visualization of liver lesions on CT, particularly on soft tissue CT windows. Adjusting the CT window to that of the liver window may help to visualize a corresponding low-attenuation lesion on CT. Second, even with intravenous contrast, FDG PET may demonstrate FDG-avid liver metastases without a corresponding lesion on CT (Fig. 12.6). This is particularly apparent when the patient has hepatic steatosis. In the setting of hepatic steatosis, the low-attenuation liver parenchyma may mask low-attenuation liver lesions which are more apparent on FDG PET.

Although much less common, it is also possible to visualize the development of liver metastases on the CT component of the PET/CT before the lesion becomes appreciably FDG avid (Fig. 12.7). The background FDG avidity of the liver may mask small or only mildly FDG-avid liver metastases. To optimize the detection of liver metastases on FDG PET/CT, view the CT images

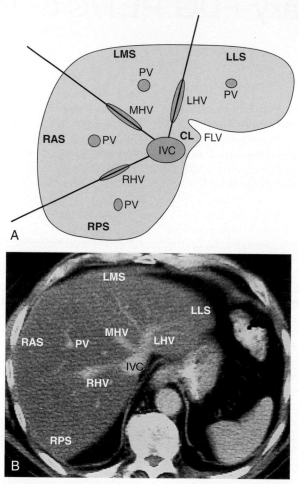

FIG. 12.1 **Hepatic Segmental Anatomy.** Diagram (A) and CT scan (B) demonstrate the anatomy of the hepatic veins that serve as landmarks for the fissures that divide the liver into lobes and segments. The hepatic and portal veins are prominent on the CT scan because the liver has diffuse fatty infiltration that lowers the CT attenuation of the liver parenchyma. *CL,* Caudate lobe; *FLV,* fissure of the ligamentum venosum; *IVC,* inferior vena cava; *LHV,* left hepatic vein; *LLS,* left lobe, lateral segment; *LMS,* left lobe, medial segment; *MHV,* middle hepatic vein; *PV,* portal veins; *RAS,* right lobe, anterior segment; *RHV,* right hepatic vein; *RPS,* right lobe, posterior segment. (Adapted from Brant W, Helms C, Webb R: *Fundamentals of body CT,* ed 2, Philadelphia, 1998, Saunders.)

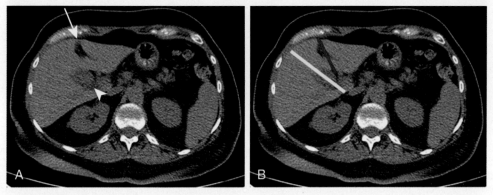

FIG. 12.2 (A) Axial noncontrast CT through the liver demonstrating the falciform ligament *(arrow)* in the gallbladder fossa *(arrow)*. (B) The same axial noncontrast CT image with the course of the left hepatic vein marked using the falciform ligament *(red line)* in the course of the middle hepatic vein approximated using the gallbladder fossa *(yellow line)*. The portion of the liver between the *red* and *yellow lines* is sometimes mistaken for a portion of the right hepatic lobe but is actually the medial segment of the left hepatic lobe.

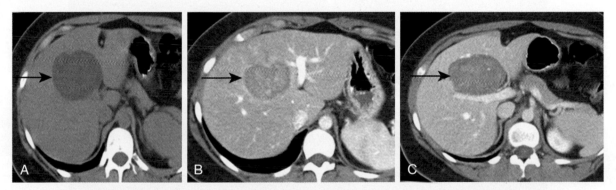

FIG. 12.3 **Differential Diagnosis for Solid Liver Lesions.** (A) Noncontrast, (B) arterial phase contrast, and (C) portal venous phase-contrast CT images of a solid enhancing liver lesion *(arrows)* in a 35-year-old woman with abdominal pain. The differential diagnosis of a solid liver lesion is broad, including both malignancies (metastasis, lymphoma, hepatocellular carcinoma [HCC], cholangiocarcinoma) and benign etiologies (hemangioma, focal nodular hyperplasia [FNH], adenoma). The liver is not cirrhotic, making HCC unlikely. Imaging characteristics of the solid liver lesion are nonspecific but are not typical for hemangioma or FNH. The lack of a history of malignancy makes metastases and lymphoma less likely. The clinical history was suggestive of adenoma. Eventually, biopsy was performed providing a diagnosis of adenoma.

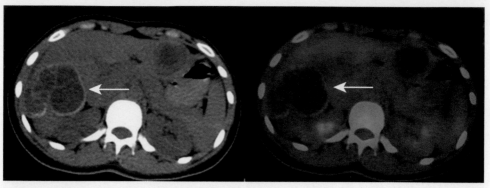

FIG. 12.4 **Differential Diagnosis for Cyst Liver Lesions.** Axial CT and fused FDG PET/CT images through a cystic liver lesion *(arrows)* in a 45-year-old woman with history of breast cancer and abdominal pain. The differential diagnosis of a cystic liver lesion is broad, including both malignancies (metastasis, hepatocellular carcinoma, cholangiocarcinoma, and biliary cystadenocarcinomas) and benign etiologies (cysts, infections, biliary hamartomas, and biliary cystadenomas). The lesion was not FDG avid, suggesting a nonactive process. The thin calcifications at the periphery of the lesion and along septae, suggesting daughter cysts, suggest an old echinococcal infection. This lesion remained stable at follow-up and was considered benign.

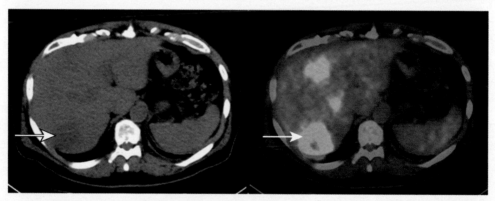

FIG. 12.5 **FDG-avid Liver Metastases from Gallbladder Cancer.** Axial CT and fused FDG PET/CT images through the liver in a patient with gallbladder cancer demonstrate multiple FDG-avid foci corresponding with low-attenuation lesions on CT *(arrows)*. As gallbladder malignancy has a propensity for metastasis to the liver; the FDG-avid liver lesions are almost certainly liver metastases. Biopsy confirmed liver metastases.

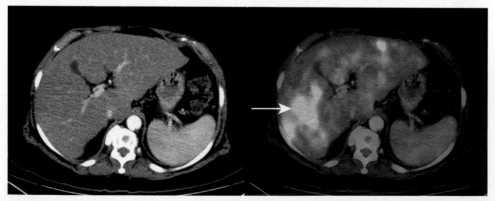

FIG. 12.6 **Liver Metastases Seen on FDG PET but Not Contrast-enhanced CT due to Hepatic Steatosis.** Axial CT and fused FDG PET/CT images through the liver in a patient with ductal breast cancer demonstrate multiple FDG-avid foci without CT correlate *(arrow)*. Note the low-background liver attenuation, consistent with hepatic steatosis. In the setting of hepatic steatosis, the low-attenuation liver parenchyma may mask low-attenuation liver lesions which are more apparent on FDG PET.

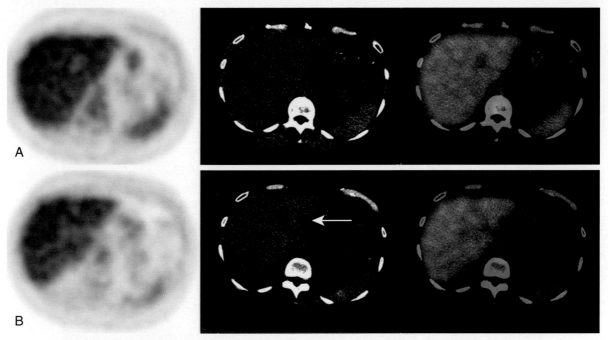

FIG. 12.7 **Liver Metastasis Seen on Noncontrast CT but Not FDG PET.** (A) Axial PET, CT, and fused PET/CT images through the liver in a patient with lobular breast cancer are unremarkable. (B) Follow-up imaging 6 months later demonstrates a new low-attenuation lesion on noncontrast CT *(arrow)*, despite no abnormalities on FDG PET. This was biopsy proven to represent a liver metastasis. Of help was setting the CT window to a narrow liver window to assist in visualizing low-attenuation liver lesions.

on a liver window, even if the CT was performed without intravenous contrast. A narrow liver window will help to visualize low-attenuation liver metastases from non- or mildly FDG-avid malignancy.

Following therapy, decreases in liver metastases may be apparent by either decreasing size on CT or FDG avidity on FDG PET (Fig. 12.8). In some scenarios, decreases in FDG avidity will better represent treatment response and decreases in size on following treatment of initially FDG-avid pancreatic lymphoma, on CT. This is particularly apparent in the setting of hepatic pseudocirrhosis (Fig. 12.9). Pseudocirrhosis is a result of successful treatment of hepatic metastases, with retraction of the liver capsule in regions of decreasing metastases. This produces a liver contour and appearance similar to that of a patient with cirrhosis but without secondary signs of cirrhosis such as splenomegaly or varices. Pseudocirrhosis is most commonly seen after treatment of patients with breast cancer. The altered morphology of a pseudocirrhotic liver may make it very difficult to determine the extent of residual malignancy on CT.

In addition, some systemic therapies may not cause liver metastases to decrease in size, but FDG avidity may still accurately reflect metabolic activity or quiescence in the lesion (Fig. 12.10). This is apparent with some immune-modulating therapies such as ipilimumab. Ipilimumab is a monoclonal antibody that helps to incite a stronger immune reaction against malignancy. These immune therapies have demonstrated substantial benefit in the treatment of melanoma, lung cancer, and other malignancies, but treatment response may not be reflected by changes in tumor size. FDG avidity may help to evaluate treatment response in patients on these immune therapies.

Interventional radiology (IR) oblations of liver metastases are another area in which FDG PET may serve to better visualize residual or recurrent malignancy than does anatomic imaging. Following ablation of liver metastases, the resulting anatomic defect is usually larger than the original metastasis and makes further evaluation of that region of liver parenchyma difficult. FDG PET is often more sensitive for the detection of

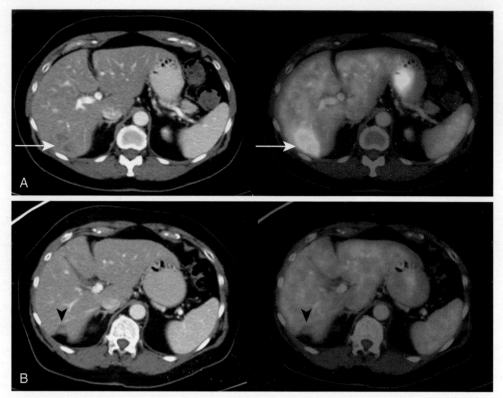

FIG. 12.8 Decreased Liver Metastases Following Therapy. (A) Axial CT and fused FDG PET/CT images through the liver in a patient with ductal breast cancer demonstrate an FDG-avid liver metastases corresponding to a low-attenuation lesions on CT *(arrows)*. (B) Axial CT and fused FDG PET/CT images following chemotherapy demonstrate a decreased metastasis both by decreased FDG avidity and by decreased size on CT *(arrowheads)*.

residual or recurrent malignancy at the site of IR oblations (Fig. 12.11).

Lymphoma

FDG PET often provides greater sensitivity for detection of active hepatic lymphoma than does anatomic imaging. After diagnosis, FDG PET provides valuable information about response to therapy in hepatic lymphoma, similar to other sites of lymphomatous involvement (Fig. 12.12). The Lugano Criteria state that (for initially FDG-avid lymphoma) posttreatment reduction of FDG avidity to less than liver background represents a complete response to treatment, whereas residual FDG avidity greater than liver background is suspicious for residual active lymphoma.

Hepatocellular Carcinoma

Individual HCC tumors vary in tumor grade. Well-differentiated HCCs are more histologically similar to normal hepatocytes, whereas poorly differentiated HCCs are more aggressive. FDG uptake in HCC correlates with tumor differentiation, with more poorly differentiated tumors tending to be more FDG avid. Because of the variability of FDG avidity in HCC, FDG PET is neither sensitive nor specific for detection of primary HCC. Contrast-enhanced CT or magnetic resonance (MR) with multiple phases of image acquisition is far more accurate for initial detection and local staging of HCC. The value of FDG PET/CT for HCC is the detection of nodal and distant metastases, in particular for subcentimeter nodal metastases and osseous metastases. Thus FDG PET/CT may assist with distant staging of HCC.

Cholangiocarcinoma

CC is a primary malignancy of the biliary ducts, which may occur within the liver or involve the extrahepatic ducts. CC most commonly occurs in the common bile duct. As is the case for HCC, FDG PET/CT is not used

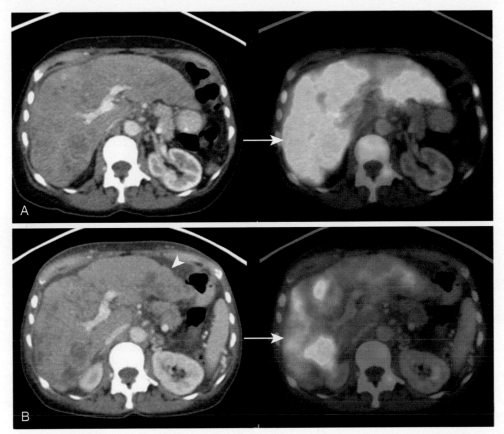

FIG. 12.9 Extent of Liver Metastasis Response to Therapy Better Visualized by FDG PET than by Contrast-enhanced CT due to Hepatic Pseudocirrhosis. (A) Axial CT and fused FDG PET/CT images through the liver in a patient with ductal breast cancer demonstrate widespread FDG-avid liver metastases *(arrow)*, many with corresponding low-attenuation lesions on CT. (B) Axial CT and fused FDG PET/CT images following chemotherapy demonstrate markedly decreased FDG-avid liver metastases *(arrow)*. It is much more difficult to appreciate the decrease in liver metastases on CT, probably because of hepatic pseudocirrhosis. Note the new nodularity of the liver margin on CT *(arrowhead)*.

for detection or local staging, where contrast-enhanced CT and MR are superior. FDG avidity of CCs will vary by histology. Nodular forms of CC tend to be more FDG avid, whereas infiltrating forms are less apparent on FDG PET. This may be due to lower cellular density in infiltrating forms of CC, so there are fewer cells per unit of volume to accumulate FDG. FDG avidity of CCs has also been shown to vary by location of the tumor. Peripherally located CCs are more apparent on FDG PET than are central/hilar lesions. As seen with other malignancies, the role of FDG PET/CT in CC is limited to the detection of unsuspected nodal and distant metastases. The role of FDG PET/CT for this has not been rigorously evaluated.

Hepatocellular Adenoma

Hepatic adenomas are unusual benign focal liver masses. Hepatic adenomas consist of benign neoplastic hepatis sites and sometimes associated Kupffer cells. Although usually solitary, adenomas may be multiple and could be mistaken for metastases on anatomic imaging. Although benign, adenomas are prone to hemorrhage. Steroids, including oral contraceptives, are risk factors for the development and growth of hepatocellular adenomas. Of use for the diagnosis of adenomas is the common presence of intracellular (microscopic) fat, which may be visualized as out-of-phase drop on T1-weighted MR images. On FDG PET/CT, most hepatic adenomas are visualized as low-attenuation lesions with

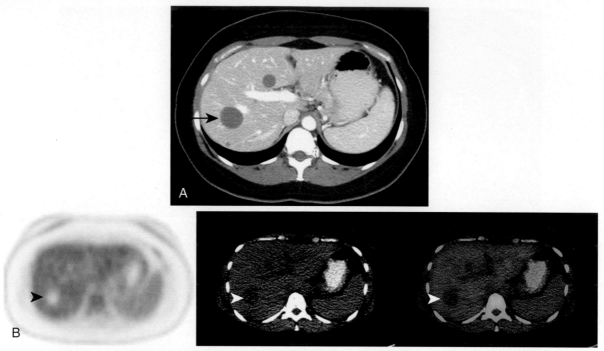

FIG. 12.10 **Treatment Response in a Patient With Metastatic Melanoma Following Ipilimumab and Nivolumab Therapy Demonstrated by FDG PET.** (A) Axial contrast-enhanced CT following therapy within the modulating agents demonstrated persistence of low-attenuation metastases *(arrow)* without significant change in size. (B) Axial PET, CT, and fused FDG PET/CT images within 1 week demonstrate the persistent low-attenuation lesions lack FDG avidity, consistent with treated disease *(arrowhead)*.

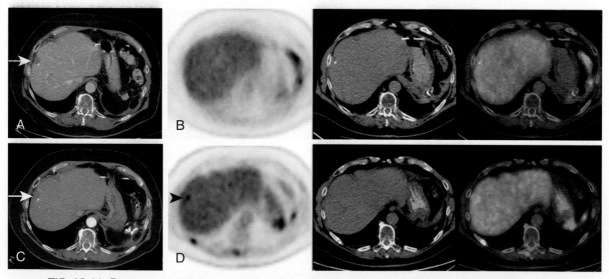

FIG. 12.11 **Recurrence of Malignancy Following Interventional Radiology Ablation of a Liver Metastasis, Better Visualized by FDG PET than by Contrast-enhanced CT.** (A) Contrast-enhanced CT demonstrates an ablation defect following ablation of a liver metastasis *(arrow)*. (B) Axial PET, CT, and fused FDG PET/CT images within 1 week demonstrate no FDG-avid foci suspicious for malignancy. (C) Follow-up contrast-enhanced CT 2 months later demonstrates no significant change *(arrow)*; however, (D) axial PET, CT, and fused FDG PET/CT images demonstrate a new focus of FDG avidity suspicious for tumor recurrence *(arrowhead)*. Biopsy demonstrated active malignancy at this site.

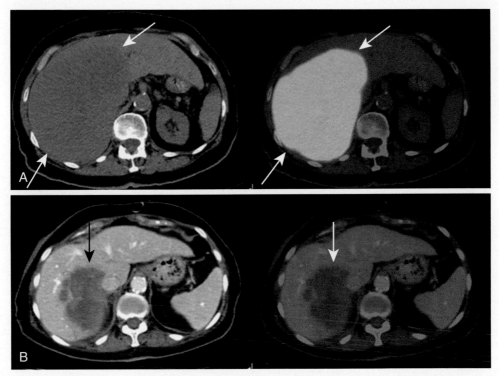

FIG. 12.12 Response to Therapy in Hepatic Lymphoma, Better Visualized by FDG PET than by CT.
(A) Axial noncontrast CT and fused PET/CT demonstrate a large FDG-avid lymphomatous hepatic mass with a corresponding low-attenuation lesion on CT *(arrows)*. (B) Axial contrast-enhanced CT and fused FDG PET/CT images following chemotherapy demonstrate decreased size and resolved FDG avidity in the mass *(arrows)*. The residual CT mass could be suspicious for residual active malignancy; however, Lugano Criteria state that residual masses with FDG avidity no greater than liver background represent treated disease, without evidence of residual active malignancy.

FDG avidity equal to background liver parenchyma. However, a small percentage of hepatic adenomas may be FDG avid and must be distinguished from malignancy (Fig. 12.13). The etiology of FDG avidity in some adenomas is unclear. If an FDG-avid hepatic lesion demonstrates T1 out-of-phase drop on MR, this is consistent with an FDG-avid hepatic adenoma because metastases should not contain intracellular fat.

Hepatic Hemangioma

Hemangiomas are the most common benign solid mass in the liver and are often incidentally discovered during imaging. Hemangiomas consist of benign blood-filled vascular spaces, lined with epithelia and containing fibrous septa. Although usually solitary, hemangiomas may be multiple and could be mistaken for metastases on anatomic imaging. On contrast-enhanced CT or MR, typical hepatic hemangiomas demonstrate characteristic peripheral nodular discontinuous enhancement with

increasing peripheral to central enhancement over time. Atypical hepatic hemangiomas may lack this characteristic appearance. On FDG PET/CT, most hepatic hemangiomas are visualized as low-attenuation lesions with FDG avidity equal to background liver parenchyma and are easily determined to be benign. However, a small percentage of hemangiomas may be FDG avid and must be distinguished from malignancy (Fig. 12.14). The etiology of FDG avidity in some hemangiomas is unclear. If an FDG-avid hepatic lesion demonstrates the peripheral nodular discontinuous enhancement characteristic of a hemangioma, this is consistent with an FDG-avid hemangioma because metastases should not demonstrate this characteristic pattern of enhancement.

Hepatic Focal Nodular Hyperplasia

FNH is the second most common form of benign liver tumor, following hemangiomas. They are also incidentally discovered during imaging. FNH is composed of

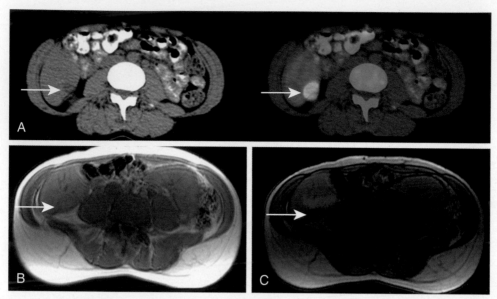

FIG. 12.13 **FDG Avidity in a Benign Hepatic Adenoma.** (A) Axial noncontrast CT and fused PET/CT in a 37-year-old woman with papillary thyroid cancer demonstrate a non–FDG-avid low-attenuation lesion in the right liver *(arrows)*. (B) Axial in-phase and (C) out-of-phase T1 magnetic resonance (MR) images demonstrate out-of-phase signal drop in the lesion *(arrows)*, representing intracellular fat in a hepatic adenoma. Without the MR images, the FDG PET/CT findings would be suspicious for a hepatic metastasis; however, metastases should not contain intracellular fat and the corresponding MR images prevented the misdiagnosis of hepatic malignancy. Although most hepatic adenomas are not FDG avid, this case is evidence that a small percentage of adenomas are avid.

all the normal histologic elements of the liver but with malformed architecture. Typical FNH lesions demonstrate well-circumscribed margins and a prominent central scar. Atypical FNH may lack the central scar and be difficult to diagnose on imaging. On FDG PET/CT, most FNH are visualized as low-attenuation lesions with FDG avidity equal to background liver parenchyma. However, a small percentage of FNH may be FDG avid and must be distinguished from malignancy. The etiology of FDG avidity in some FNH is unclear.

Hepatic Cysts

Simple hepatic cysts have uniform low attenuation, usually near water attenuation. On FDG PET, hepatic cysts are usually photopenic compared with background hepatic parenchyma.

Hepatic Infections

Bacterial abscesses usually demonstrate thickened, enhancing walls. Lesions are usually solitary but may be multiloculated. The presence of gas attenuation within the lesion on CT may help to identify areas of infection or necrosis. Old echinococcal cysts may be photopenic

on FDG PET and demonstrate calcifications along the periphery of the cyst and along septations (see Fig. 12.4).

Iatrogenic FDG Avidity in the Liver

Surgical procedures and radiation therapy may produce FDG avidity in the liver, which must be distinguished from malignancy. Surgical injury may induce FDG avidity at liver resection margins, as well as areas of hepatic retraction during surgery. External radiation ports that include the liver may induce acute radiation hepatitis. Radiation hepatitis may cause low-attenuation lesions on CT, signal abnormalities on MR, and FDG avidity on FDG PET. These abnormalities often have a linear morphology, corresponding with the radiation port. The linear morphology may help to distinguish benign radiation hepatitis from malignancy (Fig. 12.15).

GALLBLADDER

The role of FDG PET/CT in the evaluation of the gallbladder is limited. Malignant lesions involving the gallbladder include primary gallbladder malignancy, lymphoma,

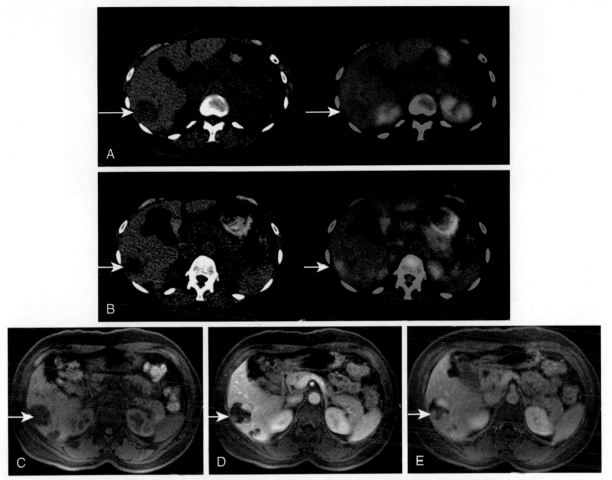

FIG. 12.14 **FDG Avidity in a Benign Hemangioma.** (A) Axial noncontrast CT and fused PET/CT in a 50-year-old woman with ductal breast cancer demonstrate a non–FDG-avid low-attenuation lesion in the right liver *(arrows)*. (B) Follow-up axial contrast-enhanced CT and fused FDG PET/CT images following chemotherapy demonstrate decreased size but new FDG avidity in the lesion *(arrows)*. (C) Axial T1 magnetic resonance (MR) prior to contrast, as well as (D) early and (E) delayed postcontrast images demonstrate nodular discontinuous enhancement with increasing peripheral to central enhancement over time *(arrows)*. This MR examination was performed in between the baseline and follow-up FDG PET/CT studies and demonstrates the hepatic lesions to be benign hemangiomas, despite FDG avidity on FDG PET/CT. Without the contrast-enhanced imaging, it would be very difficult to make this diagnosis on the noncontrast FDG PET/CT images. Although most hepatic hemangiomas are not FDG avid, this case is evidence that a small percentage of hemangiomas are avid. The availability of the contrast-enhanced MR in the patient's medical record prevented the misdiagnosis of hepatic malignancy.

and metastases, all of which are relatively rare. Inflammation of the gallbladder secondary to obstructing gallstones is a far more common pathology of the gallbladder. FDG avidity in the gallbladder should lead to evaluation and exclusion of gallbladder inflammation before the diagnosis of malignancy is made.

Gallbladder Cancer

Gallbladder cancer is a less common malignancy, for which clinical symptoms may be mistaken with benign biliary colic, and thus diagnosis is often delayed and disease advanced at diagnosis. The role of FDG PET/CT in gallbladder cancer has not been rigorously evaluated.

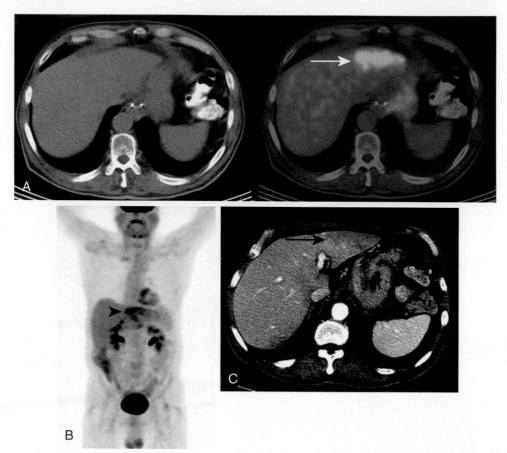

FIG. 12.15 FDG Avidity in Benign Acute Radiation Hepatitis. (A) Axial noncontrast CT and fused PET/CT in a patient with gastroesophageal (GE) malignancy treated with chemoradiation. Linear FDG avidity is visualized in the left liver *(arrow)*, directly anterior to two fiducial markers at the GE junction. (B) FDG PET maximum intensity projection (MIP) demonstrates the triangular morphology of the acute radiation hepatitis on whole-body imaging *(arrowhead)*. (C) Axial CT with contrast demonstrated a low-attenuation lesion with similar linear morphology *(arrow)*. FDG avidity in the liver of a patient with GE malignancy would raise concern for hepatic metastases; however, the linear morphology is atypical for hepatic malignancy. A history of recent radiation therapy was obtained, and a presumed diagnosis of benign radiation hepatitis was made. This linear FDG avidity resolved on follow-up imaging, without further intervention.

Most primary gallbladder malignancies are high grade and avidly take up FDG, but it is likely that anatomic imaging with contrast-enhanced CT or MR will be far more valuable for the diagnosis and local staging of primary gallbladder cancer. FDG PET/CT (as usual) may help to distant staging through the detection of nodal and distant metastases (see Fig. 12.5).

Gallbladder Metastases
Although relatively uncommon, metastases to the gallbladder do occur. The most common malignancies causing metastases to the gallbladder are melanoma and lung cancer. On CT, metastases to the gallbladder may be confused with gallstones (Fig. 12.16). Gallstones themselves are not expected to be FDG avid.

Cholecystitis
Gallbladder inflammation is most commonly secondary to impaction of a gallstone in the cystic duct or common bile duct, and this may cause extensive gallbladder FDG avidity. The FDG PET/CT images of the gallbladder itself may not clearly elucidate a benign or malignant cause for FDG avidity; however, the presence of an obstructing

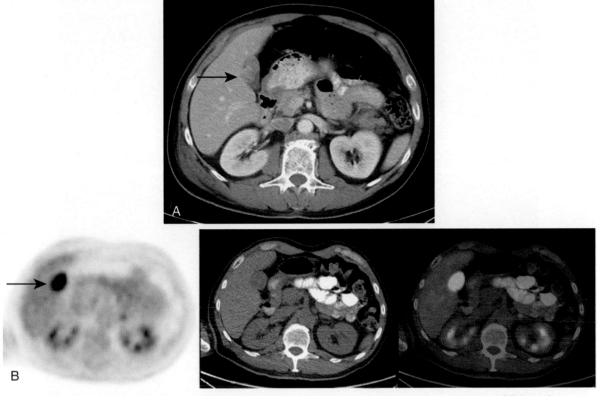

FIG. 12.16 FDG-avid Gallbladder Metastases from Melanoma. (A) Axial contrast-enhanced CT through the gallbladder in a patient with melanoma. Round structures within the gallbladder *(arrow)* were interpreted as gallstones. (B) Subsequent axial PET, noncontrast CT, and fused PET/CT demonstrate FDG avidity in the gallbladder *(arrow)*. There was no clinical evidence of acute gallbladder inflammation, thus the potential for gallbladder metastases was raised. Pathology from gallbladder resection demonstrated melanoma metastases to the gallbladder.

cystic or common bile duct stone may help to provide the diagnosis (Fig. 12.17).

Here are a few suggestions to help optimize your interpretation of FDG PET/CT of the hepatobiliary system:

1. Understand the differential for solid and cystic liver lesions. Malignant solid liver lesions include metastases, lymphoma, and primary malignancies such as HCC and CC. Benign solid liver lesions are most commonly hemangiomas, FNH, or adenomas. Malignant cystic liver lesions include metastases, HCC, CC, and biliary cystadenocarcinomas. For benign cystic liver lesions, consider cysts, infections (pyogenic, amoebic, echinococcal), biliary hamartomas (von Meyenburg complexes), and biliary cystadenomas.

2. FDG liver lesions are highly suspicious for malignancy, unless specific anatomic imaging demonstrates the lesion to be benign. A small percentage of benign hepatic hemangiomas, adenomas, and FNH will be FDG avid and can be distinguished from malignancy by characteristic anatomic imaging findings on CT, MR, or ultrasound (US).

3. Hepatic steatosis and pseudocirrhosis are two conditions that make visualization of hepatic malignancy more difficult on CT. Hepatic malignancy may be visible on FDG PET but not CT, even if the CT is contrast enhanced.

4. When reviewing FDG PET/CT images, specifically view the liver on a narrow CT liver window, even for noncontrast CT imaging. A narrow liver window will help to visualize low-attenuation liver metastases from non- or mildly FDG-avid malignancy that may be difficult or impossible to visualize on FDG PET. Hepatic malignancy may be visible on CT but not FDG PET.

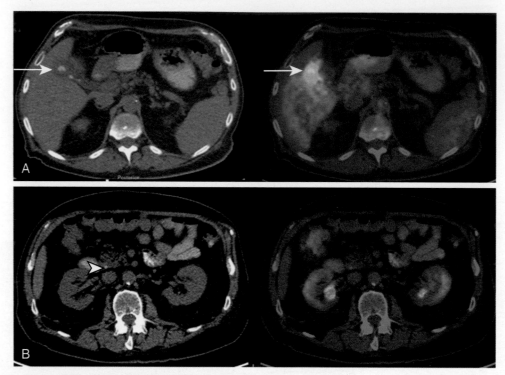

FIG. 12.17 **FDG-avid Gallbladder Inflammation.** (A) Axial noncontrast CT and fused FDG PET/CT through the gallbladder in a patient with colon cancer. The gallbladder contains multiple calcified gallstones and is FDG avid *(arrows)*. (B) Axial noncontrast CT and fused FDG PET/CT through the distal common bile duct demonstrate the common bile duct stone *(arrowhead)*. Gallstones will not be intrinsically FDG avid; however, obstructed gallstones in the cystic or common bile duct may cause gallbladder inflammation that is FDG avid.

5. It is often difficult to detect recurrent malignancy on anatomic imaging following procedures such as ablations. FDG PET/CT can provide earlier visualization of recurrent malignancy following these procedures.

6. Malignancy of the gallbladder is relatively uncommon. FDG avidity in the gallbladder may represent malignancy or gallbladder inflammation. Evaluate for corresponding CT images for obstructing biliary stones or signs of gallbladder inflammation.

SUGGESTED READINGS

Cheson, et al: Recommendations for initial evaluation, staging, and response assessment of Hodgkin and non-Hodgkin lymphoma: the Lugano classification, *J Clin Oncol* 32:3059–3068, 2014.

Maffione, et al: Diagnostic accuracy and impact on management of (18)F-FDG PET and PET/CT in colorectal liver metastasis: a meta-analysis and systematic review, *Eur J Nucl Med Mol Imaging* 42:152–163, 2015.

Parikh, et al: FDG PET/CT in pancreatic and hepatobiliary carcinomas: value to patient management and patient outcomes, *PET Clinics* 10:327–343, 2015.

Purandare, et al: Therapeutic response to radiofrequency ablation of neoplastic lesions: FDG PET/CT findings, *Radiographics* 31:201–213, 2011.

Sacks, et al: Value of PET/CT in the management of liver metastases, part 1, *AJR Am J Roentgenol* 197:W256–W259, 2011.

Sacks, et al: Value of PET/CT in the management of primary hepatobiliary tumors, part 2, *AJR Am J Roentgenol* 197:W260–W265, 2011.

Samim, et al: The diagnostic performance of 18F-FDG PET/CT, CT and MRI in the treatment evaluation of ablation therapy for colorectal livermetastases: a systematic review and meta-analysis, *Surg Oncol* 26:37–45, 2017.

Tan, et al: FDG PET/CT in the liver: lesions mimicking malignancies, *Abdom Imaging* 39:187–195, 2014.

Yoon, et al: Role of 18F-fluorodeoxyglucose positron emission tomography in detecting extrahepatic metastasis in pretreatment staging of hepatocellular carcinoma, *Oncology* 72(Suppl 1):104–110, 2007.

CHAPTER 13

Spleen on FDG PET/CT

When confronted with a focal splenic lesion, knowledge of the differential diagnosis for splenic masses is valuable (Fig. 13.1). For malignancies of the spleen, lymphoma would be most common, whereas metastases are relatively uncommon and primary splenic malignancies are rare. Benign splenic lesions encountered on fluorodeoxyglucose positron emission tomography/computed tomography (FDG PET/CT) are common and include infections, sarcoidosis, and splenic repopulation.

SPLENIC LYMPHOMA

Lymphoma is by far the most common malignancy to involve the spleen. Splenic lymphoma may manifest as splenic enlargement (splenomegaly) or solitary or multifocal lesions. FDG avidity of lymphoma ranges from no apparent FDG avidity to markedly FDG avid. The extent of FDG avidity in lymphoma tends to correlate with pathologic rate. Lymphomas with maximum standarized uptake values (SUV) greater than 20 are most often high-grade lymphomas (Fig. 13.2), whereas lymphomas with maximum SUV values less than 10 are most often low grade. This can be valuable in screening patients with low-grade lymphoma for transformation to higher-grade malignancy. Highly FDG-avid lesions would be the lesions to target for evaluation of possible high-grade malignancy. Low-grade lymphoma made be incidentally discovered during FDG PET/CT performed for another malignancy (Fig. 13.3). If the FDG avidity of low-grade lymphoma nodes is low enough, they may not be readily apparent on the FDG PET images and must be appreciated by the enlarged lymph nodes on the corresponding CT images.

As with other organ systems, FDG PET provides valuable information about response to therapy in splenic lymphoma, if the initial lymphoma was adequately FDG avid. For example, the patient in Fig. 13.3 with incidentally discovered low-grade lymphoma demonstrates only minimally FDG-avid malignancy and would not be appropriate for using FDG PET to track treatment response. If the initial lymphoma is adequately FDG avid, Lugano Criteria can be followed for evaluation of treatment response. In essence, reduction of FDG avidity to less than liver background represents a complete response to treatment, whereas residual FDG avidity greater than liver background is suspicious for residual active lymphoma.

SPLENIC METASTASES

Metastases to the spleen are relatively uncommon. The most common primary malignancies that cause metastases to the spleen are melanoma, lung, breast, and ovarian cancers. Splenic metastases may be apparent as focal FDG avidity on FDG PET, low-attenuation masses on CT, or both. Because benign causes of splenic FDG avidity (infections, sarcoid) are common, these should be considered as alternative diagnoses for FDG-avid splenic lesions.

PRIMARY SPLENIC NEOPLASMS

Primary neoplasms of the spleen are rare. Splenic hemangiomas, pathologically identical to hepatic hemangiomas, will be apparent as low-attenuation lesions on CT and probably demonstrate background FDG avidity. Malignant splenic angiosarcomas are exceedingly rare, but individual cases have been shown to be FDG avid.

GRANULOMATOSIS INFLAMMATION

Granulomatous infections such as histoplasmosis or tuberculosis, as well as noninfectious granulomatous processes such as sarcoidosis, may involve the spleen and demonstrate solitary or multifocal FDG-avid splenic foci. If FDG-avid splenic foci correspond with punctate calcifications on CT, this favors a granulomatous inflammatory process. In addition, granulomas may be seen in the lungs, hilar nodes, or liver, which would make a systemic granulomatous process highly likely.

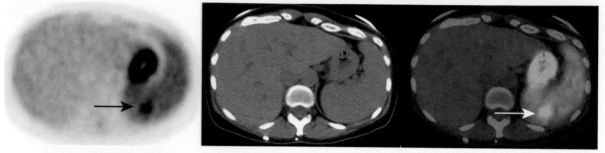

FIG. 13.1 **Differential Diagnosis for Splenic Lesions.** Axial PET, noncontrast CT, and fused PET/CT through the spleen demonstrate a focus of FDG avidity within the spleen *(arrows)*, without CT correlate. Differential diagnosis of FDG-avid splenic lesions on FDG PET/CT includes malignancies (lymphoma, metastasis, angiosarcoma) and benign etiologies (infections, sarcoidosis, splenic repopulation). This patient has a diagnosis of lymphoma, and the splenic focus is presumed lymphoma.

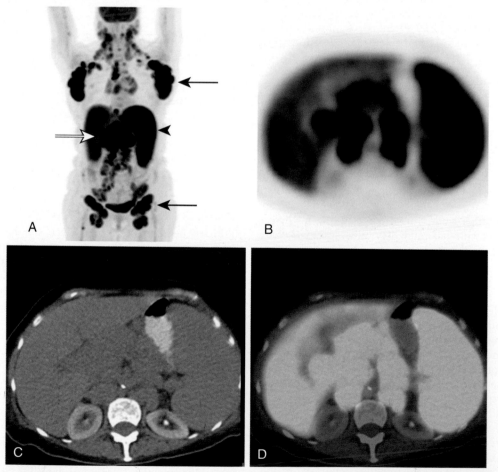

FIG. 13.2 **Marked FDG Avidity in High-grade Lymphoma.** (A and B) Axial PET, (C) axial CT, and (D) fused PET/CT images demonstrate markedly FDG-avid lymph nodes above and below the diaphragm *(arrow),* as well as splenomegaly with marked FDG avidity *(arrowhead).* Maximum standardized uptake values in this patient exceeded 20.

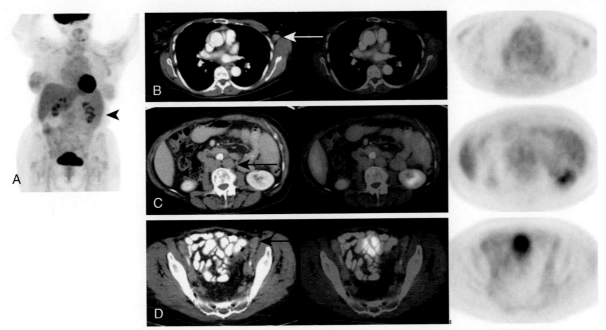

FIG. 13.3 **Incidentally Discovered Mildly FDG-avid Low-grade Lymphoma in a Patient With Breast Cancer.** (A) FDG PET maximum intensity projection (MIP) and axial CT, fused PET/CT, and PET images through the (B) chest, (C) abdomen, and (D) pelvis in a patient with a history of ductal breast cancer. No evidence of malignancy relating to breast cancer was identified. However, enlarged lymph nodes in the chest, abdomen, and pelvis *(arrows)*, as well as splenomegaly *(arrowhead)* were suspicious for a previously unknown lymphoma. The low maximum standardized uptake values (approximately 2) made the lymph nodes difficult to appreciate on FDG PET; however, they are readily apparent as enlarged nodes on CT. Axillary nodal biopsy confirmed low-grade lymphoma.

SPLENIC REPOPULATION

Oncology patients often suffer from anemia, neutropenia, or thrombocytopenia. This may be due to malignant replacement of bone marrow but is more likely due to the effects of systemic therapies such as chemotherapy. To prevent complications from anemia, neutropenia, or thrombocytopenia, many oncology patients are treated with granulocyte colony-stimulating factor (G-CSF), which promotes bone marrow and splenic repopulation. Repopulation of bone marrow and splenic tissues is often associated with elevated FDG avidity on FDG PET. There are short-acting and long-acting forms of G-CSF. Short-acting G-CSF, such as Neupogen (filgrastim), may cause FDG-avid bone marrow and splenic repopulation lasting up to 1 to 2 weeks, whereas longer-acting

formulations of G-CSF, such as Neulasta (pegfilgrastim) may cause FDG-avid changes that last 1 to 2 months. In general, FDG-avid bone marrow repopulation persists longer than FDG-avid splenic repopulation. FDG-avid bone marrow and splenic repopulation should not be confused with malignancy (Fig. 13.4). Potentially more problematic, benign elevation of bone marrow or splenic FDG avidity from bone marrow repopulation could mask underlying FDG-avid malignancy (Fig. 13.5). For a patient receiving regular G-CSF treatments, consider changing the patient to a short-acting G-CSF and then performing an FDG PET/CT examination immediately prior to the next G-CSF treatment to prevent benign bone marrow and splenic repopulation from interfering with FDG PET/CT interpretation.

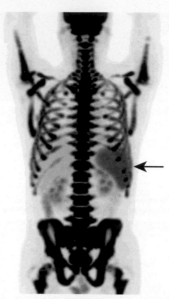

FIG. 13.4 Splenic and Bone Marrow Repopulation from Granulocyte Colony-stimulating Factors. FDG PET maximum intensity projection (MIP) demonstrates diffuse elevation of FDG avidity in the bone marrow and spleen *(arrow)*, secondary to recent treatment with granulocyte colony-stimulating factor. This may prevent evaluation for underlying FDG-avid malignancy in the bone marrow and spleen.

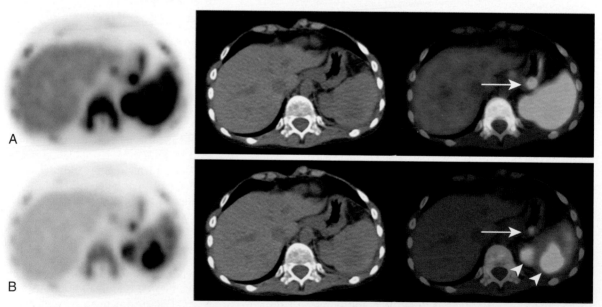

FIG. 13.5 FDG-avid Splenic Malignancy Underlying Benign FDG-avid Splenic Repopulation. (A) Axial PET, CT, and fused PET/CT images in a patient with known gastric lymphoma demonstrate FDG-avid lymphoma in the stomach *(arrow)* and diffuse FDG avidity in the bone marrow and spleen, secondary to recent granulocyte colony-stimulating factor administration. The PET images were obtained with a PET window of 0–5, meaning that all standardized uptake values greater than 5 appear as fully black on black-and-white images. (B) The same axial PET, CT, and fused PET/CT images but with a PET window of 0–10. The FDG-avid gastric lymphoma is still visible *(arrow)*, but now focal FDG-avid splenic lymphoma becomes visible *(arrowheads)*. Subtle low-attenuation splenic lesions can be seen on the corresponding CT.

Here are a few suggestions to help optimize your interpretation of FDG PET/CT of the spleen:

1. Although splenic lymphoma is common, splenic metastases are relatively rare, and primary splenic malignancies are exceedingly rare.

2. FDG avidity of lymphoma varies from markedly avid to little or no FDG avidity. This tends to correlate with lymphoma greatly, with high-grade lymphomas demonstrating marked FDG avidity and some low-grade lymphomas demonstrating little or no FDG avidity.

3. Benign causes of FDG avidity in the spleen are relatively common and include granulomatous infections, sarcoid, and splenic repopulation.

4. FDG-avid benign splenic repopulation may mask underlying FDG-avid splenic malignancy.

SUGGESTED READINGS

Cheson, et al: Recommendations for initial evaluation, staging, and response assessment of Hodgkin and non-Hodgkin lymphoma: the Lugano classification, *J Clin Oncol* 32:3059–3068, 2014.

Liu, et al: Clinical significance of diffusely increased splenic uptake on FDG-PET, *Nucl Med Commun* 30:763–769, 2009.

Ulaner, et al: Identifying and distinguishing treatment effects and complications from malignancy at FDG PET/CT, *Radiographics* 33:1817–1834, 2013.

CHAPTER 14

Pancreas on FDG PET/CT

The differential for focal pancreatic lesions depends on whether the lesion is solid or cystic. Solid pancreatic lesions include primary pancreatic adenocarcinoma, pancreatic neuroendocrine tumors (PNETs), lymphoma, and metastases. Cystic pancreatic lesions include true cysts, pseudocysts, and cystic neoplasms. Focal fluorodeoxyglucose (FDG) avidity within the pancreas is suspicious for focal pancreatic lesion. Obstruction of the pancreatic duct can result in pancreatic inflammation, such as pancreatitis, which causes longer segments of FDG avidity in the affected regions of the pancreas.

SOLID PANCREATIC LESIONS
Pancreatic Adenocarcinoma
Primary pancreatic adenocarcinomas vary widely in their FDG avidity, ranging from markedly FDG avid to not appreciable on FDG positron emission tomography (PET). Do not allow mild or lack of FDG avidity in a primary pancreatic adenocarcinoma to suggest a benign lesion, because almost all pancreatic adenocarcinomas are highly aggressive, even if not apparent on FDG PET. The variability in FDG avidity makes detection of the primary pancreatic neoplasm unpredictable on FDG PET/computed tomography (CT), and contrast-enhanced CT or magnetic resonance (MR) imaging at a pancreatic contrast phase (approximately 45 seconds) remains the mainstay for imaging primary pancreatic malignancies and determining their resectability. Pancreatic adenocarcinomas are often hypoattenuating to normal pancreatic parenchyma on contrast-enhanced CT; however, a small percentage are isoattenuating, and FDG PET may provide value in visualizing the primary pancreatic adenocarcinoma in this small percentage of patients. Overall, the detection of the primary malignancy is usually not the primary purpose of FDG PET/CT, even if the primary malignancy is FDG avid in many patients (Fig. 14.1).

As with malignancies from many other organ systems, FDG PET/CT is far more useful for the detection of nodal and distant metastases from pancreatic adenocarcinoma than for detection of the primary pancreatic malignancy. FDG avidity within borderline-sized local lymph nodes may help to raise confidence in diagnosis of nodal metastases, and FDG-avid foci within the liver of a patient with pancreatic adenocarcinoma is highly suspicious for hepatic metastases (Fig. 14.2). Peritoneal carcinomatosis may be visualized on CT, FDG PET, both (see Fig. 14.1), or neither. It is not unusual for peritoneal carcinomatosis to be detected during surgery which was occult on both CT and FDG PET.

Surgery is the only current potentially curable treatment modality for pancreatic adenocarcinoma; unfortunately, most patients present with unresectable disease. Systemic chemotherapy with or without radiation is used in most patients. Despite the method of initial therapy, most patients will have residual or recurrent malignancy within 2 years. Postsurgical changes may make detection of recurrent malignancy difficult on anatomic imaging, and FDG PET/CT has shown promise in detecting recurrent malignancy following therapy (Fig. 14.3).

Pancreatic Neuroendocrine Tumors
Neuroendocrine tumors represent a minority of pancreatic neoplasm, maybe 2%. Neuroendocrine tumors may be nonfunctioning, without secretion of hormones, or functioning, which may present with specific endocrine syndromes. The most common functioning pancreatic neuroendocrine tumor is insulinoma, followed by gastrinomas. Neuroendocrine tumors often demonstrate arterial phase enhancement on CT or MR, in contrast to pancreatic adenocarcinomas, which are usually hypoattenuating to normal pancreatic parenchyma. PNETs vary widely in their extent of FDG avidity. FDG avidity often correlates with histologic grade of a PNET, with well-differentiated PNETs demonstrating little or no FDG avidity, whereas poorly differentiated PNETs may be markedly FDG avid. Remember that this is unlike pancreatic adenocarcinomas, which also vary widely in their extent of FDG avidity but are almost always high-grade malignancies. The usefulness of FDG PET/CT for

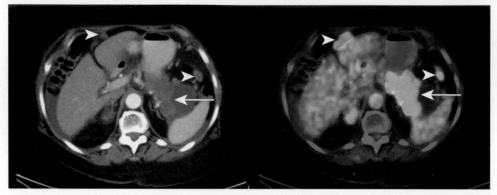

FIG. 14.1 **FDG-avid Primary Pancreatic Adenocarcinoma With FDG-avid Peritoneal Carcinomatosis.**
Axial contrast-enhanced CT and fused PET/CT through the pancreas demonstrate a large markedly FDG- avid
primary pancreatic malignancy *(arrows)*, as well as FDG-avid perineal nodules representing peritoneal carcinomatosis *(arrowheads)*. This pancreatic malignancy was markedly FDG avid; however, primary pancreatic
adenocarcinomas vary widely in FDG avidity, ranging from markedly FDG avid to no appreciable FDG avidity.

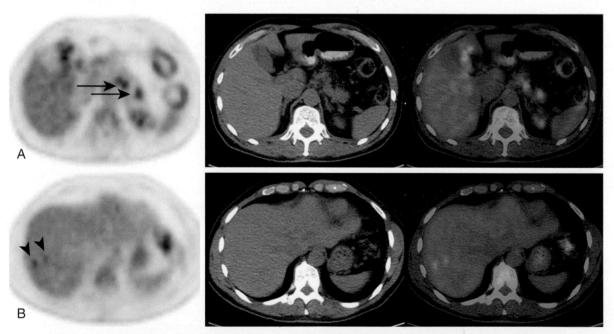

FIG. 14.2 **Primary Pancreatic Adenocarcinoma With FDG-avid Hepatic Metastases.** (A) Axial PET, CT,
and fused PET/CT through the pancreas in a patient with pancreatic adenocarcinoma demonstrate focal
FDG avidity in the pancreatic tail, probably representing a known pancreatic adenocarcinoma *(arrows)*. (B)
Axial PET, CT, and fused PET/CT through the liver demonstrate focal hepatic FDG avidity *(arrowheads)*,
without CT correlate on noncontrast CT, consistent with hepatic metastases. Further workup and biopsy
confirmed hepatic metastases.

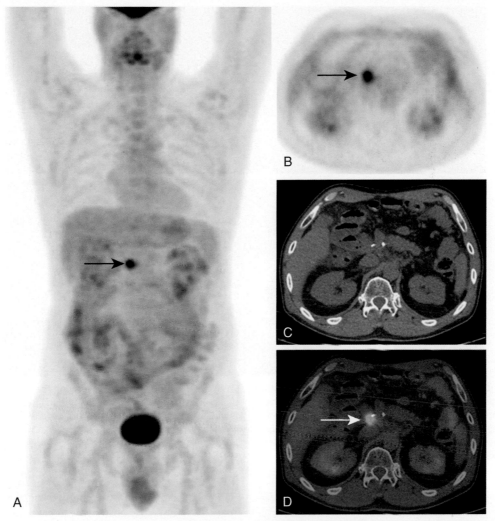

FIG. 14.3 Recurrent Pancreatic Adenocarcinoma Detected on FDG PET/CT. (A) FDG PET maximum intensity projection (MIP), (B) axial PET, (C) axial CT, and (D) fused PET/CT through the abdomen of the patient post-proximal pancreatectomy for pancreatic adenocarcinoma. FDG-avid focus *(arrows)* in the region of surgical clips on CT was subsequently proven to represent recurrent malignancy, which was not clearly evident on anatomic imaging.

detection of primary and metastatic PNETs will vary based on the extent of FDG avidity. Of note, well-differentiated PNETs with low FDG avidity may be substantially better visualized by somatostatin-based nuclear imaging, such as 18F-DOTA-octreotate (18F-DOTATATE) PET/CT or indium-111 octreotide single-photon emission computerized tomography (SPECT)/CT.

Pancreatic Lymphoma

Lymphomatous involvement of the pancreas is relatively rare, found in less than 1% of all pancreatic neoplasms.

Pancreatic lymphoma may be primary, originating in the pancreas, or secondary, originating elsewhere and secondarily involving the pancreas. Secondary pancreatic lymphoma is far more common than primary pancreatic lymphoma, and thus abnormalities elsewhere in the body, such as FDG-avid enlarged lymph nodes or splenomegaly, help to distinguish pancreatic lymphoma from other pancreatic neoplasms (Fig. 14.4). Following the treatment of initially FDG-avid pancreatic lymphoma, the Lugano Criteria are used to determine treatment response. In brief, reduction of FDG avidity to less than

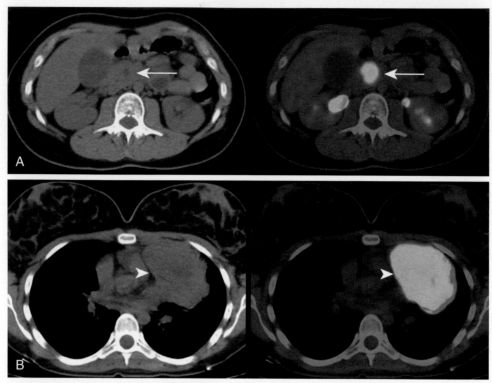

FIG. 14.4 Pancreatic and Mediastinal Lymphoma. (A) Axial CT and fused PET/CT through the pancreas demonstrate an FDG-avid soft tissue mass in the pancreatic body *(arrows)*. (B) Axial CT and fused PET/CT through the chest demonstrate a large FDG-avid mediastinal mass *(arrowheads)*. The additional findings in the chest make these findings suspicious for lymphoma with secondary involvement of the pancreas. Lymphoma was diagnosed on biopsy, and all FDG-avid lesions resolved following treatment.

liver background represents complete response to treatment, whereas residual FDG avidity greater than liver background is suspicious for residual active lymphoma.

Pancreatic Metastases

Metastases to the pancreases are also relatively rare, probably less than 2% of all pancreatic neoplasms. The primary malignancies that cause metastases to the pancreas are lung, breast, and melanoma. Metastatic disease is usually quite advanced before pancreatic metastases are recognized. They may be apparent as focal FDG avidity on FDG PET, masses on CT, or both.

CYSTIC PANCREATIC LESIONS

True Pancreatic Cysts

True pancreatic cysts are relatively rare and congenital. Multiple true pancreatic cysts may be seen in patients with autosomal dominant polycystic disease, von Hippel-Lindau syndrome, and cystic fibrosis. True pancreatic cysts demonstrate near-water attenuation on CT and are usually FDG photopenic.

Pancreatic Pseudocysts

Pancreatic pseudocysts are associated with acute or chronic pancreatitis. On CT, pseudocysts are usually near-water attenuation. Few data exist on the appearance of pseudocysts on FDG PET, although some have been noted to be FDG photopenic. If acutely inflamed, it would not be surprising to see FDG avidity.

Pancreatic Cystic Neoplasms

Cystic neoplasms are being increasingly diagnosed due to increased use and improvements in CT and MR imaging. Serous cystadenomas, mucinous cystic neoplasms, and intraductal papillary mucinous neoplasms (IPMNs) represent the vast majority of pancreatic cystic neoplasms. There are additional rare cystic neoplasms,

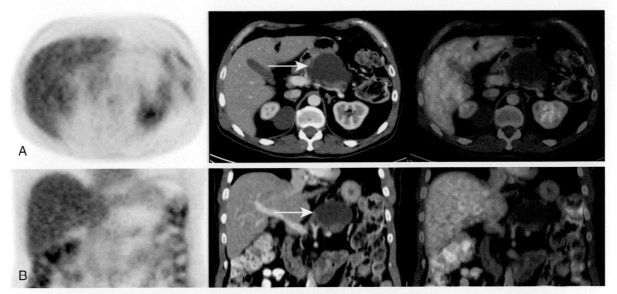

FIG. 14.5 Pancreatic Cystic Lesion. (A) Axial PET, CT, and fused PET/CT images, as well as (B) coronal axial PET, CT, and fused PET/CT images through the pancreas demonstrate a non–FDG-avid near-water attenuation cystic structure in the pancreas *(arrows)*. Differential diagnosis includes cyst, pseudocyst, and cystic neoplasm. A definitive diagnosis of pancreatic cystic lesions is often difficult to provide from imaging.

and occasionally solid pancreatic lesions may undergo cystic degeneration. Due to overlap between the appearances of different pancreatic cystic neoplasm, it is often difficult to make a definitive diagnosis (Fig. 14.5). However, an attempt should be made to differentiate categories of cystic malignancies. The diagnosis of a pseudocyst in a patient with a history of pancreatitis will prevent further workup of the lesion. Differentiating a pancreatic cystic neoplasm from a pancreatic adenocarcinoma is also crucial because the prognosis and treatment of pancreatic adenocarcinoma are dramatically different from those for pancreatic cystic neoplasms. Pancreatic cysts with solid components should be viewed as suspicious for more aggressive malignancy. After pseudocyst and cystic degeneration of a pancreatic adenocarcinoma are excluded, the management of a pancreatic cystic neoplasm can be quite variable. Management decisions, including imaging follow-up or surgical resection, may be based on the presence of symptoms, patient age, tumor size, and location.

PANCREATIC DUCTAL DILATATION
The presence of pancreatic ductal dilatation should be evaluated for on all CT scans which include the pancreas, even low-dose noncontrast CT examinations, which often

accompany FDG PET. Pancreatic adenocarcinomas may be isoattenuating to the remainder of the pancreas on CT and are sometimes not FDG avid; thus dilatation of the pancreatic duct may be the only visible manifestation of a focal pancreatic abnormality on FDG PET/CT. If pancreatic ductal dilatation is identified, this should prompt evaluation for cause. The cause of pancreatic ductal dilatation may be chronic pancreatitis, which may be evident from pancreatic calcifications, pancreatic parenchymal atrophy, or inflammatory changes adjacent to the pancreas on the CT component of FDG PET/CT (Fig. 14.6). If a cause is not evident on the FDG PET/CT images, further evaluation by MR or endoscopic evaluation may be warranted. In addition to obstructing stones, focal masses such as pancreatic adenocarcinoma (Fig. 14.7) should be considered.

PANCREATITIS
Inflammation of the pancreas (pancreatitis) is most commonly caused by gallstones or chronic alcohol use. It is diagnosed on the basis on clinical and laboratory findings. Because patients with the typical gallstone of alcohol-induced acute pancreatitis will not undergo FDG PET/CT, PET/CT images of acute pancreatitis are rare. However, occasionally the pancreatic duct may be acutely

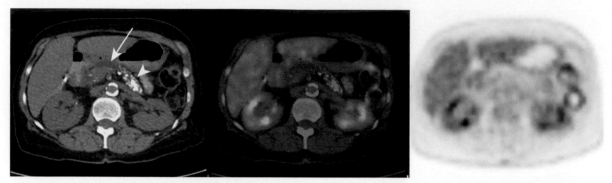

FIG. 14.6 **Pancreatic Ductal Dilatation Secondary to Chronic Pancreatitis.** Axial CT, fused PET/CT, and PET images demonstrate pancreatic ductal dilatation *(arrow)* without abnormal FDG avidity. In this case the cause of pancreatic ductal dilatation is likely chronic pancreatitis, as evidenced by pancreatic parenchymal calcifications *(arrowhead)*.

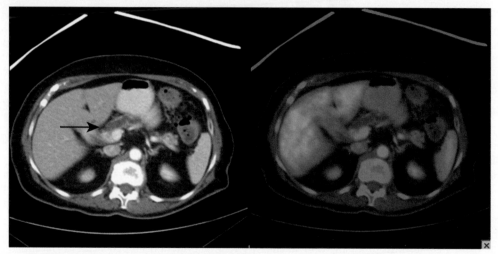

FIG. 14.7 **Pancreatic Ductal Dilatation Secondary to a Pancreatic Adenocarcinoma.** Axial CT and fused PET/CT demonstrate pancreatic ductal dilatation *(arrow)* without abnormal FDG avidity. The cause of the pancreatic ductal dilatation was not evident on FDG PET/CT images. This led to further workup, and endoscopic examination and biopsy led to diagnosis of a pancreatic adenocarcinoma. In this case the only visible manifestation of the pancreatic adenocarcinoma on FDG PET/CT was pancreatic duct dilatation.

obstructed by a malignancy, resulting in acute pancreatitis secondary to the obstructing malignancy (Fig. 14.8). When the pancreas is acutely inflamed, long segments of the pancreas may be FDG avid without a corresponding mass on CT. Indeed, the malignancy obstructing the pancreatic duct may not be visible, and the visualized extensive FDG avidity is actually inflammatory, secondary to pancreatic duct obstruction and pancreatitis.

Autoimmune pancreatitis is another uncommon cause of pancreatitis. On contrast-enhanced CT and MR, autoimmune pancreatitis may demonstrate focal or diffuse pancreatic enlargement, with a peripancreatic halo which is low attenuation on CT. On FDG PET, autoimmune pancreatitis may manifest as long segments of FDG avidity. Clues to autoimmune pancreatitis on FDG PET/CT include FDG-avid inflammation involving additional organ systems (Fig. 14.9). FDG-avid inflammation from immunoglobulin G4 (IgG4) disease may involve a wide range of organ systems, including structures in the head and neck (salivary glands, gland,

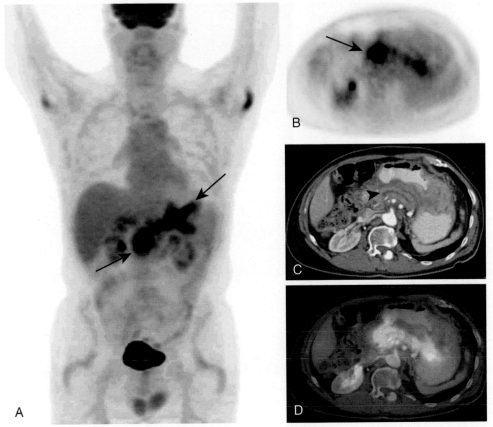

FIG. 14.8 Pancreatic Ductal Dilatation Secondary to Obstruction by a Metastasis. (A) FDG maximum intensity projection (MIP) demonstrates abnormal FDG avidity in the region of the pancreas *(arrows)* in a patient with known gastric malignancy. (B) Axial PET, (C) CT, and (D) fused PET/CT images through the pancreas demonstrate diffuse FDG avidity of the pancreas *(arrow)*, as well as pancreatic ductal dilatation *(arrowhead)*. This led to further workup, and endoscopic examination and biopsy led to diagnosis of a gastric cancer metastasis obstructing the pancreatic duct. In this case, pancreatic duct obstruction caused FDG-avid pancreatic inflammation (pancreatitis). The FDG avidity was inflammatory (pancreatitis), secondary to a pancreatic metastasis not clearly visualized on FDG PET/CT.

orbits), the nerves, lung and pleura, cardiovascular structures, multiple abdominal organs including the pancreas, genitourinary system, nodes, and skin.

Pancreatitis may also be associated with specific chemotherapies, such as vincristine (Fig. 14.10), which is a common component of chemotherapeutic regimens for many forms of lymphoma. If a patient with lymphoma responds to chemotherapy but new FDG-avid foci are apparent within the pancreas following therapy, consider investigating if vincristine was a component of the chemotherapeutic regimen.

Additional causes of pancreatic inflammation, which may manifest with FDG avidity, include pancreatic stents and postoperative changes.

Here are a few suggestions to help optimize your interpretation of FDG PET/CT of the pancreas:

1. Understand the common differentials for solid and cystic pancreatic lesions. Solid pancreatic lesions include primary pancreatic adenocarcinoma, pancreatic neuroendocrine tumors, lymphoma, and metastases. Cystic pancreatic lesions include true cysts, pseudocysts, and cystic neoplasms.

2. Focal FDG avidity within the pancreas is suspicious for a focal pancreatic malignancy. However, there are many inflammatory causes of FDG avidity, such as pancreatitis (secondary to pancreatic duct obstruction,

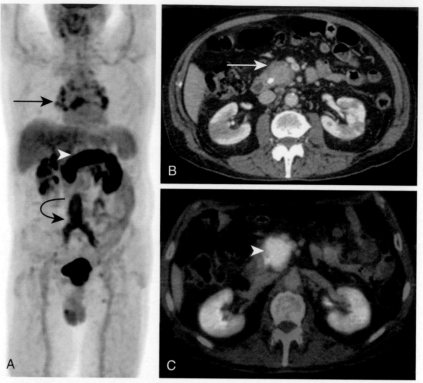

FIG. 14.9 Systemic Immunoglobulin G4 Inflammation Including Autoimmune Pancreatitis. (A) FDG maximum intensity projection (MIP) demonstrates FDG-avid inflammation involving at least the thoracic nodes *(arrow)* in the region of the pancreas *(arrowhead)* and involving the abdominal aorta *(curved arrow)*. (B) Axial CT and (C) fused PET/CT demonstrate the autoimmune pancreatitis associated with FDG avidity *(arrowhead),* as well as a low-attenuation halo on CT *(arrow)*.

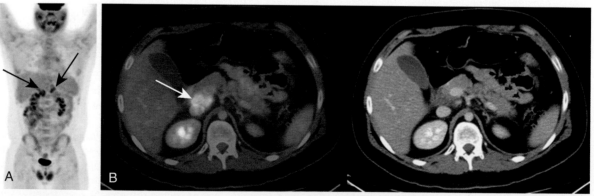

FIG. 14.10 Focal Pancreatitis Following Chemotherapy Including Vincristine. (A) FDG maximum intensity projection (MIP) demonstrates two areas of focal FDG avidity in the region of the pancreas *(arrows)*. (B) Axial fused PET/CT and CT images through the pancreatic head localize one of the FDG-avid foci to the pancreatic head *(arrow)*. This patient with T-cell blastic leukemia was treated with combination chemotherapy which included vincristine. The lymphoma above the diaphragm resolved following treatment. The new FDG-avid pancreatic foci should be recognized as an iatrogenic inflammatory effect from vincristine therapy and not malignancy.

IgG4 disease, or vincristine therapy), pancreatic stents, and postoperative changes.

3. Pancreatic ductal dilatation may be the only visible manifestation of a focal pancreatic abnormality. The pancreatic duct should be evaluated on every CT, and pancreatic duct dilatation should prompt evaluation for a cause.

4. Obstruction of the pancreatic duct can result in pancreatitis, with long segments of pancreatic FDG avidity. It is possible that a malignancy that is occult on FDG PET/CT may obstruct the pancreatic duct and then cause long segments of inflammatory FDG avidity.

SUGGESTED READINGS

Pinho, et al: PET-computed tomography and precision medicine in pancreatic adenocarcinoma and pancreatic neuroendocrine tumors, *PET Clin* 4:407–421, 2017.

Sahani, et al: State-of-the-art PET/CT of the pancreas: current role and emerging indications, *Radiographics* 32:1133–1158, 2012.

Yokoyama, et al: Intense PET signal in the degenerative necrosis superimposed on chronic pancreatitis, *Pancreas* 31:192–194, 2005.

CHAPTER 15

Adrenal Glands on FDG PET/CT

The differential diagnosis for adrenal lesions includes malignant neoplasms, benign neoplasms, and benign nonneoplastic processes. The most common adrenal malignancies by far are metastases. Additional adrenal malignancies include lymphoma, malignant pheochromocytomas, and adrenal cortical carcinomas. The most common benign adrenal neoplasms are adenomas. Additional benign adrenal neoplasms include myelolipomas, benign pheochromocytomas, and ganglioneuromas. Nonneoplastic processes that involve the adrenal gland may include physiologic adrenal fluorodeoxyglucose (FDG) avidity, adrenal hyperplasia, infections, and traumatic lesions.

ADRENAL METASTASES

The adrenal glands are a common site of metastases. The most common primary tumors causing adrenal metastases are pulmonary, gastric, and esophageal malignancies; however, a very wide range of primary malignancies may result in adrenal metastases. Adrenal metastases are usually FDG avid and are associated with corresponding adrenal masses on computed tomography (CT) (Fig. 15.1). In patients with primary malignancies with known propensity to metastasize to the adrenal glands, FDG-avid adrenal masses are suspicious for metastases until proven otherwise. FDG avidity on FDG positron emission tomography (PET) may help to highlight small adrenal metastases that could be overlooked on CT (Fig. 15.2). Although less common, early adrenal metastases or adrenal metastases from malignancies that are not highly FDG avid may not demonstrate appreciable FDG avidity. Occasionally, non–FDG-avid adrenal metastases may need to be detected on the corresponding CT images (Fig. 15.3).

ADRENAL LYMPHOMA

Similar to lymphoma of other organ systems, lymphoma involving the adrenal glands is often FDG avid. Adrenal lymphoma may be primary or secondary. The majority of adrenal lymphomas are due to secondary involvement, whereas primary adrenal lymphoma is rare (Fig. 15.4). After diagnosis, FDG PET provides valuable information about response to therapy in hepatic lymphoma, similar to other sites of lymphomatous involvement. Reduction of FDG avidity to less than liver background is considered treated lymphoma, whereas residual FDG avidity greater than liver background is suspicious for residual active lymphoma.

ADRENOCORTICAL CARCINOMA

Adrenocortical carcinomas (ACCs) are rare and highly aggressive malignancies with poor prognosis. On CT or magnetic resonance (MR), ACCs are typically large heterogeneous suprarenal masses. Data on FDG avidity of ACCs are limited; however, ACC is usually FDG avid (Fig. 15.5). Hemorrhage, necrosis, and calcifications are common. Areas of necrosis may not be appreciably FDG avid. ACC is known for rapid growth and invasion of adjacent organs and adjacent veins, such as the renal vein and inferior vena cava. Extension into the renal vein and inferior vena cava may be FDG avid.

ADENOMA

Adrenal adenomas are the most common benign adrenal neoplasm, found in up to 5% of patients on CT. Adrenal adenomas are typically small, less than 3 cm in size, and of homogenous attenuation on CT. On FDG PET the vast majority of adenomas demonstrate background FDG avidity (Fig. 15.6). Potentially problematic are the 3% to 5% of adrenal adenomas that are FDG avid and can easily be mistaken for metastases or other adrenal malignancy. Because most adrenal metastases are FDG avid and most adrenal adenomas are not, an FDG-avid adrenal mass is suspicious for malignancy until proven otherwise. CT and MR may demonstrate lesional characteristics which diagnose a benign adrenal adenoma, despite FDG avidity. For example, adenomas often contain intracellular fat, which lowers the attenuation of the lesion. An

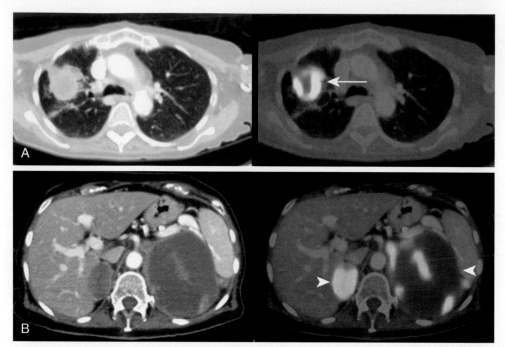

FIG. 15.1 **Adrenal Metastases Primary Lung Malignancy.** (A) Axial CT on lung window and fused PET/CT images through the chest demonstrate an FDG-avid right lung primary adenocarcinoma *(arrow)*. (B) Axial CT on soft tissue window and fused PET/CT images through the adrenals demonstrate bilateral FDG-avid adrenal masses representing adrenal metastases *(arrowheads)*.

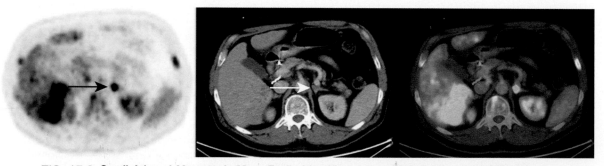

FIG. 15.2 **Small Adrenal Metastasis More Easily Identified due to FDG Avidity.** Axial PET, CT, and fused PET/CT images through the adrenals in a patient with melanoma demonstrate a small low-attenuation left adrenal nodule with marked FDG avidity representing an adrenal metastasis *(arrow)*. Hepatic and osseous metastases are also visible.

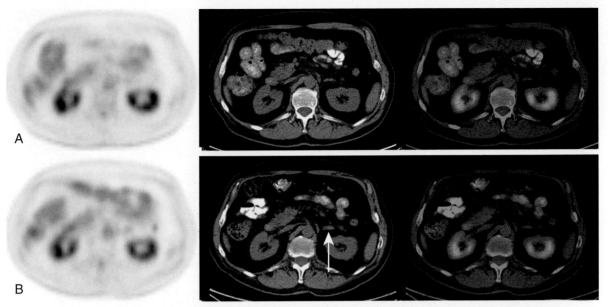

FIG. 15.3 **Early Adrenal Metastasis More Easily Identified due to Change in Adrenal Size on CT.** (A) Axial PET, CT, and fused PET/CT images through the left adrenal in a patient with early-stage lung adeno-carcinoma demonstrate a normal morphology left adrenal gland with background FDG avidity. (B) Axial PET, CT, and fused PET/CT images 6 months later demonstrate interval enlargement of the left adrenal gland on CT *(arrow)* without corresponding abnormality on FDG PET. Biopsy proved an adrenal metastasis.

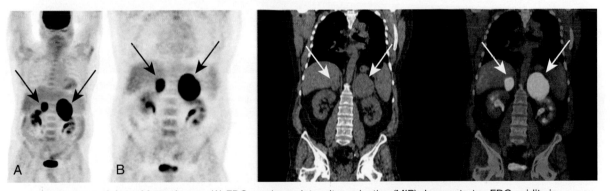

FIG. 15.4 **Adrenal Lymphoma.** (A) FDG maximum intensity projection (MIP) demonstrates FDG avidity in the region of the bilateral adrenal glands *(arrows)*. (B) Coronal PET, CT, and fused PET/CT images demonstrate FDG-avid enlarged bilateral adrenal glands *(arrows)*. No other abnormal FDG-avid foci were identified. The differential diagnosis for bilateral adrenal masses includes bilateral adrenal metastases, adrenal lymphoma, and bilateral pheochromocytoma. Biopsy demonstrated a rare primary adrenal lymphoma.

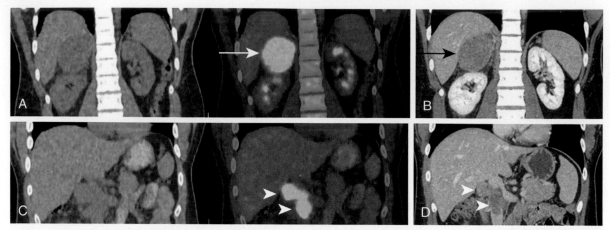

FIG. 15.5 Adrenocortical Carcinoma. (A) Coronal CT and FDG fused PET/CT demonstrate an FDG-avid right suprarenal mass, displacing the right kidney inferiorly *(arrow)*. (B) Coronal contrast-enhanced CT demonstrates the low-attenuation right suprarenal mass *(arrow)*. (C) Coronal CT and FDG fused PET/CT demonstrate growth of the FDG-avid mass through the right adrenal vein into the inferior vena cava (IVC) *(arrowheads)*. (D) Contrast-enhanced coronal CT demonstrates the low-attenuation mass through the right adrenal vein into the IVC *(arrowheads)*.

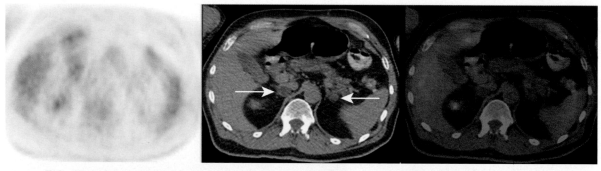

FIG. 15.6 Adrenal Adenomas. Axial PET, CT, and fused PET/CT images through the adrenal glands in a patient with base of tongue squamous cell carcinoma. There are small bilateral low-attenuation adrenal lesions *(arrows)*, with average Hounsfield units of less than 10, representing benign adrenal adenomas. Like the majority of adrenal adenomas, these demonstrate background FDG avidity.

adrenal lesion with Hounsfield units of less than 10 on unenhanced CT is a benign, lipid-rich, adrenal adenoma. Adrenal metastases should not have Hounsfield units of less than 10 on unenhanced CT. On MR, lipid-rich adrenal adenomas may demonstrate out-of-phase signal dropout, which again demonstrates that the lesion is a benign adenoma, despite FDG avidity (Fig. 15.7). Adrenal metastases should not demonstrate out-of-phase signal dropout on MR. Lipid-poor adenomas will have Hounsfield units of greater than 10 on unenhanced CT. For these lesions, contrast washout may help to demonstrate a benign adrenal adenoma, despite FDG avidity. On delayed contrast-enhanced images, adenomas typically demonstrate high levels of contrast washout. Adrenal nodules without characteristic CT or MR findings of benign adenomas may be adrenal malignancy or lipid-poor adenomas. In these cases, FDG avidity can be very helpful in distinguishing benign from malignant lesions. Adrenal nodules that are indeterminate on CT and demonstrate FDG avidity greater than that for the liver are often suspicious for adrenal malignancy. Adrenal nodules that are indeterminate on CT and demonstrate background FDG avidity are most commonly benign (Fig. 15.8).

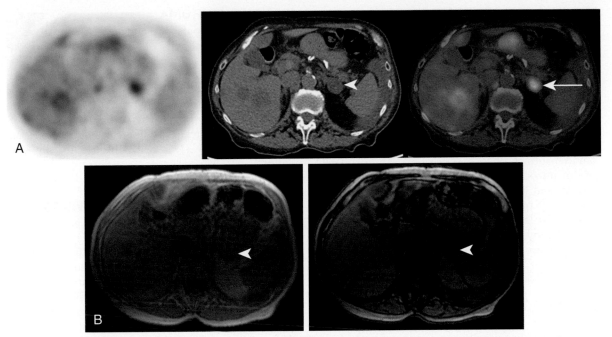

FIG. 15.7 **FDG-avid Adrenal Adenoma.** (A) Axial PET, CT, and fused PET/CT images through the adrenal glands demonstrate an FDG-avid adrenal nodule *(arrow)*. The average Hounsfield units of the nodule on noncontrast CT is 2 *(arrowhead)*, diagnosing the lesion as a benign lipid-rich adrenal adenoma, despite FDG avidity. FDG-avid hepatic metastases are also seen. (B) In-phase and out-of-phase T1-weighted magnetic resonance images demonstrate signal drop on out-of-phase images *(arrowheads)*, again diagnosing the lesion as a benign lipid-rich adrenal adenoma, despite FDG avidity.

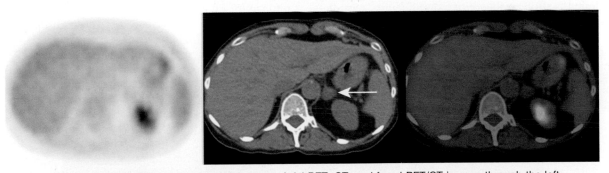

FIG. 15.8 **Non–FDG-avid Adrenal Adenoma.** Axial PET, CT, and fused PET/CT images through the left adrenal gland demonstrate adrenal nodule *(arrow)* with average Hounsfield units of 27, making this nodule indeterminate between a benign and malignant lesion on CT. The lack of FDG avidity is consistent with a benign lipid-poor adrenal adenoma. The majority of adrenal metastases are FDG avid, and the majority of adrenal adenomas demonstrate background FDG avidity. In this case the primary malignancy was a larynx squamous cell carcinoma, and there were no other suspicious lesions outside of the head/neck, adding additional weight to a benign etiology. It would be highly unlikely for a head and neck primary malignancy to first metastasize below the diaphragm.

ADRENAL PHEOCHROMOCYTOMA

Pheochromocytomas arise from the adrenal medulla. On CT or MR, pheochromocytomas typically demonstrate marked contrast enhancement. Cystic changes, hemorrhage, necrosis, and calcifications are common. On FDG PET, many but not all pheochromocytomas are FDG avid. A greater percentage of malignant pheochromocytomas are FDG avid, but in any individual case a pheochromocytomas may or may not be FDG avid. The "rule of tens" helps to remember important characteristics of pheochromocytoma. Approximately 10% of pheochromocytomas are malignant, 10% are bilateral, and 10% are extraadrenal paragangliomas. The diagnosis of pheochromocytoma is greatly assisted by clinical and laboratory evaluation in pheochromocytomas that release catecholamines, which often result in hypertension, cardiac palpitations, headaches, and hyperhidrosis.

MYELOLIPOMA

Myelolipomas are benign admixtures of hematopoietic cells and fat. They usually occur in the adrenal gland, although extraadrenal myelolipomas have been reported. On CT, macroscopic fat in myelolipomas is often visible as fat-attenuation components of the adrenal mass (Fig. 15.9). On FDG PET, most mild lipomas demonstrate no greater than background FDG avidity; however, there are reports of large myelolipomas with elevated FDG avidity. The presence of microscopic fat within the adrenal lesion is strong evidence of a myelolipoma, regardless of FDG avidity.

GANGLIONEUROMA

Ganglioneuromas are rare and benign admixtures of fully differentiated cells of the sympathetic nervous system. They may occur anywhere along the sympathetic nervous system, usually involving the adrenal gland, retroperitoneum, or mediastinum. They have nonspecific imaging findings on both CT and FDG PET and are often only diagnosed when pathology is available. Case series of adrenal ganglioneuromas demonstrate that they may be FDG avid, although usually only mildly.

PHYSIOLOGIC ADRENAL FDG AVIDITY

The adrenal glands are involved in the production of multiple hormones. The adrenal cortex is involved in production of androgens, glucocorticoids, and mineralocorticoids. The adrenal medulla produces catecholamines, which are critical to respond to stress. Needless to say, patients with cancer have multiple sources of stress. Thus, although the normal adrenal glands demonstrate FDG avidity less than liver, it is not uncommon to have elevated FDG avidity in stressed, but otherwise normal, adrenal glands (Fig. 15.10).

ADRENAL HYPERPLASIA

Cushing syndrome is caused by excessive glucocorticoids. Cushing syndrome may be adrenocorticotropic hormone (ACTH) dependent, as seen with an ACTH-secreting pituitary or other tumor, or ACTH independent, with an adrenal lesion that secretes excessive cortisol. With

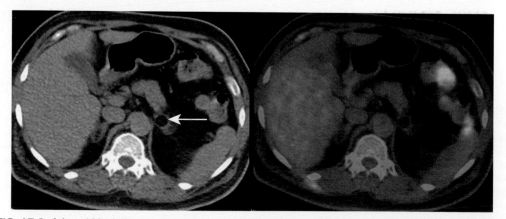

FIG. 15.9 **Adrenal Myelolipoma.** Axial CT and fused PET/CT images through the adrenal glands demonstrate an adrenal nodule with macroscopic fat on CT (arrow). This nodule demonstrates FDG avidity equal to background adrenal gland. This is diagnostic of a benign myelolipoma.

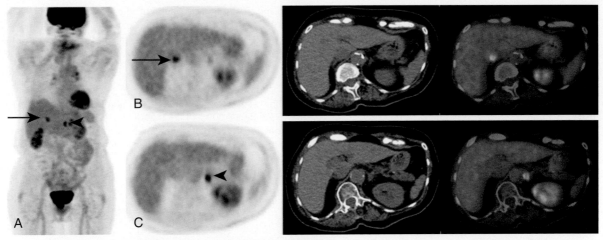

FIG. 15.10 Physiologic Elevated Adrenal FDG Avidity. (A) FDG maximum intensity projection (MIP) in a patient with anal cancer demonstrates foci of FDG avidity in the abdomen to the right *(arrow)* and left *(arrowhead)* of midline. (B) Axial PET, CT, and fused PET/CT images through the right adrenal gland demonstrate a morphologically normal adrenal gland on CT with elevated FDG avidity *(arrow)*. (C) Axial PET, CT, and fused PET/CT images through the left adrenal gland demonstrate similar findings *(arrowhead)*. Because it would be highly unusual to have bilateral adrenal metastases from anal cancer without other lesions in the abdomen or pelvis, these adrenal findings are consistent with physiologically elevated adrenal FDG avidity.

ACTH-dependent Cushing syndrome, the adrenal glands may undergo hyperplasia, evident on CT as enlargement of the glands. This may be associated with bilaterally elevated adrenal FDG avidity.

INFECTION, HEMORRHAGE, AND TRAUMA

Multiple benign processes, such as infection, hemorrhage, and trauma, produce imaging findings with much to be discriminated from malignancy on FDG PET/CT. Granulomatous infections, particularly tuberculosis, may involve the adrenal glands. Adrenal hemorrhage may occur through trauma or nontraumatic etiologies such as stress or underlying neoplasms. Acute adrenal infection or hemorrhage may be FDG avid, mimicking malignancy. Chronic processes may develop calcifications, which help to clarify the chronicity of the lesion. Chronic processes may retain FDG avidity, particularly granulomatous infections.

ADRENAL COLLISION TUMORS

Collision tumors are an admixture of two different neoplastic processes. This may include an admixture of a benign and a malignant process. Coexisting benign and malignant neoplasms and a single adrenal gland could provide a significant diagnostic dilemma. Fortunately, collision tumors are very rare. The separate components of the collision tumor follow CT and FDG PET findings of the individual neoplastic processes.

Here are a few suggestions to help optimize your interpretation of FDG PET/CT of the adrenal gland:

1. Understand the common differential for adrenal masses, including malignancies (metastases, lymphoma, malignant pheochromocytomas, and cortical carcinomas) and benign neoplasms (lipid-rich and lipid-poor adenomas, myelolipomas, benign pheochromocytomas, and ganglioneuromas).

2. Most benign adrenal neoplasms demonstrate background FDG avidity; however, a small percentage of adenomas and other benign neoplasms are FDG avid.

3. Characteristic CT and MR findings of lipid-rich adenomas are diagnostic of a benign lesion, despite FDG avidity. Adrenal malignancy should *not* have Hounsfield units of less than 10 on unenhanced CT. Adrenal malignancy should not demonstrate out-of-phase signal dropout on MR. These two characteristics of lipid-rich adrenal adenomas can help to prevent calling a benign adrenal adenoma a metastasis for the 3% to 5% of adenomas that are FDG avid.

4. The presence of macroscopic fat in an adrenal lesion is consistent with a myelolipoma, despite presence or absence of FDG avidity.

5. Most adrenal malignancies demonstrate elevated FDG avidity; however, in a small percentage of cases, changes on CT may be suspicious for adrenal malignancy in the absence of FDG avidity.

SUGGESTED READINGS

Ansquer, et al: 18F-FDG PET/CT in the characterization and surgical decision concerning adrenal masses: a prospective multicentre evaluation, *Eur J Nucl Med Mol Imaging* 37:1669–1678, 2010.

Boland, et al: Characterization of adrenal masses by using FDG PET: a systematic review and meta-analysis of diagnostic test performance, *Radiology* 259:117–126, 2011.

Brady, et al: Adrenal nodules at FDG PET/CT in patients known to have or suspected of having lung cancer: a proposal for an efficient diagnostic algorithm, *Radiology* 250:523–530, 2009.

Dong, et al: (18)F-FDG PET/CT of adrenal lesions, *AJR Am J Roentgenol* 203:245–252, 2014.

Wong, et al: Molecular imaging in the management of adrenocortical cancer: a systematic reivew, *Clin Nucl Med* 41:e368–e382, 2016.

CHAPTER 16

Gastrointestinal Tract on FDG PET/CT

The gastrointestinal (GI) tract poses challenges for interpretation on 18F-fluorodeoxyglucose positron emission tomography/computed tomography (FDG PET/CT). The esophagus, stomach, and small and large bowel may all demonstrate physiologic FDG avidity, and physiologic FDG avidity may be even more intense than a coexisting malignancy. The areas of physiologic FDG avidity on imaging at one time point may not be the same as the areas of physiologic FDG avidity at another time point. Benign inflammatory etiologies such as esophagitis and gastritis may also be FDG avid. Medications, such as metformin, may induce substantial FDG benign avidity in the colon. These sources of benign FDG avidity may obscure underlying FDG-avid malignancy and may also be mistaken for malignancy.

The differential diagnosis of lesions along the GI tract is similar for the different organs, although the frequency of each type of malignancy will vary at the different organ sites. The differential diagnosis of a malignancy includes primary tumors, lymphoma, and metastases. Primary malignancies of the GI tract include squamous and adenocarcinomas, neuroendocrine tumors (carcinoid), and mesenchymal malignancies (GI stromal tumors [GISTs] or rare leiomyosarcomas). Involvement of multiple sites along the GI tract, as well as corresponding widespread nodal enlargement, favors lymphoma. Lymphoma may also be suggested by "aneurysmal dilation" of bowel lumen, rather than narrowing of the lumen, which is more typical with other genitourinary (GU) tract malignancies. Benign lesions of the GI tract which may be FDG avid include esophagitis and gastritis from stomach acid, infections, ischemia, radiation inflammation, and idiopathic bowel diseases (Crohn disease and ulcerative colitis).

An important concept is to define the GI tract FDG avidity as focal or nonfocal. Another important concept is to correlate the FDG avidity in the GI tract with corresponding findings on the CT images. Small focal FDG avidity in the GI tract without a CT correlate may be physiologic or represent a lesion which is occult on CT, and thus further evaluation may be warranted. If a small focus of FDG avidity corresponds with a polyp or mass on CT, a lesion is confirmed and further evaluation is warranted. Nonfocal FDG avidity (such as large segments of FDG-avid GI tract), without CT correlate, are probably physiologic. Large segments of FDG avidity in the GI tract associated with wall thickening or mass on CT are abnormal, and further evaluation is warranted.

Oral contrast will help to distend the lumen of the GI tract, which helps to visualize wall thickening and masses. Oral contrast is a valuable component of CT and PET/CT studies when the GI tract is a focus of investigation and should be included whenever possible. Some investigators also include intravenous contrast because contrast enhancement will help to visualize enhancing bowel wall masses as well as distant metastases.

ESOPHAGUS

The most common malignancies of the esophagus are squamous and adenocarcinomas. Endoscopy and endoscopic ultrasound are the most accurate means of staging a primary esophageal malignancy. On CT the primary esophageal cancer may be visualized as wall thickening or a focal mass. If the malignancy causes obstruction, then the esophagus may be dilated proximal to the malignancy. If advanced, the mass may demonstrate direct invasion of structures adjacent to the esophagus. Both squamous and adenocarcinomas of the esophagus usually demonstrate high FDG avidity; however, mucinous and signet ring histologies often have lower FDG avidity. A primary esophageal malignancy may be visualized on FDG PET, CT, or both. Small primary esophageal malignancies may not be visible on either FDG PET or CT.

Esophageal cancer demonstrates lymphatic spread to local lymph nodes, usually in the mediastinum for upper esophageal malignancies and also in upper abdominal nodes for lower esophageal malignancies. FDG PET/CT has demonstrated value for the detection of local subcentimeter nodal metastases from esophageal

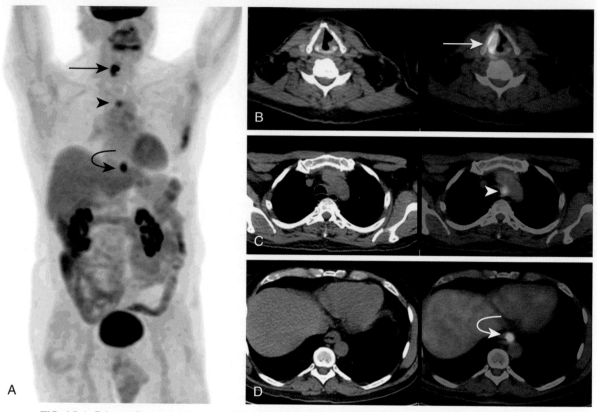

FIG. 16.1 **Primary Esophageal Cancer With Mediastinal Nodal Metastasis Causing Vocal Cord Paralysis.** (A) FDG PET maximum intensity projection (MIP) demonstrating FDG avidity in the neck *(arrow)*, upper chest *(arrowhead)*, and lower chest *(curved)*. (B) Axial CT and fused PET/CT through the neck demonstrate that the neck avidity corresponds with asymmetric right vocalis musculature *(arrow)*. (C) Axial CT and fused PET/CT through the upper chest demonstrate an FDG-avid lymph node adjacent to the aortic arch *(arrowhead)*. (D) Axial CT and fused PET/CT through the lower chest demonstrate FDG-avid distal esophageal wall thickening *(curved arrow)*. The FDG-avid distal esophageal wall thickening represents the known primary esophageal malignancy. The FDG-avid periaortic node is a thoracic nodal metastasis. The asymmetric right vocal cord FDG avidity is actually physiologic, whereas the absent left vocal cord avidity and keyhole shape of the left vocal cord are evidence of left-sided vocal cord paralysis. The left recurrent laryngeal nerve loops under the aortic arch and was probably involved by the nodal metastasis, resulting in left vocal cord paralysis.

cancer which may be overlooked on anatomic imaging. Nodal metastases in the mediastinum may involve the vagus or recurrent laryngeal nerves, resulting in vocal cord paralysis (Fig. 16.1).

Hematogenous spread to any site is possible, with the most common hematogenous metastases being seen in the liver. Contrast-enhanced CT is the standard imaging modality for evaluation of distant metastases; however, FDG PET/CT may demonstrated unsuspected distant metastases not visualized on anatomic imaging, resulting in upstaging of malignancy and alterations in therapeutic management.

Following therapy of esophageal cancer, FDG PET/CT may help to visualize therapy response (Fig. 16.2). It is important to realize that treatment response in solid tumor such as esophageal cancer cannot be compared with treatment response in lymphoma. For lymphoma, residual FDG avidity below liver background is considered treated disease. For solid tumors such as esophageal cancer, reduction of FDG avidity correlates with treatment response, but complete response cannot be distinguished from partial response. Low-volume residual malignancy may be present, despite reduction to background FDG avidity. Tissue sampling would be

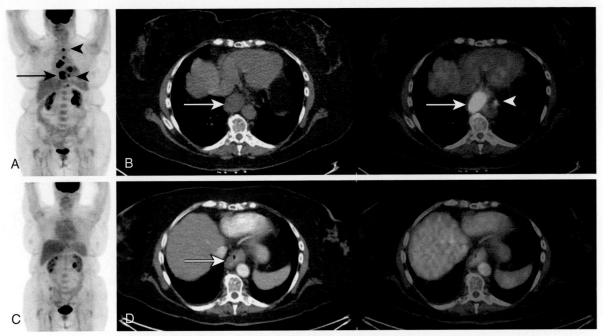

FIG. 16.2 Primary Esophageal Cancer Before and Following Chemoradiotherapy. (A) FDG PET maximum intensity projection (MIP) demonstrates multiple FDG-avid lesions in the thorax and upper abdomen (*arrow* and *arrowheads*). (B) Axial CT and fused PET/CT through the distal esophagus demonstrate the FDG-avid thickened distal esophagus (*arrows*) representing the primary esophageal malignancy, as well as an FDG-avid nodal metastasis (*arrowhead*). (C) Following chemoradiotherapy, FDG PET MIP demonstrates resolution of all FDG-avid lesions. (D) Axial CT and fused PET/CT following chemotherapy demonstrates decreased distal esophageal wall thickening (*arrow*) and resolution of FDG-avid lesions. It is important to remember that, in a solid tumor such as esophageal cancer, reductions of FDG avidity to background cannot distinguish complete pathologic response from partial pathologic response. Thus small-volume residual malignancy is often present despite background FDG avidity.

needed to distinguish partial from complete pathologic response.

The most common malignancies of the esophagus are primary esophageal squamous and adenocarcinomas; however, it is important to remember that the differential for malignant esophageal masses also includes less common esophageal neuroendocrine tumors, mesenchymal tumors, lymphoma, and metastases.

The esophagus may demonstrate physiologic or inflammatory FDG avidity, which must be distinguishing malignancy. In some cases, corresponding CT can help to distinguish benign from malignant esophageal FDG avidity. Small focal areas of FDG avidity may represent esophageal malignancy even without any CT correlate. However, larger segmental areas of FDG avidity are usually accompanied by wall thickening or mass on CT if they are malignant. Larger segmental areas of FDG avidity in the esophagus, without corresponding CT abnormality, are often physiologic or inflammatory. For example, this may be seen with postradiation esophagitis (Fig. 16.3).

If FDG avidity is associated with wall thickening or mass on CT, the FDG avidity is not physiologic. These findings may be malignant or benign (e.g., inflammatory conditions such as Barrett esophagus) (Fig. 16.4). Barrett esophagus is a chronic inflammatory condition secondary to gastric reflux. Endoscopy and biopsy may be needed for workup of incidental FDG avidity in the esophagus to distinguish between benign and malignant etiologies.

STOMACH

Adenocarcinomas are the most common malignancies of the stomach. Endoscopy and biopsy are the most accurate means for diagnosis of a primary gastric malignancy. On CT, the primary gastric malignancy may

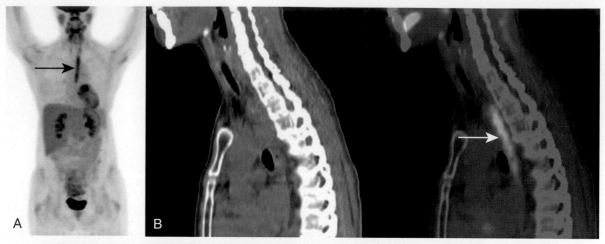

FIG. 16.3 Benign FDG-avid Postradiation Esophagitis. (A) FDG PET maximum intensity projection (MIP) demonstrates a long segment of linear FDG avidity in the mid-chest *(arrow)*. (B) Sagittal CT and fused PET/CT through the chest demonstrate that the linear FDG avidity corresponds with the esophagus *(arrow)*, without mass or wall thickening on CT. As this patient has received radiation therapy to the esophagus, and the linear segmental FDG avidity is probably benign postradiation esophagitis.

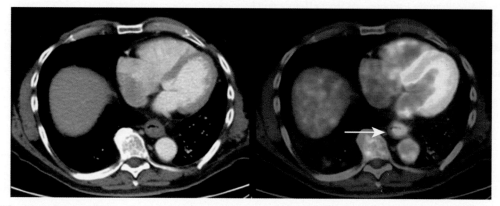

FIG. 16.4 Benign FDG-avid Esophageal Wall Thickening Associated With Barrett Esophagus. Axial CT and fused PET/CT through the chest demonstrate focal FDG-avid wall thickening in the distal esophagus *(arrow)*. The differential for this finding includes both benign esophagitis and esophageal malignancies. Endoscopy and biopsy were performed, and pathology demonstrated benign Barrett esophagus without evidence of malignancy.

be visualized as wall thickening or focal mass. An undistended stomach may seem to have gastric wall thickening or a mass which actually does not exist, and these "pseudotumors" must be distinguished from true masses. In a stomach distended with gastric contents or oral contrast, the evaluation of wall thickening or focal masses is more reliable. On FDG PET, focal FDG avidity may be seen at the site of the primary malignancy; however, FDG PET is not sensitive for the detection of a primary gastric malignancy. This is particularly true for mucinous and signet ring histologies, which demonstrate lower FDG avidity. Overall, primary gastric malignancy may be visualized on FDG PET, CT, or both, whereas small primary gastric malignancies may not be visible on either FDG PET or CT.

Gastric malignancies demonstrate lymphatic spread to local lymph nodes, usually beginning with perigastric nodes, then extending of the regional nodes along the

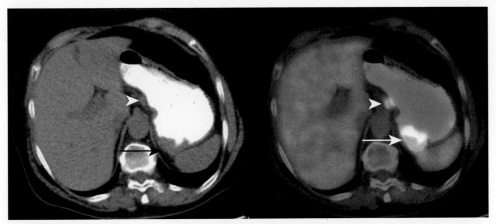

FIG. 16.5 **Gastric Adenocarcinoma With Subcentimeter Perigastric Lymph Node Metastasis.** Axial CT and fused PET/CT through the stomach demonstrate focal FDG-avid gastric wall thickening *(arrows)*, as well as an FDG-avid subcentimeter perigastric node *(arrowhead)*. The differential for a gastric mass includes adenocarcinoma, carcinoid, gastrointestinal stromal tumors, lymphoma, metastasis, and inflammatory causes. Endoscopy and biopsy proved a primary gastric adenocarcinoma. The FDG-avid perigastric node is suspicious for a nodal metastasis, despite subcentimeter size.

celiac artery and its branches. FDG PET, like CT, has demonstrated low sensitivity for the detection of gastric lymph node metastases; thus a lack of FDG-avid or enlarged nodes on FDG PET/CT does not exclude regional nodal metastases. FDG PET has relatively higher specificity for detection of nodal metastases within draining nodal basins and may identify subcentimeter nodes suspicious for metastases which are overlooked on anatomic imaging (Fig. 16.5). Nodal drainage to the thoracic duct may result in left supraclavicular nodal metastases, which are considered distant metastases.

Hematogenous spread to any site is possible, with the most common hematogenous metastases being seen in the peritoneum and liver. Contrast-enhanced CT is the standard imaging modality for evaluation of distant metastases from primary gastric malignancies. The value of FDG PET/CT in the initial systemic staging of gastric malignancy has not been proven.

Following therapy, FDG PET/CT may help to visualize therapy response. FDG PET may be able to distinguish responders from nonresponders following chemotherapy or radiation therapy. FDG PET cannot distinguish complete pathologic response from partial pathologic response in gastric malignancies. This is due to physiologic and inflammatory FDG avidity in the stomach, as well as inability for FDG PET to sensitively visualize small-volume residual malignancy.

Gastric adenocarcinomas are aggressive with high rates of recurrence. The most common sites of recurrence for gastric malignancies are at the resection margins, peritoneum, and liver. There may be value for FDG PET/CT in the evaluation of recurrent gastric malignancy.

The most common malignancy of the stomach is adenocarcinoma; however, it is important to remember that the differential for gastric masses also includes less common gastric carcinoids, GISTs (Fig. 16.6), lymphoma, and metastases (Fig. 16.7). In some cases, FDG PET/CT may demonstrate gastric wall thickening without significant FDG avidity. Thus gastric wall thickening may be the only sign of a gastric malignancy (Fig. 16.8). Endoscopy and biopsy may be needed for workup of incidental focal FDG avidity or wall thickening in the stomach.

The stomach may demonstrate physiologic or inflammatory FDG avidity, which must be distinguished from malignancy (Fig. 16.9). In some cases the corresponding CT can help to distinguish benign from malignant gastric FDG avidity. Small focal areas of FDG avidity may be benign (Fig. 16.10) or represent a gastric lesion which is occult on CT. Larger segmental areas of FDG avidity in the stomach are normally accompanied by wall thickening or mass on CT if malignant. Larger segmental areas of FDG avidity without corresponding CT abnormality are probably benign. If FDG avidity is associated with wall thickening or mass on CT, then the FDG avidity is not physiologic. Unfortunately, the PET/CT findings of benign and malignant gastric processes demonstrate substantial overlap. Endoscopy and biopsy may be

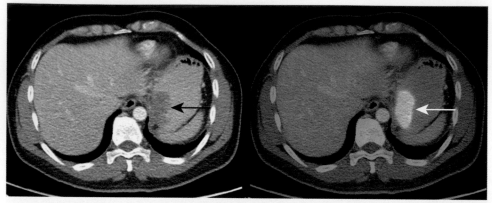

FIG. 16.6 Gastrointestinal Stromal Tumors (GISTs). Axial CT and fused PET/CT through the stomach demonstrate focal FDG-avid gastric wall mass *(arrows)*. Endoscopy and biopsy proved a primary gastric GIST. The imaging features may be identical in a gastric adenocarcinoma or other gastric masses.

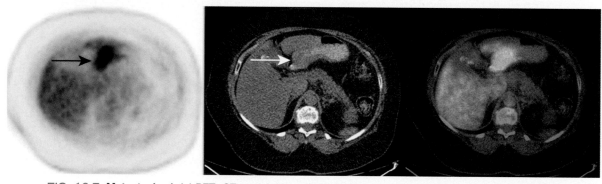

FIG. 16.7 Metastasis. Axial PET, CT, and fused PET/CT images through the stomach in a patient with breast cancer demonstrate focal FDG avidity and possible gastric wall thickening *(arrows)*. Differential includes both benign and malignancy etiologies. Endoscopy and biopsy proved metastatic breast cancer to the stomach.

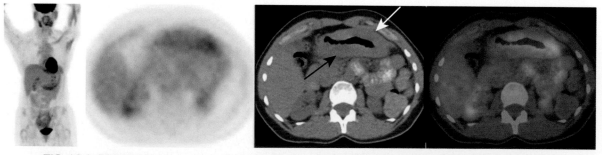

FIG. 16.8 FDG PET Maximum Intensity Projection in a Patient With Lobular Breast Cancer Demonstrates No Suspicious Focal FDG Avidity. Axial PET, CT, and fused PET/CT images through the stomach demonstrate substantial gastric wall thickening *(arrows)* without focal FDG avidity. Differential for the gastric wall thickening includes both benign and malignancy etiologies. Endoscopy and biopsy proved metastatic breast cancer to the stomach.

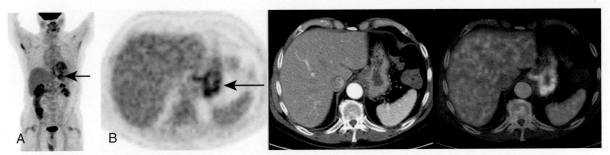

FIG. 16.9 **Physiologic Gastric FDG Avidity.** (A) FDG PET maximum intensity projection (MIP) demonstrates FDG avidity in the region of the distal esophagus and proximal stomach *(arrow)*. (B) Axial PET, CT, and fused PET/CT images through the stomach demonstrate segmental FDG avidity in the stomach *(arrow)* without corresponding abnormality of the corresponding CT images. Physiologic FDG avidity in the stomach is common, may be intense, is usually nonfocal, and should not have a corresponding abnormality on CT.

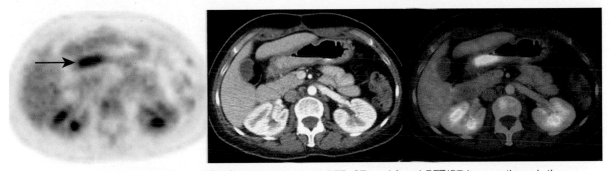

FIG. 16.10 **FDG Avidity from Benign Gastritis.** Axial PET, CT, and fused PET/CT images through the stomach in a patient with breast cancer demonstrate focal FDG avidity in the stomach without corresponding abnormality of the corresponding CT images *(arrow)*. Differential includes both benign and malignancy etiologies. Due to the focal nature of the FDG avidity, endoscopy and biopsy were performed, which demonstrated chronic inflammation without evidence of malignancy. Compare this case with Fig. 16.7. The imaging findings are nearly identical, and endoscopy with biopsy was needed to distinguish between benign and malignant etiologies of focal gastric FDG avidity.

needed to distinguish between benign and malignant etiologies of gastric FDG avidity or wall thickening.

SMALL BOWEL

Small bowel malignancies are uncommon. When they do occur, primary small bowel malignancies include adenocarcinomas, carcinoids, and GISTs. Evaluation of a primary small bowel lesion is often difficult because endoscopy from above does not reach farther than the proximal small bowel and colonoscopy from below visualizes only the very distal small bowel. On CT a primary small bowel malignancy may be visualized as wall thickening or a focal mass. On FDG PET, small

bowel malignancy may demonstrate focal FDG avidity. A primary small bowel malignancy may be visualized on FDG PET, CT, both, or neither.

Small bowel malignancies demonstrate lymphatic spread to local draining lymph nodes (Fig. 16.11). Similar to other organ systems, FDG PET/CT may help to detect subcentimeter nodal metastases which may be overlooked on anatomic imaging. For carcinoids, metastatic mesenteric masses may be confused for the primary malignancy.

Primary small bowel malignancies may demonstrate hematogenous spread. Most common sites of distant metastases of small bowel adenocarcinomas are the peritoneum and liver. Although most GISTs are benign,

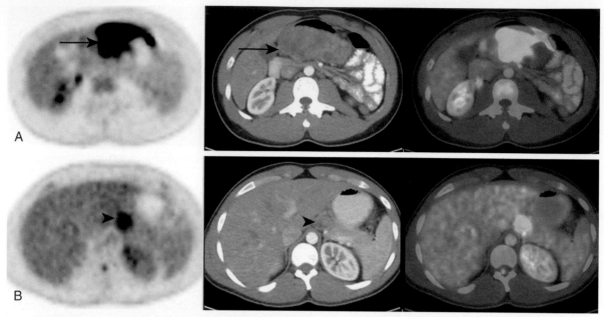

FIG. 16.11 **Small Bowel Gastrointestinal Stromal Tumors (GISTs) With Perigastric Nodal Metastasis.** (A) Axial PET, CT, and fused PET/CT images through the stomach demonstrate an FDG-avid gastric mass *(arrows)*. (B) Axial PET, CT, and fused PET/CT images slightly more superiorly demonstrate an FDG-avid perigastric node *(arrowheads)*, consistent with nodal metastasis. These findings may be seen with small bowel adenocarcinoma, carcinoid, or GIST, as well as with lymphoma or metastases. Biopsy of the bowel mass demonstrated a GIST.

when malignant, they metastasize most frequently to the peritoneum, liver, lung, and bone. Contrast-enhanced CT is the standard imaging modality for evaluation of distant metastases. The value of FDG PET/CT in detecting unsuspected distant metastases at initial diagnosis of small bowel tumors has not been established.

FDG PET/CT may help to visualize therapy response in small bowel primary malignancies. As with the rest of the GI tract, low-volume residual malignancy may be present despite background FDG avidity, and thus FDG PET cannot distinguish between partial and complete therapeutic responses. Of particular importance is the role of FDG PET/CT in the evaluation of treatment response of GISTs. Most GISTs have characteristic mutations in the tyrosine kinase Kit or a homologous tyrosine kinase. The targeted tyrosine kinase inhibitors imatinib and sunitinib are used to treat GISTs with tyrosine kinase mutations and often result in substantial tumor response. GIST response to imatinib and sunitinib may paradoxically occur with tumor enlargement. Response to imatinib and sunitinib therapy measured by FDG avidity has been shown to be more accurate than response measurements based on size criteria.

In addition to primary small bowel malignancies, the small bowel may be involved by lymphoma or metastases. Involvement of multiple sites along the GI tract, as well as widespread nodal enlargement, favors lymphoma (Fig. 16.12). Lymphoma may also be suggested by "aneurysmal dilation" of bowel lumen (Fig. 16.13). Most other small bowel malignancies cause narrowing of the lumen. Metastases to be small bowel are relatively uncommon but occur with primary malignancies from the GI and GU tracts, as well as lung, breast, and melanoma malignancies. Melanoma metastases may act as lead points causing small bowel intussusception (Fig. 16.14).

The small bowel often demonstrates benign physiologic or inflammatory FDG avidity. The corresponding CT images can sometimes help to distinguish benign from malignant small bowel FDG avidity. Small focal areas of FDG avidity may represent tumors which are occult on CT (Fig. 16.15). However, larger segmental areas of FDG avidity are usually accompanied by wall thickening or mass on CT if malignant. If FDG avidity is associated with wall thickening or mass on CT, the FDG avidity is not physiologic. FDG-avid small bowel

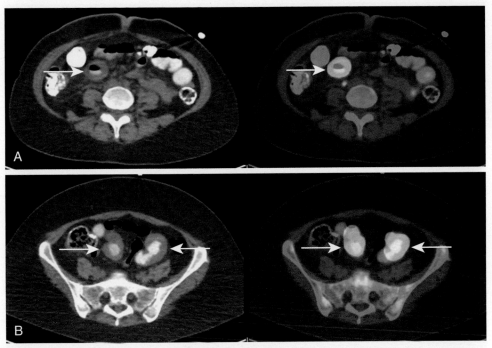

FIG. 16.12 **Multifocal Small Bowel Lymphoma.** Axial CT and fused PET/CT images through the (A) abdomen and (B) pelvis demonstrate multiple sites of FDG-avid bowel wall thickening *(arrows)* in this patient with small bowel lymphoma.

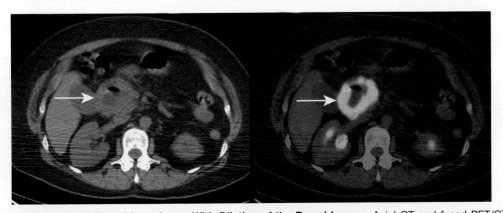

FIG. 16.13 **Small Bowel Lymphoma With Dilation of the Bowel Lumen.** Axial CT and fused PET/CT images through the abdomen demonstrate FDG-avid bowel wall thickening *(arrows)*. Despite circumferential bowel wall thickening, the bowel lumen is dilated, rather than narrowed. This is a feature which favors lymphoma.

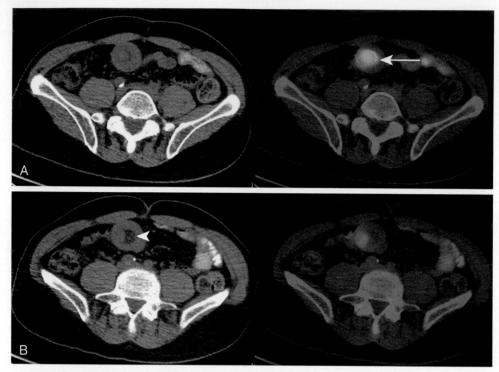

FIG. 16.14 Small Bowel Metastasis Causing Intussusception. (A) Axial CT and fused PET/CT images through the pelvis in a patient with melanoma demonstrate an FDG-avid small bowel mass *(arrow)*, representing a small bowel metastasis. (B) Axial CT and fused PET/CT images from an adjacent level demonstrate fat attenuation within the lumen of the small bowel *(arrowhead)*, representing intussuscepted mesenteric fat.

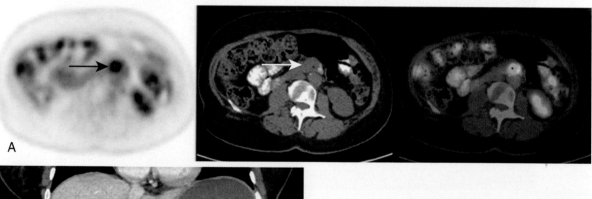

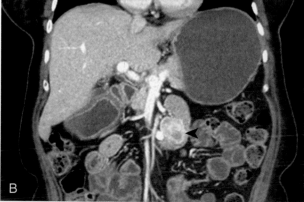

FIG. 16.15 Incidental Small Bowel Gastrointestinal Stromal Tumors (GISTs) Detected as Focal FDG Avidity on FDG PET/CT. (A) Axial PET, CT, and fused PET/CT images through the abdomen demonstrate focal FDG avidity in the duodenum *(arrows)*. The presence of corresponding mass or wall thickening is unclear due to underdistension. The focal nature of the FDG avidity in a patient with known malignancy leads to further evaluation with contrast-enhanced CT. (B) Coronal contrast-enhanced CT demonstrates an enhancing mass at the location of the focal FDG avidity in the duodenum *(arrowhead)*. The differential includes primary small bowel malignancy and metastasis. Pathology demonstrated an incidental small bowel GIST.

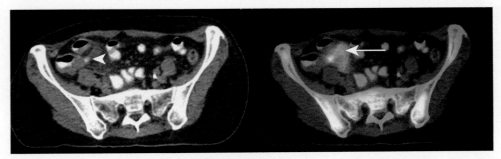

FIG. 16.16 Incidental Appendicitis on FDG PET/CT. Axial CT and fused PET/CT images through the pelvis demonstrate focal FDG avidity in the appendix *(arrow)*. Corresponding CT image demonstrates an appendicolith *(arrowhead)*. Upon questioning, the patient complained of right lower quadrant abdominal pain. Subsequent surgery and pathology documented appendicitis.

wall thickening/mass may be malignant or benign (e.g., with Crohn disease or postradiation inflammation).

APPENDIX

FDG avidity in the appendix may be physiologic, inflammatory, or malignant. Again, correlation with CT images can help to discriminate physiologic FDG avidity from other causes. Appendiceal wall thickening or mass may be seen on the CT component of PET/CT for primary appendiceal malignancies (adenocarcinoma, cystadenocarcinomas, and neuroendocrine tumors), lymphoma, and metastases. FDG avidity in the appendix may be inflammatory. In patients with abdominal pain and an appendicolith on CT, FDG PET/CT has even led to the diagnosis of appendicitis (Fig. 16.16).

COLORECTAL

The most common malignancy of the colon is adenocarcinoma. Colonoscopy and biopsy are used to make the diagnosis of colorectal masses. For T staging of the primary malignancy, colonic primaries are assessed on CT, whereas rectal primaries are most accurately T staged with magnetic resonance. Endoscopic ultrasound may also be used for T staging rectal malignancies. On CT, primary colon malignancies may be visualized as wall thickening or a focal mass. Luminal stenosis is common and if severe enough may cause obstruction. If advanced, the mass may demonstrate extramural extension into the pericolonic fat. Adenocarcinomas of the colon often demonstrate high FDG avidity; however, mucinous adenocarcinomas often have lower FDG avidity. The primary colorectal malignancy may be visualized on FDG PET, CT, or both. Small primary colorectal malignancies may not be visible on either FDG PET or CT.

Given the high incidence of primary colorectal malignancies, they may be incidentally detected on FDG PET/CT scans performed for another malignancy (Fig. 16.17). Incidental focal colonic FDG avidity without CT correlate may be further evaluated by colonoscopy or by imaging follow-up. If the FDG-avid focus resolves on follow-up, the avidity was probably physiologic. If the FDG avid focus is persistent, there is probably an underlying CT occult lesion, and colonoscopy can be performed for further evaluation. Incidental focal colonic FDG avidity which is associated with a polyp (Fig. 16.18) or wall thickening (Fig. 16.19) on CT confirms an abnormality, and colonoscopy can be performed for further evaluation. The need for colonoscopy workup will depend on the clinical scenarios of the patient. In a patient with nonresponding metastatic pancreatic cancer, the workup of an incidental FDG-avid colonic focus may not be clinically relevant. In a patient with treated lymphoma, an incidentally discovered FDG-avid colonic focus is more likely to represent a clinically relevant issue.

Colorectal cancer demonstrates lymphatic spread to local lymph nodes, along mesenteric drainage pathways. FDG PET/CT may detect subcentimeter nodal metastases overlooked on anatomic imaging. Conversely, CT may also identify nodal metastases which are not apparent on FDG PET (Fig. 16.20). FDG-avid, enlarged, *or* rounded lymph nodes in the appropriate mesenteric drainage pathway of a primary colonic malignancy should be considered suspicious for nodal metastases, even if apparent on only one imaging modality, FDG PET or CT.

Hematogenous spread from colon adenocarcinoma to any site is possible, with the most common hematogenous metastases being seen in the liver. Contrast-enhanced CT is the standard imaging modality for evaluation of distant metastases. The value of FDG PET/

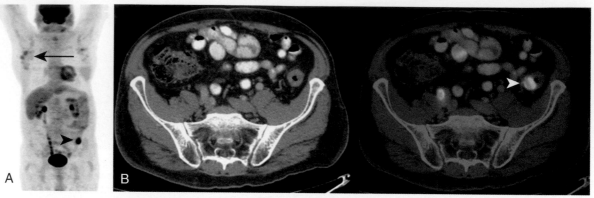

FIG. 16.17 **Incidental Colon Cancer Detected on FDG PET/CT for a Patient With Lymphoma.** (A) FDG PET maximum intensity projection (MIP) demonstrates mildly FDG-avid lymph nodes above and below the diaphragm *(arrow)*, as well as focal FDG avidity in the left pelvis *(arrowhead)*. (B) Axial CT and fused PET/CT images localize the left pelvic focus to the descending colon *(arrowhead)*. Colonoscopy was performed for further evaluation, and biopsy proved a previously unknown primary colon adenocarcinoma.

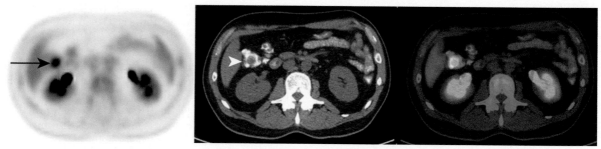

FIG. 16.18 **Incidental Colon Cancer Detected on FDG PET/CT for a Patient With Esophageal Cancer.** Axial PET, CT, and fused PET/CT images demonstrate focal FDG avidity in the right abdomen, corresponding to ascending colon *(arrow)*. CT demonstrates a corresponding polyp within the ascending colon at the site of FDG avidity *(arrowhead)*, confirming the FDG avidity is abnormal and not physiologic. Colonoscopy was performed for further evaluation, and biopsy proved a previously unknown primary colon adenocarcinoma.

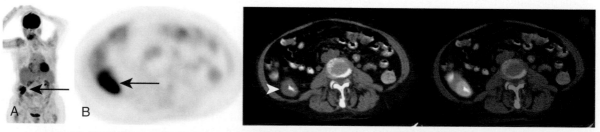

FIG. 16.19 **Incidental Colon Cancer Detected on FDG PET/CT for a Patient With Plasmacytoma.** (A) FDG PET maximum intensity projection (MIP) demonstrates focal FDG avidity in the right abdomen *(arrow)*. (B) Axial PET, CT, and fused PET/CT images demonstrate the focal avidity localizes to the ascending colon and corresponds with wall thickening on CT *(arrowhead)*, confirming the FDG avidity is abnormal and not physiologic. Colonoscopy was performed for further evaluation, and biopsy proved a previously unknown primary colon adenocarcinoma.

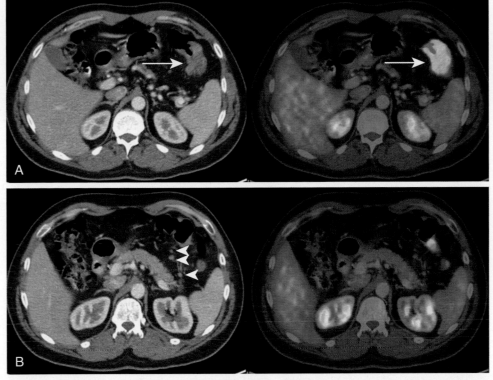

FIG. 16.20 Primary Colon Malignancy With Mesenteric Nodal Metastases Not Appreciable on FDG PET. (A) Axial CT and fused PET/CT through the abdomen demonstrate an FDG-avid left colon mass *(arrows)*, representing a primary colonic adenocarcinoma. (B) Axial CT and fused PET/CT in an adjacent level demonstrate subcentimeter rounded lymph nodes *(arrowheads)* in the expected mesenteric drainage pathway of the colon cancer, which represent nodal metastases despite no corresponding finding on FDG PET.

CT in detecting unsuspected distant metastases at initial diagnosis of colon cancer has not been established.

Following therapy, FDG PET/CT may help to visualize therapy response but cannot distinguish between complete and partial responses even if FDG-avidity decreases to background levels.

Colonic adenocarcinomas have reasonably high rates of recurrence. The most common sites of recurrence for colonic malignancies are the resection margin, peritoneum, and liver. Although there is no definite proof of value for FDG PET/CT in evaluating colon adenocarcinoma recurrence, FDG PET/CT may detect recurrent malignancy overlooked on anatomic imaging (Fig. 16.21).

The most common primary malignancy of the colon is adenocarcinoma; however, it is important to remember that the differential diagnosis for malignant esophageal masses also includes less common esophageal neuroendocrine tumors, GIST, lymphoma, and metastases. As with GISTs elsewhere in the GI tract, FDG PET/CT

demonstrates more accurate evaluation of response to the targeted tyrosine kinase inhibitors imatinib and sunitinib than response measurements based on size criteria (Fig. 16.22).

The colon may demonstrate physiologic or inflammatory FDG avidity, which must be distinguished from malignancy. Inflammatory processes involving the colon include inflamed diverticula, infections, ischemia, and idiopathic bowel disease (ulcerative colitis and Crohn disease). In some cases the corresponding CT can help to distinguish benign from malignant FDG avidity. As previously discussed, small focal areas of FDG avidity without any CT correlate may represent colon malignancy. A small focal area of FDG avidity without CT correlate may also be physiologic or inflammatory, such as related to diverticula (Fig. 16.23). A benign FDG-avid focus related to a diverticulum should resolve on follow-up imaging. If the focus is persistent on follow-up imaging, then colonoscopy could be considered for further

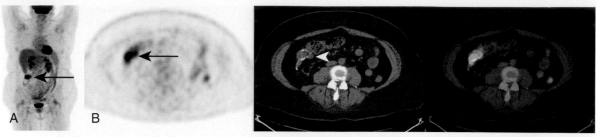

FIG. 16.21 **Recurrent Colon Adenocarcinoma at the Colonic Anastomosis Visualized by FDG PET.**
(A) FDG PET maximum intensity projection (MIP) in a patient with colonic adenocarcinoma post–right
hemicolectomy demonstrates focal FDG avidity in the right abdomen *(arrow)*. (B) Axial PET, CT, and fused
PET/CT through the abdomen demonstrate the FDG focus localizes to the colonic anastomosis *(arrow)*
without evidence of mass or wall thickening on CT *(arrowhead)*. The differential for the FDG avidity includes
physiologic and malignant etiologies. Colonoscopy was performed for further evaluation, and biopsy proved
recurrent colon adenocarcinoma.

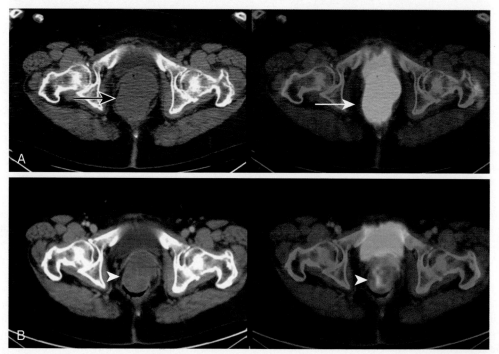

FIG. 16.22 **Rectal Gastrointestinal Stromal Tumors (GISTs) With Imatinib Therapy Response Is Better
Visualized by Change in FDG Avidity Than by Change in Tumor Size.** (A) Axial CT and fused PET/CT
through the abdomen demonstrate an FDG-avid rectal mass *(arrows)*, representing a primary rectal GIST.
(B) Axial CT and fused PET/CT following imatinib therapy demonstrate minimal decrease in size but marked
decrease in FDG avidity *(arrowheads)*. Successful treatment response to imatinib therapy was better visualized
on FDG PET than by change in size on CT.

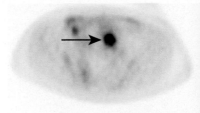
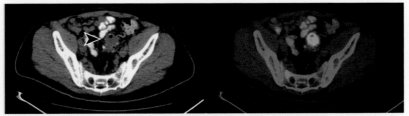

FIG. 16.23 **Benign FDG-avid Colonic Diverticula.** Axial PET, CT, and fused PET/CT through the pelvis demonstrate an FDG-avid focus *(arrow)* that correlates with a diverticulum on CT *(arrowhead)*. This is probably a benign diverticulum and it resolved on follow-up imaging.

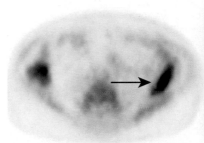
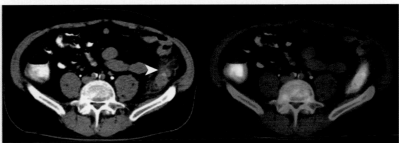

FIG. 16.24 **Benign FDG-avid Inflamed Colonic Diverticula.** Axial PET, CT, and fused PET/CT through the pelvis demonstrate an FDG-avid focus *(arrow)* that correlates with a diverticulum and adjacent inflammatory changes on CT *(arrowhead)*. This is probably a benign inflamed diverticulum and it resolved on follow-up imaging.

evaluation. Inflamed diverticula may result in inflammatory changes extending into the adjacent mesentery (Fig. 16.24). Again, this should resolve on follow-up imaging, and if persistent, colonoscopy could be considered for further evaluation. Note that FDG-avid diverticula are referred to here as inflamed diverticulum, rather than as diverticulitis. This nomenclature was chosen because diverticulitis is a clinical diagnosis of pain associated with inflamed diverticula. In the absence of abdominal pain, referring to FDG-avid diverticula as diverticulitis is inaccurate and could lead to a diagnostic label that the patient does not deserve. Longer segmental areas of FDG avidity in the colon are usually accompanied by wall thickening or mass on CT if malignant. Longer segmental areas of FDG avidity in the colon without corresponding CT abnormality are probably benign. Active idiopathic bowel disease (ulcerative colitis and Crohn disease) is often associated with long segments of FDG avidity. This may correlate with segments of wall thickening on CT. When chronic, edema in the bowel wall results in "bowel wall stratification" with low-attenuation submucosal edema sandwiched between soft tissue attenuation mucosa and muscularis layers (Fig. 16.25). When the entire colon demonstrates FDG avidity and there is no corresponding wall thickening on CT, this is often related to diabetic medications such as metformin (Fig. 16.26). If the entire colon demonstrates FDG avidity and correlates with thickening of the entire colon on CT, consider an infectious etiology such as *Clostridium difficile* colitis (Fig. 16.27). When necessary, colonoscopy and biopsy could be considered for workup of colonic FDG avidity of unclear etiology.

ANUS

The anus is composed of epithelium surrounded by multiple muscular sphincters. The anal sphincter complex may demonstrate substantial physiologic FDG avidity (Fig. 16.28). In a patient with no suspicion of anal malignancy, symmetric FDG avidity in the anal sphincter without corresponding CT abnormality is physiologic. In a patient with suspicion of anal malignancy, this FDG avidity cannot be so easily dismissed as only

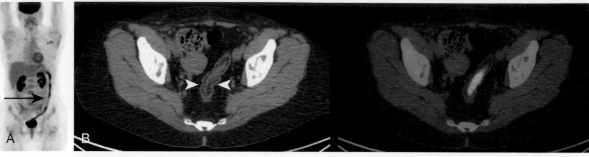

FIG. 16.25 **FDG Avidity Associated With Ulcerative Colitis.** (A) FDG PET maximum intensity projection (MIP) demonstrating a long segment of FDG avidity in the left colon *(arrow)*. (B) Axial CT and fused PET/CT through the pelvis demonstrate that the segmental FDG avidity corresponds to left colon with mural stratification. The edematous submucosa is visualized as a low-attenuation stripe in the bowel wall *(arrowheads)*. This is a CT finding corresponding to chronic inflammation in this patient with known ulcerative colitis.

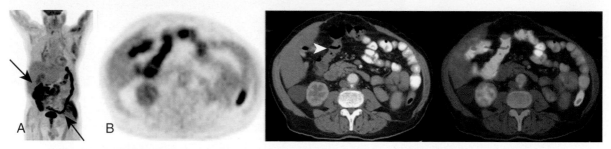

FIG. 16.26 **FDG Avidity in the Entire Colon Related to Metformin Medication Use.** (A) FDG PET maximum intensity projection (MIP) demonstrating FDG avidity in the entire colon *(arrows)*. (B) Axial PET, CT, and fused PET/CT through the abdomen demonstrate FDG avidity in the entire colon but no corresponding abnormality on CT *(arrowhead)*. This patient takes metformin, a diabetic medication which may cause FDG avidity in the colon without CT correlate.

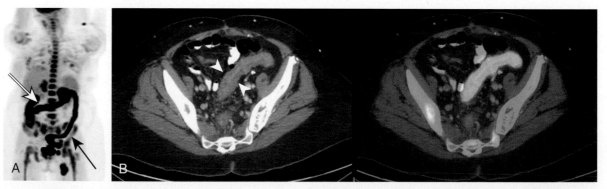

FIG. 16.27 **FDG-avid Bowel Wall Thickening in the Entire Colon in a Patient with *Clostridium difficile* Colitis.** (A) FDG PET maximum intensity projection (MIP) demonstrating FDG avidity in the entire colon *(arrows)*. (B) Axial CT and fused PET/CT through the abdomen demonstrate FDG avidity in the entire colon, which correlates with wall thickening of the entire colon on CT *(arrowheads)*. This patient subsequently had stool culture–proven *C. difficile* colitis. Compare with Fig. 16.26. The FDG findings in the colon are nearly identical. It is the corresponding presence or absence of CT wall thickening that discriminates the imaging findings of a patient taking metformin and the patient with *C. difficile* colitis.

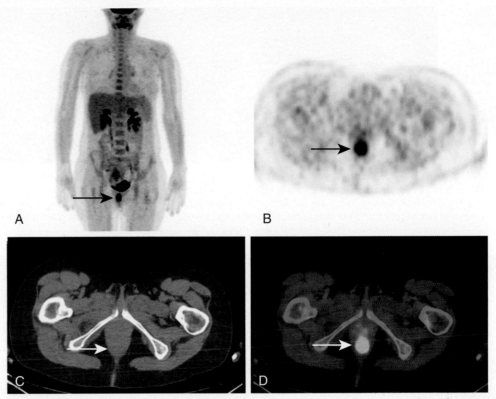

FIG. 16.28 Physiologic FDG Avidity in the Anal Sphincter. (A) FDG PET maximum intensity projection (MIP) in a patient with treated lymphoma demonstrates FDG avidity overlying the lower pelvis *(arrow)*. (B) Axial PET, (C) CT, and (D) fused PET/CT through the lower pelvis demonstrate that the focal FDG avidity localizes to the anus and is symmetric in respect to the anal sphincter, and there is no corresponding CT abnormality *(arrows)*. This represents benign physiologic FDG avidity in the anal sphincter.

physiologic. The CT component of the PET/CT may assist with differentiating benign and malignant FDG avidity in the anus. If the FDG avidity is asymmetric to the anal sphincter on CT, then the avidity is not physiologic. CT may also demonstrate a mass lesion (Fig. 16.29). In cases of unclear interval FDG avidity, manual physical examination could be performed to evaluate for a mass.

Lymphatic drainage of a primary anal malignancy depends on its relationship to the dentate (or pectinate) line which divides lower squamous mucosa from non-squamous mucinous above. Tumors above the dentate line usually drain to perirectal nodes, whereas tumors below the dentate line usually drain to inguinal and femoral nodes. FDG PET/CT may detect subcentimeter nodal metastases overlooked on anatomic imaging (Fig. 16.30). Conversely, CT may also identify nodal metastases which are not apparent on FDG PET.

FDG-avid, enlarged, *or* rounded lymph nodes in the appropriate drainage pathway of an anal cancer should be considered suspicious for nodal metastases, even if apparent on only one imaging modality, FDG PET or CT.

Hematogenous spread from anal cancer to any site is possible, with the most common hematogenous metastases being seen in the liver. Contrast-enhanced CT is the standard imaging modality for evaluation of distant metastases. The value of FDG PET/CT in detecting unsuspected distant metastases at initial diagnosis of anal cancer has not been established.

Curvilinear FDG avidity extending from the anal canal and toward the ischiorectal fossae or skin surface may be seen in patients with benign rectal tracts or fistulas (Fig. 16.31). A corresponding soft tissue tract will be seen on CT.

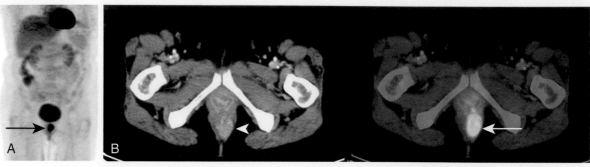

FIG. 16.29 FDG-avid Primary Anal Malignancy. (A) FDG PET maximum intensity projection (MIP) in a patient with known anal malignancy demonstrates FDG avidity overlying the lower pelvis *(arrow)*. (B) Axial CT and fused PET/CT through the lower pelvis demonstrate that the focal FDG avidity localizes to the anus but is asymmetric in respect to the anal sphincter *(arrow)* and corresponds with an enhancing left anal mass on CT *(arrowhead)*. This represents the primary anal malignancy.

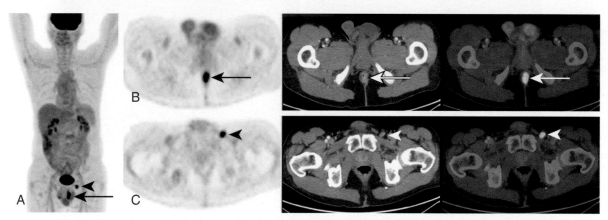

FIG. 16.30 FDG-avid Primary Anal Malignancy With FDG-avid Inguinal Nodal Metastasis. (A) FDG PET maximum intensity projection (MIP) in a patient with known anal malignancy demonstrates FDG avidity overlying the lower pelvis *(arrow),* as well as another more superior focus *(arrowhead)*. (B) Axial PET, CT, and fused PET/CT through the lower pelvis demonstrate that the focal FDG avidity localizes to the anus but is asymmetric in respect to the anal sphincter *(arrows)*. This represents the primary anal malignancy. (C) Axial PET, CT, and fused PET/CT through a more superior plane localize this additional focus to a subcentimeter left inguinal node *(arrowheads)*. Although subcentimeter FDG-avid inguinal nodes are commonly seen and are often inflammatory, in a patient with anal cancer they are suspicious for nodal metastasis. This node was biopsy proven to be a nodal metastases.

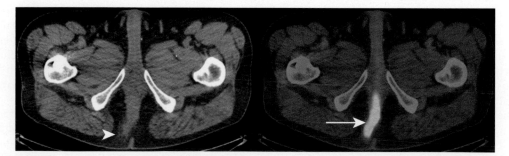

FIG. 16.31 Benign FDG-avid Ischiorectal Tract. Axial CT and fused PET/CT through the lower pelvis demonstrate a curvilinear FDG-avid soft tissue density *(arrow)* with adjacent soft tissue stranding in fat *(arrowhead)*. This patient has papillary thyroid cancer and no evidence of malignancy below the diaphragm. The FDG soft tissue in the ischiorectal fossa represents a benign inflammatory ischiorectal tract.

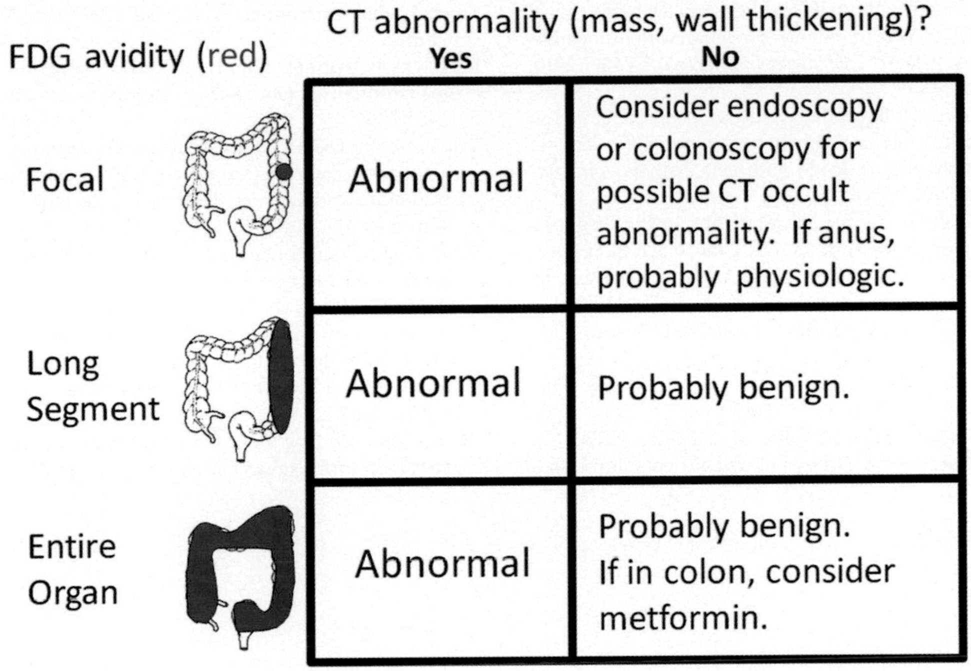

FDG avidity (red)	CT abnormality (mass, wall thickening)? Yes	CT abnormality (mass, wall thickening)? No
Focal	Abnormal	Consider endoscopy or colonoscopy for possible CT occult abnormality. If anus, probably physiologic.
Long Segment	Abnormal	Probably benign.
Entire Organ	Abnormal	Probably benign. If in colon, consider metformin.

FIG. 16.32 Evaluation of the gastrointestinal (GI) tract on FDG PET/CT, considering the morphology of the FDG avidity (focal, segmental, entire organ) and the presence/absence of wall thickening/mass on CT. Diagrams of the colon are provided, but this could apply to any organ of the GI tract. If there is wall thickening or mass on CT, the FDG avidity is abnormal, not physiologic. The abnormality may be benign (infectious, ischemic, idiopathic) or malignant in etiology. If there is no corresponding CT abnormality, long segments of FDG avidity are probably physiologic/benign. Small foci of FDG avidity may represent processes that are occult on CT. Consider follow-up examination to confirm resolution or endoscopy/colonoscopy for further evaluation.

To help optimize your interpretation of FDG PET/CT for the GI tract, evaluate:

1. Is the FDG avidity focal or nonfocal (segmental or involves the entire organ)?

2. Is there a corresponding CT abnormality (wall thickening or mass)?

Then consider the diagrams in Fig. 16.32 for an oversimplification of how to combine FDG PET and CT findings in the GI tract to determine if the finding is normal or abnormal. Of course, each situation will need to be evaluated individually.

SUGGESTED READINGS

Agarwal, et al: FDG PET/CT in the management of colorectal and anal cancers, *AJR Am J Roentgenol* 203:1109–1119, 2014. PMID: 25341152.

Agress, et al: Detection of clinically unexpected malignant and premalignant tumors with whole-body FDG PET: histopathologic comparison, *Radiology* 230:417–422, 2004. PMID: 14699176.

Antoch, et al: Comparison of PET, CT, and dual-modality PET/CT imaging for monitoring of imatinib (STI571) therapy in patients with gastrointestinal stromal tumors, *J Nucl Med* 45:357–365, 2004. PMID: 15001674.

Cronin, et al: Utility of positron emission tomography/CT in the evaluation of small bowel pathology, *Br J Radiol* 85:1211–1221, 2012. PMID: 22919004.

Ferri, et al: Perioperative docetaxel, cisplatin, and 5-fluorouracil (DCF) for locally advanced esophageal and gastric adenocarcinoma: a multicenter phase II trial, *Ann Oncol* 23:1512–1517, 2012. PMID: 22039085.

Fuster, et al: Is there a role for PET/CT with esophagogastric junction adenocarcinoma?, *Clin Nucl Med* 40:e201–e207, 2015. PMID: 25546207.

Ishimori, et al: Detection of unexpected additional primary malignancies with PET/CT, *J Nucl Med* 46:752–757, 2005. PMID: 15872346.

Kei, et al: Incidental finding of focal FDG uptake in the bowel during PET/CT: CT features and correlation with histopathologic results, *AJR Am J Roentgenol* 194:W401–W406, 2010. PMID: 20410385.

Li, et al: Fluorine-18-fluorodeoxyglucose positron emission tomography to evaluate recurrent gastric cancer after surgical resection: a systematic review and meta-analysis, *Ann Nucl Med* 30:179–187, 2016.

Malibari, et al: PET/computed tomography in the diagnosis and staging of gastric cancers, *PET Clin* 10:311–326, 2015.

Moon, et al: Prediction of occult lymph node metastasis by metabolic parameters in patients with clinically N0 esophageal squamous cell carcinoma, *J Nucl Med* 55:743–748, 2014.

Prabhakar, et al: Bowel hot spots at PET-CT, *Radiographics* 27:145–159, 2007. PMID:17235004.

Purandare, et al: Incremental value of 18F-FDG PET/CT in therapeutic decision-making of potentially curable esophageal adenocarcinoma, *Nucl Med Commun* 35:864–869, 2014.

Reavey, et al: Normal patterns of 18F-FDG appendiceal uptake in children, *Petiatr Radiol* 44:398–402, 2014. PMID: 24287869.

Rymer, et al: FDG PET/CT can assess the response of locally advanced rectal cancer to neoadjuvant chemoradiotherapy: evidence from meta-analysis and systematic review, *Clin Nucl Med* 41:371–375, 2016.

Schmidt, et al: Value of functional imaging by PET in esophageal cancer, *J Natl Compr Canc Netw* 13:239–247, 2015. PMID: 25691614.

Treglia, et al: Clinical significance of incidental focal colorectal (18)F-fluorodeoxyglucose uptake: our experience and a review of the literature, *Colorectal Dis* 14:174–180, 2012. PMID: 21689289.

Van den Abbeele: The lessons of GIST–PET and PET/CT: a new paradigm for imaging, *Oncologist* 13(Suppl 2):8–13, 2008.

CHAPTER 17

Peritoneum on FDG PET/CT

The peritoneum is a membranous lining of the abdominal cavity and organs. The parietal peritoneum lines the abdominal cavity, whereas the visceral peritoneum lines the intraperitoneal organs. Between layers of the peritoneum is the peritoneal cavity, a potential space. This potential space is normally not identifiable on imaging studies, unless the space becomes filled with fluids, air, or masses. Masses in the peritoneum include both benign and malignant etiologies. Malignancies involving the peritoneum include metastases, lymphoma, and primary malignancies such as mesothelioma and desmoplastic round cell tumor. Benign peritoneal masses include infections and omental infarcts.

PERITONEAL METASTASES

The most common peritoneal malignancy is metastatic disease. The most common primary malignancies to cause peritoneal metastases are colon, ovary, pancreas, and stomach (the "COPS"), although nearly any primary malignancy may result in peritoneal metastases when advanced. Diffuse peritoneal metastases are often referred to as peritoneal carcinomatosis. When peritoneal carcinomatosis is noted and a primary malignancy has not been identified, check the COPS for masses or wall thickening. On computed tomography (CT), peritoneal metastases may present as nodules or thickening of the peritoneal membranes and mesentery or thickening/implants along the surface of the bowel or abdominal organs and may often be accompanied by peritoneal free fluid. Peritoneal metastases may be 18F-fluorodeoxyglucose (FDG) avid and if avid may identify sites of disease not appreciated on anatomic imaging. Overall, peritoneal metastases may be seen on both FDG positron emission tomography (PET) and CT (Fig. 17.1), FDG PET only (Fig. 17.2), or CT only (Fig. 17.3) and unfortunately may be present even when not identified on either CT or FDG PET. Diffuse peritoneal carcinomatosis may be occult on all known imaging modalities but then identified during surgical exploration.

There are multiple peritoneal reflections which invaginate into the abdominal organs. Examples include the falciform ligament and fissure for the ligamentum venosum along the surface of the liver, as well as the splenic hilum. If possible, differentiate between peritoneal metastases on these peritoneal invaginations from parenchymal organ metastases (Fig. 17.4). Often, parenchymal organ metastases have a different clinical significance from peritoneal metastases. An unusual peritoneal metastasis is the Sister Mary Joseph "node" (Fig. 17.5). This is a peritoneal metastasis that protrudes out of the umbilicus. Sister Mary Joseph was an assistant at St. Mary's Hospital in Rochester, Minnesota, who noticed that patients with abdominal malignancies who developed a nodule at the umbilicus had very poor prognoses. The term was subsequently eponymously named for Sister Mary Joseph.

PRIMARY PERITONEAL MALIGNANCIES

Primary peritoneal malignancies are far less common than peritoneal metastases. These rare malignancies include peritoneal mesothelioma (Fig. 17.6) and desmoplastic round cell tumor (Fig. 17.7). Peritoneal mesothelioma usually is found in older patients, whereas desmoplastic round cell tumor is more common in teenagers and young adults. Both demonstrate multiple peritoneal masses that are typically highly FDG avid. Desmoplastic round cell tumor may demonstrate metastases in nodes and parenchymal liver. Again, it is important to distinguish peritoneal metastases on these peritoneal invaginations from parenchymal organ metastases.

Following treatment of peritoneal malignancy, residual masses may represent viable tumor and/or treated residual scar tissue. It is often difficult to distinguish these two possibilities on anatomic imaging. FDG PET/CT may help to localize areas of residual metabolically active malignancy, aiding in evaluation of residual disease and, if necessary, helping to identify the best location of residual masses to biopsy (Fig. 17.8).

Text continued on p. 176

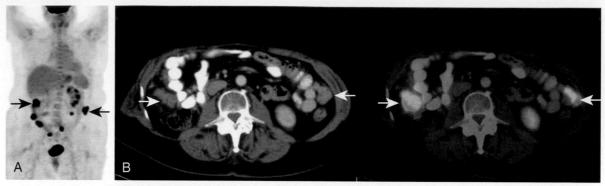

FIG. 17.1 **Peritoneal Metastases Seen on Both FDG PET and CT.** (A) FDG PET maximum intensity projection (MIP) in a patient with endometrial cancer posthysterectomy demonstrates multiple FDG-avid foci overlying the abdomen *(arrows)*. (B) Axial CT and fused FDG PET/CT images through the abdomen demonstrate multiple FDG-avid peritoneal soft tissue masses which represent peritoneal metastases *(arrows)*.

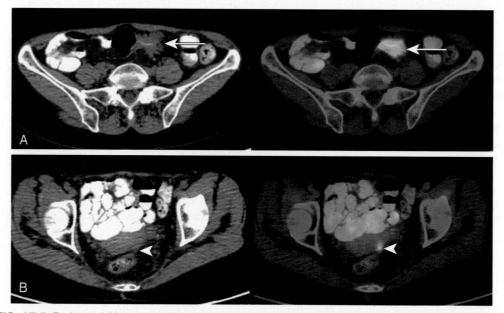

FIG. 17.2 **Peritoneal Metastases More Readily Visualized on FDG PET Than on CT.** (A) Axial CT and fused FDG PET/CT images through the pelvis in a patient with colon cancer demonstrate the FDG-avid transverse colon mass causing luminal narrowing *(arrows)*. (B) Axial CT and fused FDG PET/CT images through the lower pelvis demonstrate an FDG-avid tiny soft tissue mass *(arrowheads)*. At surgery this was one of many peritoneal metastases. The FDG PET draws attention to the peritoneal metastasis on the CT, which would be very easily overlooked on CT alone.

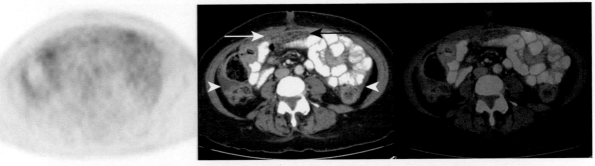

FIG. 17.3 **Peritoneal Metastases More Readily Visualized on CT Than on FDG PET.** Axial PET, CT, and fused FDG PET/CT images through the abdomen in a patient with lobular breast cancer demonstrate soft tissue implants in the peritoneum *(arrows)*. In addition, peritoneal free fluid in seen in the paracolic gutters *(arrowheads)*. These CT findings are consistent with peritoneal metastases, despite no abnormal foci on FDG PET. Fluid sampling confirmed peritoneal malignancy.

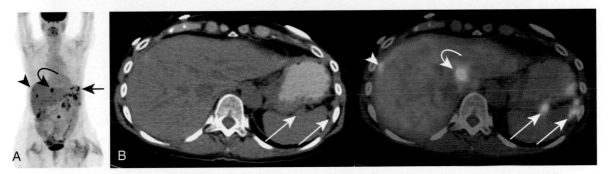

FIG. 17.4 **Peritoneal metastases, Not Parenchymal Liver Metastasis.** (A) FDG PET maximum intensity projection (MIP) in a patient with ovarian cancer posthysterectomy demonstrates multiple FDG-avid foci overlying the abdomen *(arrow, arrowhead,* and *curved arrow)*. (B) Axial CT and fused FDG PET/CT images through the abdomen demonstrate multiple peritoneal metastases adjacent to the spleen which are visible on both CT and FDG PET *(arrows)*, an FDG-avid peritoneal metastasis overlying the liver without CT correlate *(arrowhead)*, and an FDG-avid peritoneal metastasis in the fissure for the ligamentum venosum without CT correlate *(curved arrow)*. The metastasis in the fissure for the ligamentum venosum should be recognized as a peritoneal metastasis along a peritoneal reflection, rather than a parenchymal liver metastasis. Patients with ovarian cancer metastases to the liver parenchyma have a worse prognosis than patients with only peritoneal metastases.

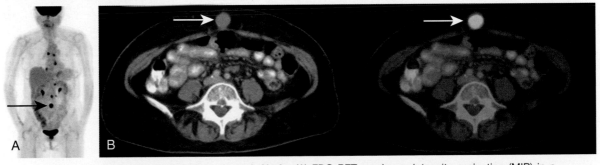

FIG. 17.5 **FDG-avid Sister Mary Joseph Node.** (A) FDG PET maximum intensity projection (MIP) in a patient with ovarian cancer post-hysterectomy demonstrates multiple FDG-avid metastases, including one overlying the mid-abdomen *(arrow)*. (B) Axial CT and fused FDG PET/CT images through the mid-abdomen demonstrate an FDG-avid soft tissue nodule in the umbilicus *(arrows)*, representing a Sister Mary Joseph node, a peritoneal metastasis that protrudes out of the umbilicus.

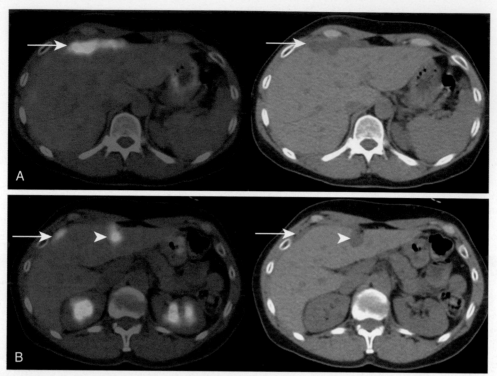

FIG. 17.6 **Primary Peritoneal Mesothelioma.** (A) Axial CT and fused FDG PET/CT images in a patient with primary peritoneal mesothelioma demonstrate FDG-avid peritoneal soft tissue masses on the liver surface *(arrows)*. (B) Axial CT and fused FDG PET/CT images at a lower level demonstrate additional FDG-avid peritoneal soft tissue on the liver surface *(arrows)*, as well as FDG-avid soft tissue along the falciform ligament *(arrowheads)*. The malignancy along the falciform ligament is peritoneal disease, not parenchymal liver disease.

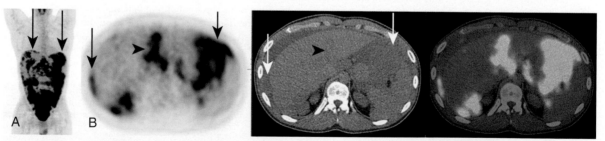

FIG. 17.7 **Peritoneal Desmoplastic Round Cell Tumor.** (A) FDG PET maximum intensity projection (MIP) in a patient with desmoplastic round cell tumor demonstrates widespread abnormal FDG avidity beneath the diaphragm *(arrows)*. (B) Axial CT and fused FDG PET/CT images through the liver demonstrate multiple FDG-avid peritoneal soft tissue masses and peritoneal free fluid *(arrows)* representing peritoneal malignancy. There is also FDG-avid soft tissue insinuating along the fissure for the ligamentum venosum *(arrowheads)*, which represents additional peritoneal malignancy, not parenchymal liver malignancy.

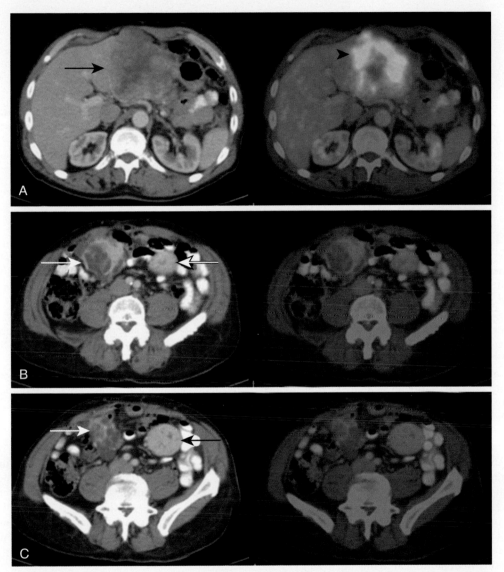

FIG. 17.8 FDG PET Aids in Localizing Metabolically Active Residual Malignancy Following Therapy.
(A–C), Selected axial CT and fused FDG PET/CT images through the abdomen of a patient with malignant fibrous tumor of the peritoneum following chemotherapy. CT images demonstrate multiple residual peritoneal masses *(arrows)* which may represent viable malignancy or postchemotherapy scars. Fused FDG PET/CT images demonstrate that the anterior peritoneal mass at the level of the liver is FDG avid *(arrowhead)* and suspicious for residual active malignancy, whereas other masses demonstrate background FDG avidity, more likely to represent posttherapy scar. FDG PET/CT helped to select the most metabolically active location of tumor for biopsy, which proved residual active malignancy.

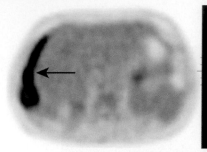
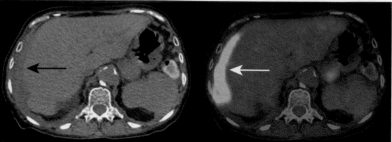

FIG. 17.9 Perihepatic Infections Collection Mimicking Malignancy. Axial PET, CT, and fused FDG PET/CT images through the abdomen of a patient with lung cancer and no known malignancy outside of the chest demonstrate FDG-avid soft tissue overlying the right liver *(arrows)*. Peritoneal metastases should be considered. However, this patient has a known history of recent perforated stercoral ulcer of the right colon, and the localized right peritoneal FDG-avid soft tissue is consistent with this history.

BENIGN PERITONEAL PROCESSES

There are multiple benign processes that can mimic malignancy in the peritoneum on FDG PET/CT. Infections and abscesses in the peritoneum may appear as FDG-avid soft tissue collections (Fig. 17.9). Causes of peritoneal infections/abscesses include bowel perforations from diverticula and appendicitis, as well as pelvic inflammatory disease. Tuberculous peritonitis may have an identical FDG PET/CT appearance to peritoneal carcinomatosis. If large enough, abscesses may only be avid in the periphery, although centrally necrotic tumors may also demonstrate only peripheral FDG avidity. Postsurgical changes can result in FDG-avid peritoneal inflammation which mimics malignancy. For example, surgical manipulation of the peritoneal cavity may result in mesenteric infarcts. The presence of fat on CT may greatly assist in distinguishing benign mesenteric/peritoneal infarcts from malignancy. Mesenteric infarcts often have both fat and soft tissue attention components on CT. Unless the patient has a rare liposarcoma or malignant teratoma, the presence of fat within the lesion strongly favors a benign process such as a mesenteric infarct, rather than peritoneal malignancy (Fig. 17.10). Uncommon benign neoplasms, such as desmoids, may also be identified in the peritoneum.

Physiologic FDG avidity from the bowel and urinary tract may be mistaken for a more ominous finding. Careful correlation with the corresponding CT images will help to minimize overcalling physiologic FDG avidity

as disease; however, even with careful CT correlation, artifacts arising from patient motion, respiration, and movement of internal organs between acquisition of CT and FDG PET images could result in imaging findings that are difficult to appropriately identify.

Here are a few suggestions to help optimize your interpretation of the peritoneum on FDG PET/CT:

1. The differential diagnosis of peritoneal masses/lesions includes both malignant (metastases, lymphoma, primary peritoneal malignancies) and benign (bowel perforations, pelvic inflammatory disease) etiologies.

2. Peritoneal carcinomatosis may be visible on both FDG PET and CT, appreciated on FDG PET only, appreciated on CT only, or be occult on both FDG PET and CT and identified during surgical exploration.

3. Primary malignancies that are only mildly or non–FDG avid may produce peritoneal metastases that need to be recognized on the corresponding CT images.

4. If possible, differentiate between peritoneal malignancy on peritoneal invaginations along intraabdominal organs and intrinsic parenchymal organ metastases. The clinical significance of peritoneal disease and parenchymal organ disease is often different.

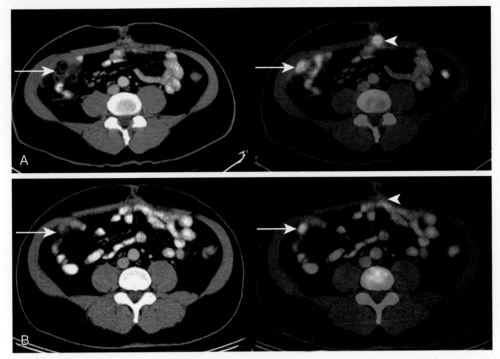

FIG. 17.10 **FDG-avid Mesenteric Infarction.** This patient had a small bowel mass which was resected and pathology demonstrated lymphoma. An FDG PET/CT was then ordered for systemic staging. (A) Axial CT and fused FDG PET/CT images through the abdomen demonstrate an FDG-avid mixed soft tissue and fat attenuation lesion in the right abdominal cavity *(arrows)*. Although the FDG avidity raises the possibility of additional lymphoma, the presence of fat within the lesion strongly favors a benign process such as a mesenteric infarct, which could have been caused during surgery. FDG avidity at the site of the midline abdominal incision, without a corresponding CT mass, is also inflammatory *(arrowhead)*. (B) Axial CT and fused FDG PET/CT images at the same level on a follow-up PET/CT demonstrate decreasing FDG avidity and mixed soft tissue/fat mass *(arrows)*. Given no interval therapy, this represents a resolving benign mesenteric infarct. The inflammatory avidity at the abdominal incision has resolved *(arrowhead)*.

SUGGESTED READINGS

Anthony, et al: Spectrum of (18)F-FDG PET/CT appearances in peritoneal disease, *AJR Am J Roentgenol* 193:W523–W529, 2009. PMID: 19933627.

De Gaetano, et al: Imaging of peritoneal carcinomatosis with FDG PET-CT: diagnostic patterns, case examples and pitfalls, *Abdom Imaging* 34:391–402, 2009. PMID: 18446399.

DeMeo, et al: Anatomic CT demonstration of the peritoneal spaces, ligaments, and mesenteries: normal and pathologic processes, *Radiographics* 15:755–770, 1995. PMID: 7569127.

Dromain, et al: Staging of peritoneal carcinomatosis: enhanced CT vs. PET/CT, *Abdom Imaging* 33:87–93, 2008. PMID: 17632751.

Dubreuil, et al: 18F-FDG-PET/CT of peritoneal tumors: a pictorial essay, *Nucl Med Commun* 38:1–9, 2017. PMID: 27820721.

Meyers, et al: The peritoneal ligaments and mesenteries: pathways of intraabdominal spread of disease, *Radiology* 163:593–604, 1987.

Schmidt, et al: Peritoneal carcinomatosis in primary ovarian cancer staging: comparison between MDCT, MRI, and 18F-FDG PET/CT, *Clin Nucl Med* 40:371–377, 2015. PMID: 25783507.

Wahl: Why nearly all PET of abdominal and pelvic cancers will be performed as PET/CT, *J Nucl Med* 45(Suppl 1):82S–95S, 2004.

CHAPTER 18

Urinary Tract on FDG PET/CT (Kidneys, Ureters, Bladder)

The urinary tract is one the most difficult organ systems of the body to evaluate on F18-fluorodeoxyglucose positron emission tomography/computed tomography (FDG PET/CT). This is because of physiologic excretion of FDG through the kidneys, ureters, and bladder. FDG in urine may hide FDG-avid malignancy or be mistaken for FDG-avid malignancy. Combine this with the fact that neoplasms of the urinary tract are often only mildly FDG avid, and you can see why careful attention must be paid to both the FDG PET and CT components of an FDG PET/CT to prevent mistakes.

KIDNEY

There are two paired kidneys in the retroperitoneum of the abdomen. However, there are multiple congenital anomalies which result in an unexpected location or absence of a kidney. These congenital anomalies should be recognized on FDG PET/CT images to prevent misinterpretation. In a case of renal agenesis, only one kidney will be visualized on the FDG maximum intensity projection (MIP) and cross-sectional images. With a horseshoe kidney, the kidneys will be fused in the midline. As opposed to normal separate kidneys which normally lie superomedial to inferolateral, the inferior poles with a horseshoe kidney will be directed medially (Fig. 18.1). Crossed fused renal ectopia is a less common congenital anomaly where the kidneys are fused and lie on one side of the spine (Fig. 18.2). With crossed fused renal ectopia there will be two collecting systems and two ureters arising from the fused kidney.

Renal masses have a different differential diagnosis depending on whether they are solid or cystic. The differential diagnosis for solid renal masses includes primary renal neoplasms (renal cell carcinoma [RCC], oncocytoma, transitional cell carcinoma [TCC], angiomyolipoma [AML]), as well as renal lymphoma and renal metastases. In children, solid renal masses are uncommon, but when they occur they are most often Wilms tumors. Cystic renal masses include simple cysts, complicated cyst, multilocular cystic nephroma, cystic RCC, and renal abscesses/infections.

Renal Cell Carcinoma

The majority of solid renal masses in adults are RCC. There are multiple histologic subtypes of RCC, the most common being clear cell carcinoma, with the majority of the remainder being papillary or chromophobe RCC. On CT, RCC may be hypointense, isointense, or hyperintense to normal renal parenchyma. Following intravenous contrast administration, RCC demonstrates variable intensities of enhancement, with clear cell subtypes usually enhancing more avidly. Hemorrhage, necrosis, and/or calcifications are common. On FDG PET, RCC ranges from markedly FDG avid to FDG avidity equal to background renal parenchyma. Even when an RCC is FDG avid, urine within the collecting system of the kidney may obscure the RCC. The RCC may be more apparent on CT images than on FDG PET, particularly if intravenous contrast has been administered. Sometimes, it is only an abnormality in renal contour or change in size of a renal mass which allows detection of RCC on FDG PET/CT (Fig. 18.3). Because RCCs are increasingly being detected incidentally on imaging examinations, it is important to combined findings from the kidneys on both FDG PET and CT to prevent missing lesions. Metastases from RCC may be more FDG avid than the primary malignancy (Fig. 18.4). RCC metastases are most commonly pulmonary and osseous, although any organ may be involved. Local nodal metastases in the retroperitoneum are also common. RCC may grow directly into the renal vein and then into more central veins. Expansion, enhancement, or FDG avidity in the local veins is suspicious for direct venous extension.

Oncocytoma

Oncocytoma is a benign solid renal tumor. Unfortunately, it is usually difficult to distinguish an oncocytoma from

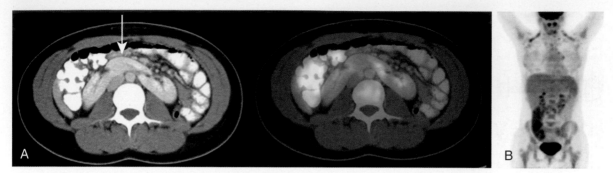

FIG. 18.1 **Horseshoe Kidney.** (A) Axial CT with intravenous contrast and fused PET/CT images through the level of the kidneys demonstrate fusion of the kidneys in the midline *(arrow)*, representing a horseshoe kidney. (B) FDG maximum intensity projection (MIP) demonstrates inferior poles of the kidneys are directed medially.

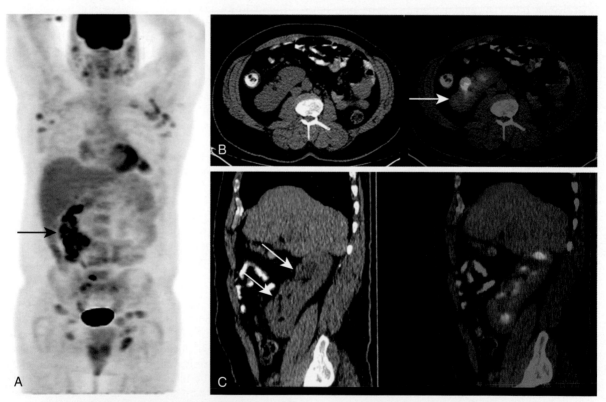

FIG. 18.2 **Crossed Fused Renal Ectopia.** (A) FDG maximum intensity projection (MIP) in a patient with low-grade lymphoma demonstrates a single enlarged kidney to the right spine *(arrow)*. (B) Axial CT and fused PET/CT images demonstrate single renal unit *(arrow)*. (C) Sagittal CT and fused PET/CT images through the crossed fused renal ectopia demonstrate two renal hila for two collecting systems *(arrows)*.

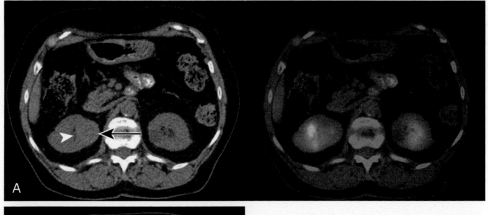

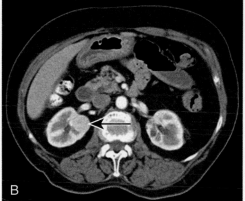

FIG. 18.3 **Minimally FDG-avid Renal cell Carcinoma (RCC) Visualized by Abnormal Renal Contour on CT.** (A) Axial CT and fused FDG PET/CT images through the kidneys. The right kidney demonstrates an abnormal contour with a subtle abnormal curvature at the kidney surface *(arrow)* and convex border in the renal hilum *(arrowhead)*. (B) Comparison with a contrast-enhanced scan from 3 years prior demonstrates interval growth of a solid renal mass *(arrow)* which was pathologically proven to be RCC.

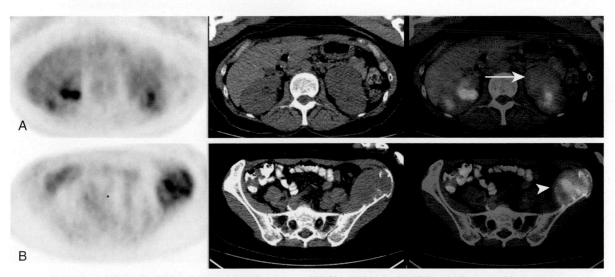

FIG. 18.4 **Minimally FDG-avid Renal Cell Carcinoma (RCC) with Markedly FDG-avid Osseous Metastases.** (A) Axial PET, CT, and fused FDG PET/CT images through the kidneys demonstrates an exophytic renal mass with only minimal FDG avidity, best visualized due to the abnormal renal contour *(arrow)*. (B) Axial PET, CT, and fused FDG PET/CT images through the pelvis demonstrate a markedly FDG-avid left iliac wing osseous metastasis with soft tissue component *(arrowhead)*. It is not uncommon for metastases from RCC to be more FDG avid than the primary malignancy.

an RCC on imaging, thus tissue sampling is usually required to make the diagnosis. On CT, oncocytomas are usually isointense or hyperintense to normal renal parenchyma. Enhancement is common. The presence of a central stellate scar may suggest an oncocytoma, but this is not sufficiently accurate to rely upon. On FDG PET, oncocytomas demonstrate FDG avidity that varies from background renal parenchyma to markedly FDG avid, similar to RCC, and thus FDG PET cannot distinguish an oncocytoma from an RCC.

Transitional Cell Carcinoma

TCCs are malignant tumors of the renal collecting system epithelium. TCCs may be found in the kidneys, ureters, or bladder, with the bladder being the most common site. On CT, TCCs may be visualized as soft tissue masses causing a filling defect or distortion within the collecting system or the lumen of the ureter or bladder. Enhancement is usually mild. Calcifications are uncommon. On FDG PET, TCCs demonstrate FDG avidity that varies from background to marked FDG avidity. As TCCs occur in the lining of the collecting system, obscuration by FDG in urine is common, and thus comparison with the findings is essential for localizing these tumors. When the TCC is less FDG avid than FDG in the urine, CT findings may be the only evidence of the lesion (Fig. 18.5). TCCs are known for drop metastases, with primary malignancies in the kidney collecting system resulting in drop metastases in the ipsilateral ureter or the bladder (Fig. 18.6).

Angiomyolipoma

AMLs are benign tumors composed of blood vessels ("angio"), smooth muscle ("myo"), and fat ("lipoma"). Renal AMLs are associated with tuberous sclerosis and lymphangioleiomyomatosis. When macroscopic fat is visible in a renal lesion on CT, then the diagnosis is almost always AML (Fig. 18.7). However, some AMLs do not contain enough macroscopic fat to be apparent on CT, and thus they can be confused with other solid renal neoplasms. In addition, rarely RCCs may engulf renal hilar fat, which may be confused with an AML. Large AMLs may be accompanied by feeding blood vessels. On FDG PET, FDG uptake is usually low.

Wilms Tumor

Wilms tumor, or nephroblastoma, is a rare renal malignancy that typically occurs in young children. A solid renal mass in a young child is suspicious for a Wilms tumor. On ultrasound or CT, Wilms tumors are often heterogeneous masses, with hemorrhage, necrosis, and calcifications being common. On FDG PET, Wilms tumors usually demonstrate FDG avidity.

Renal Lymphoma

Renal involvement with lymphoma is common and, like other renal masses, may be overlooked on FDG PET due to obscuration by FDG in the urine (Fig. 18.8). As in other organ systems, low-grade lymphoma may be minimally if at all FDG avid, whereas high-grade lymphoma is usually markedly FDG avid. On CT, renal lymphoma may present as solitary renal masses, multiple renal masses, or diffuse infiltration of the kidneys which may cause renal enlargement. Renal lymphoma is usually hypoattenuating compared with normal renal parenchyma, particularly following contrast administration. FDG PET/CT provides valuable information about the response of lymphoma to therapy, similar to other sites of lymphomatous involvement. Following Lugano Criteria, reduction of FDG avidity to less than liver background

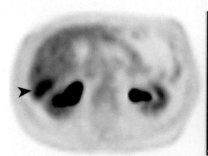 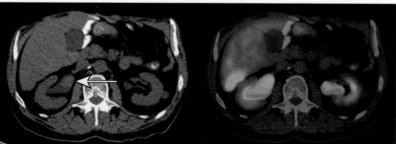

FIG. 18.5 Renal Collecting System Transitional Cell Carcinoma (TCC) is Best Visualized on the CT Component of FDG PET/CT. Axial PET, CT, and fused FDG PET/CT images through the kidneys demonstrate a high attenuation mass in the right renal collecting system *(arrow)* which represents the primary TCC. The TCC is difficult to appreciate on any window setting of the FDG PET. An FDG-avid hepatic metastasis *(arrowhead)* is also identified.

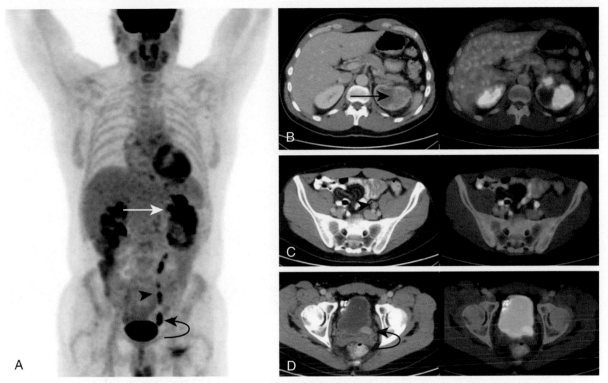

FIG. 18.6 **Renal Transitional Cell Carcinoma (TCC) with Drop Metastases Visualized on the CT Component of an FDG PET/CT.** (A) FDG maximum intensity projection (MIP) demonstrates FDG avidity along the course of the left kidney and ureter (*arrow, arrowhead,* and *curved arrow*). These foci could easily be mistaken for FDG in the urine of the collecting system. Axial CT and fused FDG PET/CT images through the (B) left kidney, (C) left ureter, and (D) left ureterovesicular junction demonstrate that the FDG-avid foci correspond with enhancing soft tissue masses, rather than urine within the collecting system. In (B) FDG avidity corresponds with the primary TCC, visible as a soft tissue mass *(arrow)*. In (C) FDG avidity corresponds with enhancing soft tissue thickening of the ureter *(arrowhead)*, representing a drop metastasis. In (D) FDG avidity corresponds with enhancing soft tissue at the ureterovesicular junction *(curved arrow)*, representing another drop metastasis. This demonstrates that FDG-avid malignancy involving the urinary tract can easily be misinterpreted as physiologic FDG in urine.

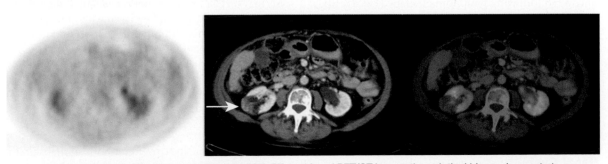

FIG. 18.7 **Angiomyolipoma (AML).** Axial PET, CT, and fused PET/CT images through the kidneys demonstrate a mixed fat and soft tissue attenuation mass in the right kidney, diagnostic of an AML *(arrow)*. Like most AMLs, this one demonstrates minimal to any FDG avidity.

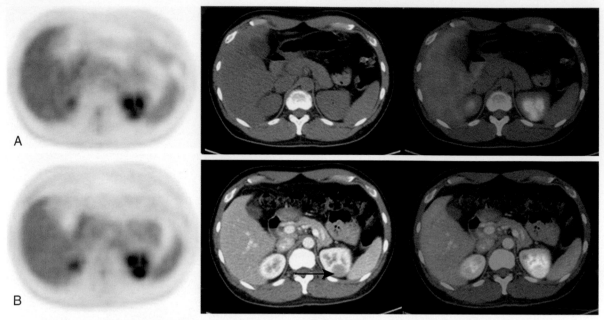

FIG. 18.8 Renal Lymphoma Obscured by Urine on FDG PET. (A) Axial PET, CT, and fused PET/CT images through the kidneys appear to demonstrate normal FDG within the urine of the kidney collecting systems. (B) Axial PET, CT, and fused PET/CT images, obtained with intravenous contrast within 1 month of the first PET/CT, demonstrate a low-attenuation mass in the left kidney *(arrow)*. The FDG avidity associated with this mass is now appreciated to be due to renal lymphoma, rather than FDG in urine. These two FDG PET/CT examinations performed before initiation of lymphoma therapy demonstrate the potential to overlook an FDG-avid renal mass as physiologic FDG in the urine.

represents treated malignancy (Fig. 18.9), whereas residual FDG avidity greater than liver background is suspicious for residual active lymphoma. An FDG-avid renal mass in a patient with lymphoma is most likely to be renal lymphoma; however, other renal neoplasms are not excluded. For instance, if most FDG-avid lesions resolve following treatment of lymphoma, yet a renal lesion persists, this may be a second unrelated neoplasm uncovered following lymphoma therapy (Fig. 18.10).

Renal Metastases

Renal metastases usually, but not always, occur in the setting of diffuse metastatic disease. The most common primary malignancies which metastasize to the kidneys are lung, breast, melanoma, and colorectal in origin. On CT, renal metastases are often multiple in bilateral. On FDG PET, renal metastases are often FDG avid (Fig. 18.11).

Renal Cysts

Renal cysts are common benign findings on imaging studies. If the cyst demonstrates near-water attenuation

(0 ± 15 Hounsfield units) with an imperceptible wall, this is probably a simple cyst. Simple cysts are photopenic on FDG PET. If the cyst demonstrates internal septations, calcifications, or greater than water attenuation, then it is more likely a complicated cyst. Complicated cyst may be involved with hemorrhage or infection. Bosniak criteria may be used to help classify cysts with septations, solid components, or enhancement on CT. Complicated cysts may be FDG avid, but not malignant. If the kidneys are bilaterally enlarged and replaced with multiple cysts, the patient may have an inherited condition known as autosomal dominant polycystic disease (ADPD). ADPD causes multiple parenchymal cysts, most commonly involving the kidneys, liver, and pancreas (Fig. 18.12). Patients usually present in adulthood with hypertension and/or renal failure.

Renal Infections

Renal infections include pyelonephritis and abscesses. On CT, inflammation associated with renal infections may cause renal enlargement and/or perinephric soft tissue stranding. Following intravenous contrast, focal

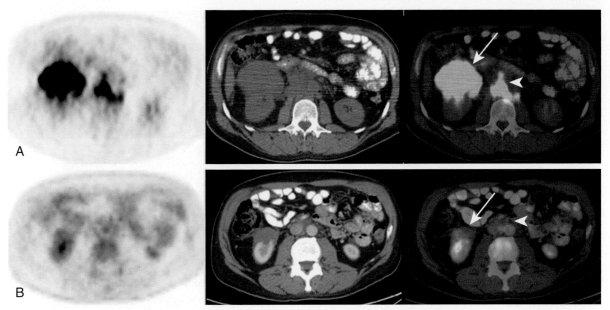

FIG. 18.9 **Renal Lymphoma Before and After Chemotherapy.** (A) Axial PET, CT, and fused PET/CT images through the kidneys demonstrate an FDG-avid right kidney mass *(arrow)* and FDG-avid retroperitoneal lymph nodes *(arrowhead)* in a patient with lymphoma. (B) Axial PET, CT, and fused PET/CT images following chemotherapy demonstrate decreased size and FDG avidity of the renal mass *(arrow)* and retroperitoneal lymph nodes *(arrowhead)*. Residual FDG avidity of the renal mass and lymph nodes is less than liver background (not shown), representing treated disease.

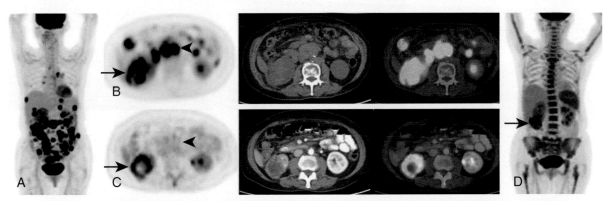

FIG. 18.10 **FDG-avid Renal Cell Carcinoma Revealed Following Treatment of Lymphoma.** (A) FDG maximum intensity projection (MIP) of a patient with biopsy-proven lymphoma demonstrates multiorgan system lymphoma involvement. (B) Axial PET, CT, and fused PET/CT images through the kidneys of this patient demonstrate an FDG-avid right kidney mass *(arrow),* as well as FDG-avid retroperitoneal lymph nodes *(arrowhead)*. (C) Axial PET, CT, and fused PET/CT images following chemotherapy demonstrate resolution of nodal lymphoma *(arrowhead)* but persistence of the FDG-avid right renal mass *(arrow)*. (D) FDG MIP of the patient following chemotherapy demonstrates resolution of almost all FDG-avid masses, except the FDG-avid right renal mass *(arrow)*. Bone marrow and splenic repopulation are also visualized following chemotherapy. The right renal mass was subsequently biopsied and proven to be a renal cell carcinoma. This case demonstrates how persistence of a lesion following therapy, when all other lesions resolve, may be due to an unrelated secondary malignancy.

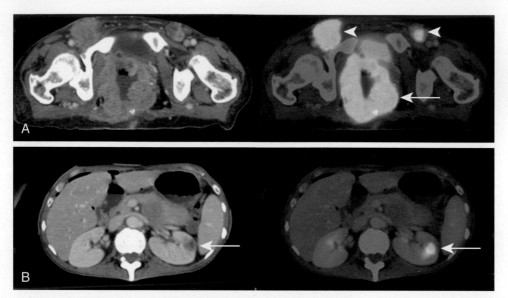

FIG. 18.11 **Renal Metastasis.** (A) Axial CT and fused PET/CT images through the kidneys of a patient with primary anal cancer *(arrow)* and bilateral inguinal nodal metastases *(arrowheads)*. (B) Axial CT and fused PET/CT images through the kidneys demonstrate an FDG-avid renal mass *(arrows)* which was biopsy-proven to be a renal metastasis.

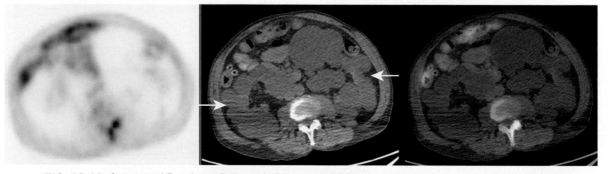

FIG. 18.12 **Autosomal Dominant Polycystic Disease (ADPD).** Axial PET, CT, and fused PET/CT images through the kidneys of a patient with ADPD. Note the bilateral renal enlargement and replacement with multiple cysts *(arrows)*. No FDG is seen in the renal collecting systems because renal failure has prevented formation of urine.

areas of decreased parenchymal enhancement may be evident. Few data are available on FDG avidity of renal infections; however, active infection may be FDG avid and need to be distinguished from malignancy.

BLADDER
Bladder Cancer
Bladder cancer is the most common malignancy of the urinary tract. Most bladder cancers are TCCs, with a

minority representing squamous cell and adenocarcinomas. As with renal and ureter lesions, masses and the bladder may be difficult to appreciate on FDG PET due to obscuration by FDG in the urine. The CT component of the FDG PET/CT should be scrutinized for bladder wall thickening and masses which may only be apparent on CT (Fig. 18.13). The FDG component of the FDG PET/CT is usually far more valuable in the detection of nodal and distant metastases than for the primary bladder malignancy (Fig. 18.14). In patients with

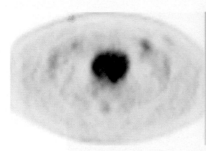
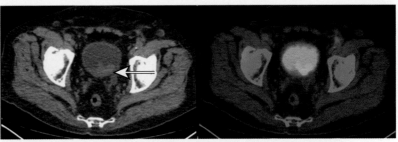

FIG. 18.13 **Bladder Cancer Apparent as a Mass on the CT Component of FDG PET/CT.** Axial PET, CT, and fused PET/CT images through the bladder demonstrate a posterior bladder wall irregular mass *(arrow)* representing a primary bladder malignancy. The bladder mass demonstrates FDG avidity lower than the adjacent urine, making the lesion more apparent on the CT component of the FDG PET/CT.

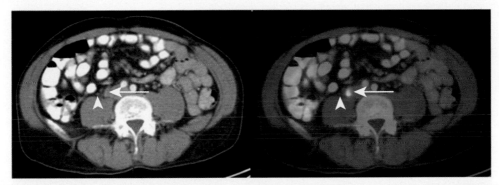

FIG. 18.14 **Subcentimeter Nodal Metastasis in a Patient with Bladder Cancer Detected on the FDG PET Component of FDG PET/CT.** Axial CT and fused PET/CT images through the lower abdomen demonstrate a subcentimeter short axis right common iliac node which is FDG avid *(arrows)*, suspicious for nodal metastasis. Note this FDG focus is not coming from the right ureter, which is located more lateral to the lymph node *(arrowheads)*. This case demonstrates how lesion localization with CT can help to distinguish malignant FDG-avid lesions from benign FDG in the ureter.

advanced local bladder malignancy under consideration for radical surgical resection, FDG PET/CT may demonstrate unsuspected distant metastatic disease, which alters patient management. The most common sites of metastases from bladder carcinoma are nodal metastases and distant osseous and pulmonary metastases.

Bladder Diverticula Versus Pericystic Nodes/Masses

Bladder malignancies often directly spread to the perivesicular fat and metastasize to local pelvic lymph nodes. Perivesicular nodes are not uncommon. The perivesicular region is also commonly involved with bladder diverticula. Due to FDG in the urine, bladder diverticula could be mistaken for perivesicular nodes, and vice versa. Often, correlation with the CT component of FDG PET/CT helps to distinguish FDG-avid perivesicular nodes from urinary FDG in bladder diverticula. If the CT

demonstrates that the perivesicular lesion is near-water attenuation or has a luminal connection to the bladder, the FDG-avid finding is probably bladder diverticula (Fig. 18.15). Conversely, if the perivesicular lesion is soft tissue attenuation, the FDG-avid finding is probably a pericystic node/mass (Fig. 18.16). Evaluation of the CT component of FDG PET/CT can also help to distinguish bladder diverticula from more ominous masses in the scenario of bladder hernias (Fig. 18.17).

Urachal Lesions

The urachus is an embryonic remnant of the allantois, a connection between the fetal urinary bladder and the umbilical cord. Failure of the urachus to close may result in urachal remnant. The remnant may be located anywhere from the umbilicus to the anterior bladder in the midline. A potentially confusing finding on FDG PET/CT is an FDG-avid focal or linear lesion anterior to

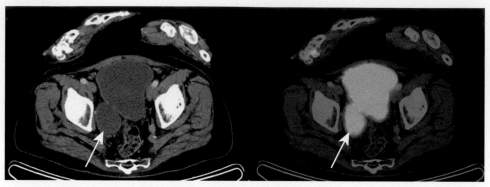

FIG. 18.15 **Bladder Diverticula.** Axial CT and fused PET/CT images through the bladder demonstrate an FDG-avid perivesicular lesion *(arrows)*. This CT component demonstrates the lesion has near-water attenuation, similar to bladder contents, and represents bladder diverticula.

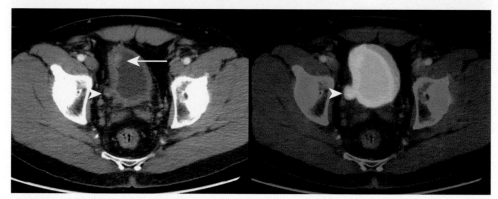

FIG. 18.16 **Perivesicular Nodal Metastasis.** Axial CT and fused PET/CT images through the bladder demonstrate right bladder wall thickening *(arrow)* on CT, which is obscured on FDG PET due to FDG in urine. There is also a right perivesicular lesion which is FDG avid *(arrowheads)*. This CT component demonstrates the perivesicular lesion has soft tissue attenuation and represents a perivesicular nodal metastasis.

the bladder, which represents an inflamed or malignant urachal remnant (Fig. 18.18). It may not be possible to distinguish urachal inflammation from malignancy on imaging.

A final comment about the urinary tract: Account for the kidneys and bladder on the FDG maximum intensity projection (MIP) images of all FDG PET/CT scans. Unusual locations or fusions of the kidneys, as described at the beginning of this chapter, will be evident on the FDG MIP images and should be reported. If the kidneys or bladder cannot be visualized, there may have been a surgical removal or the patient may suffer from renal failure (Fig. 18.19).

Here are a few suggestions to help optimize your interpretation of FDG PET/CT of the urinary tract:

1. FDG in urine may hide FDG-avid malignancy or be mistaken for FDG-avid malignancy. It is necessary to correlate FDG findings with the corresponding CT to help determine if FDG corresponds to urine of a soft tissue lesion.

2. The differential diagnosis for solid renal masses includes RCC, oncocytoma, TCC, AML, lymphoma, and metastases. The presence of macroscopic fat on CT is usually diagnostic of AML. TCCs arise from the collecting system epithelium and are usually centered along this epithelium. It is usually not possible to distinguish RCC and oncocytoma on imaging, and thus pathology is usually necessary. All of these lesions have variable FDG avidity which may be obscured by FDG in adjacent urine.

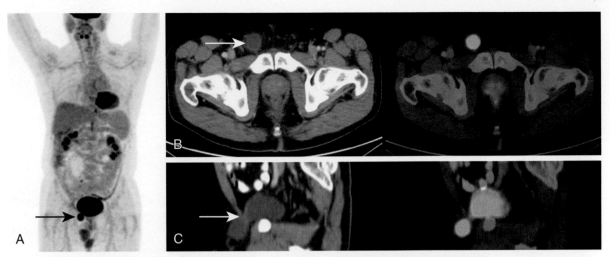

FIG. 18.17 **Bladder Hernia.** (A) FDG maximum intensity projection (MIP) in a patient with lymphoma demonstrates an FDG-avid focus in the right inguinal region *(arrow)*. (B) Axial CT and fused PET/CT images through the pelvis demonstrate an FDG-avid lesion in the right inguinal region *(arrow)*, which could easily be mistaken for an FDG-avid lymph node. The CT component demonstrates that the lesion is near-water attenuation. Lymph nodes are normally soft tissue attenuation. (C) Coronal CT infused PET/CT images demonstrate the lesion connects with the bladder through an inguinal hernia *(arrow)*. This case demonstrates how corresponding CT images can help to distinguish FDG in urine from more ominous lesions.

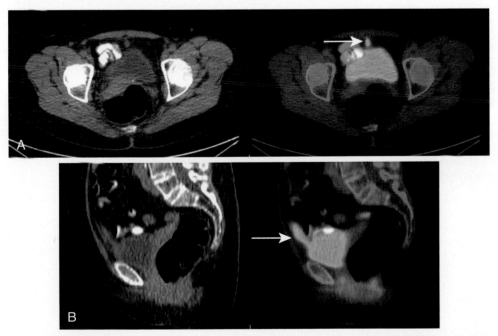

FIG. 18.18 **Urachal Lesion.** (A) Axial CT and fused PET/CT images through the bladder demonstrate an FDG-avid lesion anterior to the bladder in the midline *(arrow)*. (B) Sagittal CT and fused PET/CT images demonstrate a linear FDG-avid lesion arising from the anterior bladder and extending superiorly *(arrow)*. This is in the expected location of a urachal remnant. FDG avidity in a urachal remnant could represent FDG in urine, inflammation, or malignancy. The CT component demonstrates that the lesion is soft tissue in attenuation, thus excluding FDG in urine from the differential diagnosis. On pathology this was an inflamed urachal remnant.

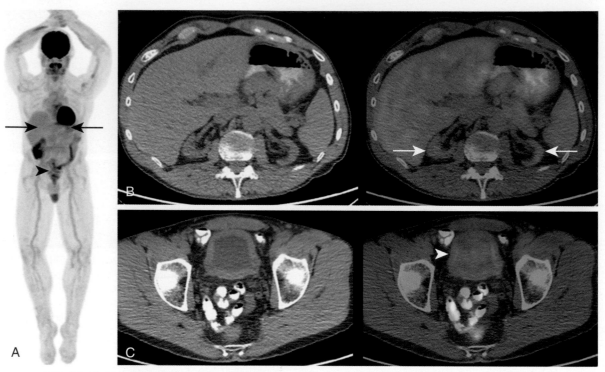

FIG. 18.19 **Renal Failure.** (A) FDG maximum intensity projection (MIP) in a patient with myeloma demonstrates absence of suspected FDG kidneys in the urinary tract, including the kidneys *(arrows)* and bladder *(arrowhead)*. (B) Axial CT and fused PET/CT images through the kidneys demonstrate small kidneys without FDG in the collecting systems *(arrows)*. (C) Axial CT and fused PET/CT images through the bladder demonstrate absence of FDG in the urine *(arrowhead)*. This patient has renal failure and does not produce urine.

SUGGESTED READINGS

Ferda, et al: 18F-FDG-PET/CT in potentially advanced renal cell carcinoma: a role in treatment decisions and prognosis estimation, *Anticancer Res* 33:2665–2672, 2013.

Goodfellow, et al: Role of fluorodeoxyglucose positron emission tomography (FDG PET)-computed tomography (CT) in the staging of bladder cancer, *BJU Int* 114:389–395, 2014.

Høilund-Carlsen PF, et al: FDG in urologic malignancies, *PET Clin* 9:457–468, 2014.

Kibel, et al: Prospective study of [18F]fluorodeoxyglucose positron emission tomography/computed tomography for staging of muscle-invasive bladder carcinoma, *J Clin Oncol* 27:4314–4320, 2009.

Lawrentschuk, et al: Functional imaging of renal cell carcinoma, *Nat Rev Urol* 7:258–266, 2010.

Rioja, et al: Role of positron emission tomography in urological oncology, *BJU Int* 106:1578–1593, 2010.

Uslu, et al: Value of 18F-FDG PET and PET/CT for evaluation of pediatric malignancies, *J Nucl Med* 56:274–286, 2015.

Zukotynski, et al: PET/CT and renal pathology: a blind spot for radiologists? Part 1, primary pathology, *AJR Am J Roentgenol* 199:W163–W167, 2012.

Zukotynski, et al: PET/CT and renal pathology: a blind spot for radiologists? Part 2–lymphoma, leukemia, and metastatic disease, *AJR Am J Roentgenol* 199:W168–W174, 2012.

CHAPTER 19

Female Pelvis on FDG PET/CT

The female pelvis can be difficult to evaluate on 18F-fluorodeoxyglucose positron emission tomography/computed tomography (FDG PET/CT). The endometrium and ovaries may demonstrate physiologic FDG avidity. Benign leiomyomata of the myometrium may be FDG avid. In addition, physiologic FDG avidity in the adjacent bowel and urinary tract may obscure FDG-avid ovarian or uterine lesions. Nevertheless, FDG PET/CT has demonstrated value for detecting unsuspected nodal and distant metastases in ovarian and uterine malignancies, as well as for evaluation of treatment response and detection of recurrent malignancy.

PHYSIOLOGIC FDG AVIDITY IN THE FEMALE REPRODUCTIVE TRACT

Physiologic FDG avidity has been observed in the endometrium, fallopian tubes, and ovaries. In premenopausal women, FDG avidity in the endometrium is most likely physiologic (Fig. 19.1). Likewise, in premenopausal women, FDG avidity in the ovary/adnexa is likely physiologic (Fig. 19.2). Physiologic FDG avidity in the adnexa may be unilateral or bilateral. In studies with intravenous contrast, a corresponding ring of enhancement may be seen in the adnexa, representing a corpus luteum cyst (Fig. 19.3). Corpus luteum cysts often demonstrate physiologic FDG avidity. Physiologic FDG avidity is also expected in the adnexa of patients who have undergone ovarian hyperstimulation for oocyte retrieval (Fig. 19.4). Hyperstimulated ovaries may be seen on CT as enlarged adnexa with multiple low-attenuation cystic lesions separated by soft tissue septae. In young women with pelvic malignancy, beware of surgically transposed ovaries with physiologic FDG avidity in unexpected locations. If radiation is planned for the pelvis, the ovaries may be surgically transposed to remove them from the radiation port, to preserve their function and fertility (Fig. 19.5). Transposed ovaries may be unilateral or bilateral. In some cases, adjacent surgical clips will provide evidence of transposed ovaries.

OVARY

Ovarian Cancer

Ovarian cancer is one of the most common gynecologic malignancies. The primary malignancy in the adnexa has direct communication with the peritoneum and direct spread with peritoneal disease is common. Ovarian cancer may also demonstrate lymphatic spread to lymph nodes and hematogenous spread to multiple organ systems. Most patients are usually diagnosed with advanced disease. Disease burden in ovarian cancer may be followed by tumor markers in the serum, as well as by imaging.

The imaging techniques of choice for visualizing and local staging of a primary ovarian malignancy are ultrasound and magnetic resonance (MR). FDG PET/CT may complement these imaging modalities through the detection of FDG avidity in the adnexa. Although FDG avidity in the adnexa of premenopausal patients is often physiologic, FDG avidity in the adnexa or postmenopausal patients is abnormal and may prompt further workup (Fig. 19.6). There is no standardized uptake value (SUV) threshold to distinguish malignant from benign adnexal lesions; however, in general, malignant adnexal lesions demonstrate greater FDG avidity.

The imaging technique of choice for visualization and staging of nodal and distant metastases from ovarian malignancy is contrast-enhanced CT. Peritoneal carcinomatosis may be visualized as increased peritoneal opacities on CT. Lymphatic spread of ovarian cancer is most common to the pelvic and retroperitoneal nodes; however, extension to the inguinal and thoracic nodes also occurs, and enlarged nodes in any of these nodal basins may be suspicious for nodal metastases. Distant metastases involve multiple organ systems, most commonly lung, bone, and liver. FDG PET/CT may complement contrast-enhanced CT by detection of unsuspected FDG-avid metastases, such as nodal metastases or implants which are subcentimeter in size and thus overlooked on anatomic imaging (Fig. 19.7). The vaginal cuff is a common site of malignancy recurrence following hysterectomy. Postsurgical changes at the vaginal cuff

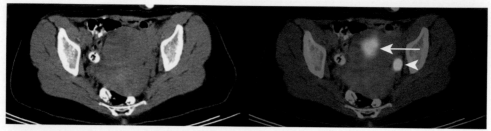

FIG. 19.1 **Physiologic FDG Avidity in the Endometrium and Ovary.** Axial CT and fused FDG PET/CT images in a 39-year-old woman demonstrate FDG avidity in the central uterus *(arrow)*, representing physiologic endometrial avidity. There is also an FDG-avid focus in the left adnexa *(arrowhead)*, representing physiologic ovarian avidity. These foci should not be confused with FDG-avid malignancy.

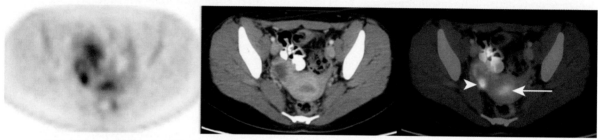

FIG. 19.2 **Physiologic FDG Avidity in the Endometrium and Ovary.** Axial CT and fused FDG PET/CT images in a 15-year-old woman with Hodgkin lymphoma of the mediastinum demonstrate FDG avidity in the central uterus *(arrow)*, corresponding with low-attenuation endometrium on CT, representing physiologic endometrial avidity. There is also an FDG-avid focus in the right adnexa *(arrowhead)*, corresponding with a low-attenuation right adnexal cyst on CT, representing physiologic ovarian avidity. These foci should not be confused with FDG-avid malignancy.

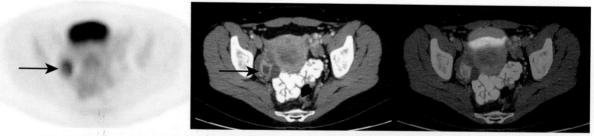

FIG. 19.3 **Physiologic FDG Avidity in an Ovarian Corpus Luteum Cyst.** Axial PET, CT, and fused FDG PET/CT images in a 36-year-old woman demonstrate FDG avidity in the right adnexa *(arrows)*, corresponding with a low-attenuation right adnexal cyst with a ring-enhancing corpus luteum cyst on CT.

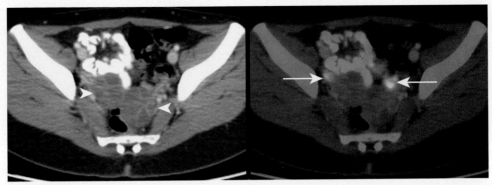

FIG. 19.4 Physiologic FDG avidity in bilateral hyperstimulated ovaries in preparation for oocyte retrieval in a 21-year-old woman with lymphoma above the diaphragm. Axial contrast-enhanced CT and fused FDG PET/CT demonstrate FDG avidity in the bilateral adnexa *(arrows)*. Corresponding CT images demonstrate the typical appearance of hyperstimulated ovaries with ovarian enlargement and multiple cysts *(arrowheads)*. This patient is not undergoing ovarian hyperstimulation in preparation for oocyte retrieval and storage prior to chemotherapy. These foci should not be confused with FDG-avid lymphoma, which would increase the patient's lymphoma stage.

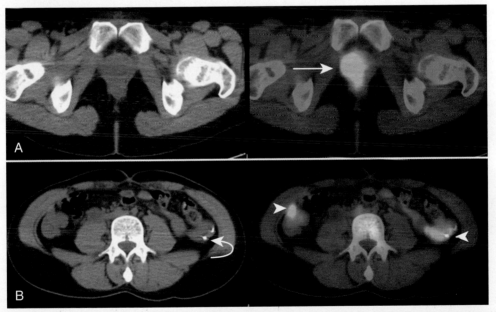

FIG. 19.5 **Physiologic FDG Avidity in Transposed Ovaries in a 33-Year-Old Woman with Vaginal Carcinoma.** (A) Axial CT and fused FDG PET/CT demonstrate the FDG-avid primary vaginal malignancy *(arrow)*. (B) Axial CT and fused PET/CT images demonstrate bilateral lower abdominal FDG-avid foci *(arrowheads)*. These represent ovaries that have been transposed from the pelvis up into the lower abdomen. This patient has planned radiation therapy, and the ovaries are transposed out of the radiation port to preserve fertility. Surgical clips seen on the corresponding CT *(curved arrow)* provide localization for transposed the ovaries.

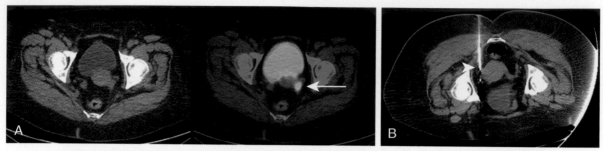

FIG. 19.6 **FDG-avid Unsuspected Primary Ovarian Malignancy.** (A) Axial CT and fused FDG PET/CT in a 69-year-old woman with adenocarcinoma of unknown primary demonstrate FDG avidity in the left adnexa *(arrow)*. FDG avidity in the adnexa is abnormal in a postmenopausal patient and prompted further workup. (B) Prone axial CT image from a CT-guided biopsy of the left adnexa demonstrates the biopsy needle in the left adnexa *(arrowhead)*. Pathology demonstrated a primary serous ovarian cancer.

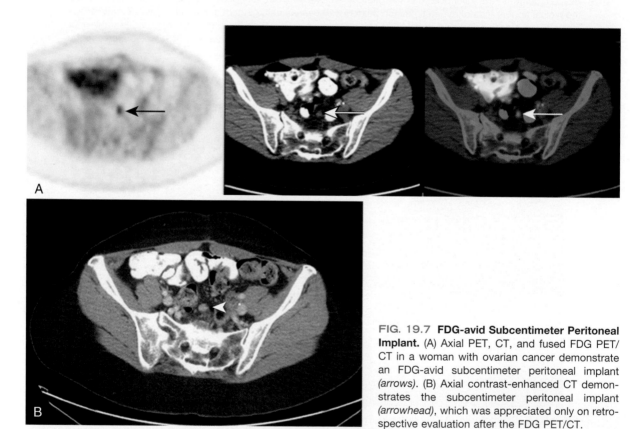

FIG. 19.7 **FDG-avid Subcentimeter Peritoneal Implant.** (A) Axial PET, CT, and fused FDG PET/CT in a woman with ovarian cancer demonstrate an FDG-avid subcentimeter peritoneal implant *(arrows)*. (B) Axial contrast-enhanced CT demonstrates the subcentimeter peritoneal implant *(arrowhead)*, which was appreciated only on retrospective evaluation after the FDG PET/CT.

may obscure recurrent malignancy at this location on CT but may be more readily appreciated on FDG PET (Fig. 19.8). Peritoneal implants may be visible on CT, FDG PET, both, or neither. Small peritoneal implants are difficult to visualize on current imaging modalities and may only be identified during surgical exploration.

It is important to remember that peritoneal reflections along the liver surface, such as the falciform ligament, may be involved with peritoneal malignancy. Implants along peritoneal reflections should be recognized as peritoneal malignancy, rather than hepatic parenchymal disease (Fig. 19.9). Patients with hepatic parenchymal

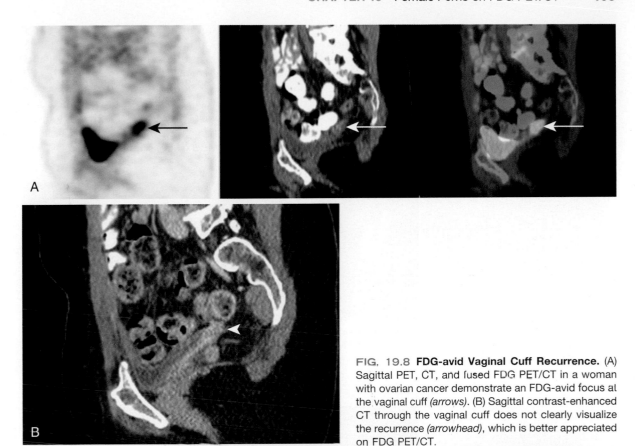

FIG. 19.8 FDG-avid Vaginal Cuff Recurrence. (A) Sagittal PET, CT, and fused FDG PET/CT in a woman with ovarian cancer demonstrate an FDG-avid focus at the vaginal cuff *(arrows)*. (B) Sagittal contrast-enhanced CT through the vaginal cuff does not clearly visualize the recurrence *(arrowhead)*, which is better appreciated on FDG PET/CT.

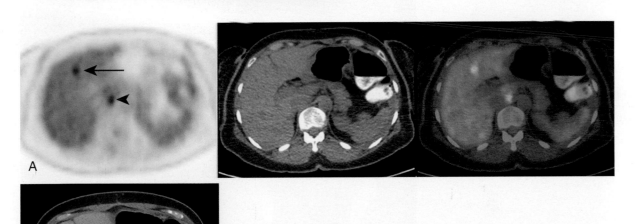

FIG. 19.9 Peritoneal Implants Along the Falciform Ligament. (A) Axial PET, CT, and fused FDG PET/CT in a woman with ovarian cancer demonstrate an FDG-avid focus along the falciform ligament *(arrow)*. This is a peritoneal implant along the falciform ligament, rather than a hepatic parenchymal metastasis. There is also an FDG-avid focus posterior to the liver *(arrowhead)* which may represent a hepatic surface implant or small lymph node. (B) Axial contrast-enhanced CT performed on the same day failed to visualize these FDG-avid implants.

disease have a worse prognosis than do patients with disease along peritoneal reflections. There is evidence that FDG PET can predict response to systemic therapy of ovarian cancer metastases. Following treatment, FDG PET/CT may have higher sensitivity for detecting recurrent malignancy than serum tumor markers such as cancer antigen 125 or CT alone.

As discussed in other organ systems, not all malignancies will be FDG avid. There are multiple histologic subtypes of ovarian cancer, which vary in the extent of their FDG avidity. Mucinous malignancies may be mildly or non–FDG avid, and thus the extent of malignancy may need to be recognized on the corresponding CT images (Fig. 19.10).

The ovary/adnexa may also be involved by metastatic disease or lymphoma. Primary malignancies of stomach, colon, and breast may metastasize to the adnexa, so called Krukenberg metastases (Fig. 19.11). An FDG-avid

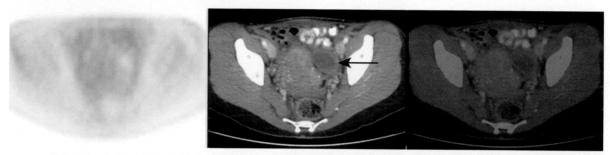

FIG. 19.10 **Non–FDG Avid Peritoneal Implant in a Patient with Newly Diagnosed Mucinous Ovarian Cancer.** (A) Axial PET, CT, and fused FDG PET/CT in a woman with ovarian cancer demonstrate a low-attenuation mucinous peritoneal implant on CT *(arrow)*, which represents malignancy despite lack of FDG avidity.

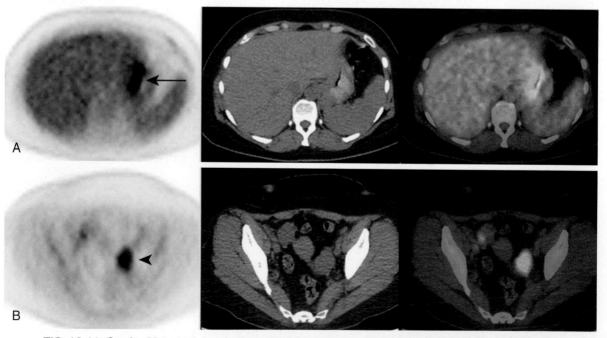

FIG. 19.11 **Ovarian Metastasis in a Patient with Primary Gastric Malignancy.** (A) Axial PET, CT, and fused FDG PET/CT through the stomach in a woman with primary gastric malignancy demonstrate the FDG-avid primary malignancy *(arrow)*. (B) Axial PET, CT, and fused FDG PET/CT through the pelvis demonstrate an enlarged FDG-avid left adnexa *(arrowhead)*, which was subsequently proven to be an adnexal metastasis.

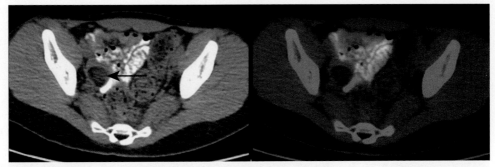

FIG. 19.12 **Benign Ovarian Teratoma.** Axial CT and fused FDG PET/CT demonstrating mixed fat and soft tissue lesion in the right adnexa *(arrow)*, which is diagnostic of an ovarian teratoma.

adnexal mass in a patient with another primary malignancy could thus represent a metastasis or primary adnexal lesion.

Benign Ovarian Lesions

Benign ovarian/adnexal masses are commonly encountered, particularly in premenopausal patients. These benign ovarian lesions, including teratomas, fibromas, endometriomas, and functional cysts, may be FDG avid and confused with malignancy. In general, FDG-avid adnexal lesions on FDG PET/CT can be further evaluated by ultrasound or MR for better characterization of the lesion. If an adnexal lesion contains macroscopic fat on the CT component of FDG PET/CT, they can usually be diagnosed as a benign teratoma (Fig. 19.12).

ENDOMETRIUM
Endometrial Cancer

Endometrial cancer is the most common gynecologic malignancy in the United States. In premenopausal women, FDG avidity in the endometrium is probably physiologic. However, in postmenopausal women, FDG avidity in the endometrium is abnormal, and ultrasound should be considered for further evaluation and to exclude an endometrial malignancy (Fig. 19.13).

The imaging technique of choice for visualizing and local staging of a primary endometrial malignancy is MR. T2-weighted MR imaging will visualize the low T2 signal junctional zone, which, if intact, excludes myometrial invasion. Interruption of the low T2 junctional zone is evidence of myometrial invasion. This determination cannot be made on FDG PET/CT (Fig. 19.14). The primary malignancy may also extend directly into the cervix, vagina, and adnexa, all of which are evaluable by MR imaging.

For visualization and staging of nodal and distant metastases in patients with endometrial cancer, both contrast-enhanced CT and FDG PET/CT have demonstrated value. FDG PET/CT has demonstrated the best sensitivity for identification of pelvic and retroperitoneal nodal metastases, as well as distant metastases. Similar to FDG PET/CT in patients with ovarian cancer, in patients with endometrial malignancy FDG PET/CT may demonstrate FDG-avid nodal metastases which are subcentimeter in size and thus overlooked on anatomic imaging, as well as FDG-avid vaginal cuff/peritoneal implants. Following therapy, recurrent endometrial cancer is most common in lymph nodes and the vaginal cuff, sites where FDG PET/CT may provide higher sensitivity than CT alone.

Benign Endometrial FDG Avidity

As previously discussed, in premenopausal women, FDG avidity in the endometrium is probably physiologic. Benign FDG avidity may also be associated with intrauterine devices (Fig. 19.15). When uncertainty exists, FDG avidity in the endometrium can be further evaluated by pelvic ultrasound.

MYOMETRIUM
Myometrial Leiomyomata

The most common myometrial neoplasm is by far the benign uterine leiomyoma. Leiomyomata may demonstrate background uterine FDG avidity but may also be significantly FDG avid (Fig. 19.16). Leiomyoma may be singular or multiple and may result in significant uterine enlargement (Fig. 19.17). Given the high prevalence of benign uterine leiomyomata and the low prevalence of other myometrial lesions, almost all FDG-avid foci in the myometrium will turn out to be benign myometrial

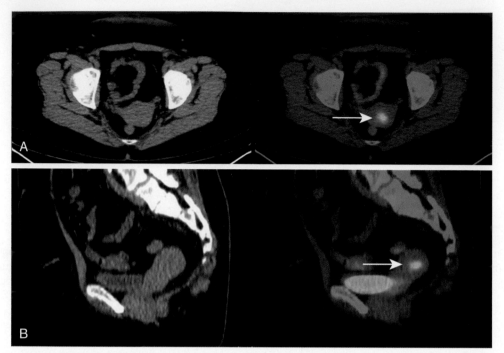

FIG. 19.13 **Unsuspected Endometrial Cancer Detected on FDG PET/CT.** (A) Axial and (B) sagittal CT and fused FDG PET/CT images in a 65-year-old woman with lymphoma demonstrate FDG avidity within the central uterus *(arrows)*, probably the endometrium. Because she was postmenopausal, ultrasound was ordered for further evaluation, leading to biopsy and diagnosis of a previously unknown endometrial carcinoma.

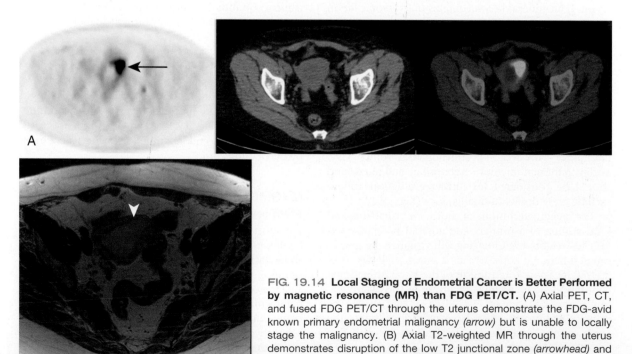

FIG. 19.14 **Local Staging of Endometrial Cancer is Better Performed by magnetic resonance (MR) than FDG PET/CT.** (A) Axial PET, CT, and fused FDG PET/CT through the uterus demonstrate the FDG-avid known primary endometrial malignancy *(arrow)* but is unable to locally stage the malignancy. (B) Axial T2-weighted MR through the uterus demonstrates disruption of the low T2 junctional zone *(arrowhead)* and the finding of myometrial invasion allows local staging of the endometrial malignancy.

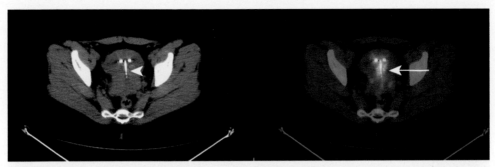

FIG. 19.15 **Benign FDG Avidity Associated with an Intrauterine Device.** Axial CT and fused FDG PET/CT through the uterus demonstrate FDG avidity in the central uterine endometrium *(arrow)*, associated with a high-attenuation T-shaped intrauterine device *(arrowhead)*.

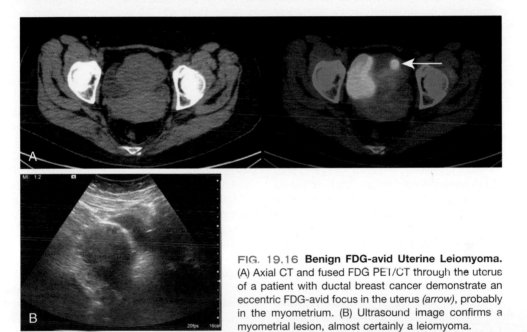

FIG. 19.16 **Benign FDG-avid Uterine Leiomyoma.** (A) Axial CT and fused FDG PET/CT through the uterus of a patient with ductal breast cancer demonstrate an eccentric FDG-avid focus in the uterus *(arrow)*, probably in the myometrium. (B) Ultrasound image confirms a myometrial lesion, almost certainly a leiomyoma.

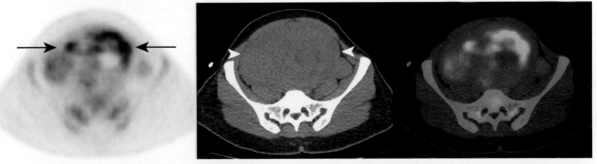

FIG. 19.17 **Benign FDG-avid Myometrial Leiomyomata.** Axial PET, CT, and fused FDG PET/CT through the uterus of a patient with ductal breast cancer demonstrate a markedly enlarged uterus *(arrowheads)* containing multifocal FDG-avid lesions *(arrows)*. Although the uterine enlargement and FDG avidity may first appear concerning, these are almost certainly benign myometrial leiomyomata in a patient with no previously known uterine malignancy.

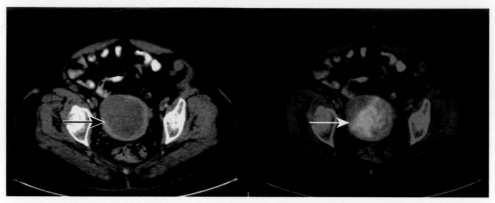

FIG. 19.18 Malignant Myometrial Leiomyosarcoma. Axial CT and fused FDG PET/CT images through the uterus of a patient known uterine leiomyosarcoma demonstrate an FDG-avid low-attenuation mass replacing the majority of the uterus *(arrows)*. Uterine leiomyosarcoma are extremely rare primary malignancies and unlikely to be incidentally detected on FDG PET/CT.

leiomyomata. When uncertainty exists, FDG avidity in the myometrium can be further evaluated by pelvic ultrasound.

Myometrial Leiomyosarcoma

Uterine leiomyosarcomas are extremely rare primary malignancies which are usually markedly FDG avid (Fig. 19.18). Uterine leiomyosarcoma is most often diagnosed incidentally following a hysterectomy for a presumed benign uterine process. They are extremely aggressive malignancies with high rates of metastases and poor prognosis. It is not possible to distinguish malignant leiomyosarcomas from the far more common benign leiomyomata on FDG PET/CT imaging. Given that the incidence of leiomyosarcoma is almost literally one in a million, an incidentally discovered FDG-avid myometrial lesion is still highly unlikely to be a myometrial leiomyosarcoma. There are published criteria for distinguishing a malignant leiomyosarcoma from benign leiomyomas on MR; however, making this distinction is extremely difficult and best left to experts in pelvic MR imaging.

CERVIX
Cervical Carcinoma

In the United States the mortality from cervical cancer has significantly declined due to Pap smear screening and early detection; however, worldwide, cervical cancer remains the leading cause of cancer mortality in women.

FDG avidity in the cervix is abnormal and should prompt further evaluation. It may be difficult to separate cervical FDG avidity from urine in the adjacent bladder at PET window settings typically used during evaluation

of FDG PET/CT. Altering the PET window setting to a higher maximum window level may, in some cases, assisted visualizing an FDG-avid cervical malignancy as distinct from excreted FDG in the adjacent bladder urine (Fig. 19.19).

The imaging technique of choice for visualizing and local staging of a primary endometrial malignancy is MR, with the T2 sequence usually the most helpful for visualizing and local staging of the primary cervical malignancy. FDG PET/CT plays a limited role in T staging for cervical cancer.

For visualization and staging of nodal and distant metastases in patients with cervical cancer, both contrast-enhanced CT and FDG PET/CT have demonstrated value. FDG PET/CT has demonstrated the best sensitivity for identification of pelvic and retroperitoneal nodal metastases, as well as distant metastases. Similar to FDG PET/CT in patients with ovarian cancer, in patients with cervical malignancy, FDG PET/CT may demonstrate FDG-avid nodal metastases which are subcentimeter in size and thus overlooked on anatomic imaging (Fig. 19.20). Following therapy, recurrent cervical cancer is most common in lymph nodes and the vaginal cuff, sites where FDG PET/CT may provide higher sensitivity than does CT alone.

Not all cervical malignancies will be FDG avid. Mucinous cervical malignancies may be mildly or non–FDG avid, and thus the extent of malignancy may need to be recognized on the corresponding CT images (Fig. 19.21).

Although uncommon, the cervix may also be involved by metastatic disease or lymphoma (Fig. 19.22). The most common primary malignancies resulting in metastases

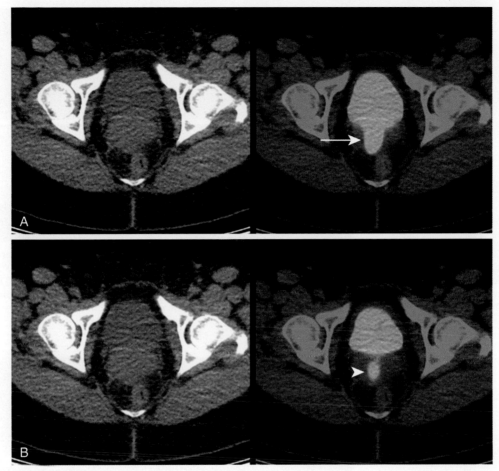

FIG. 19.19 **Altering the PET Window Level to Help Distinguish a Primary Cervical Malignancy from Urine in the Adjacent Bladder.** (A) Axial CT and fused FDG PET/CT images through bladder and cervix in a patient with known cervical cancer demonstrate FDG avidity in the cervix *(arrow)* which is contiguous with excreted FDG in bladder urine. (B) Axial CT and fused FDG PET/CT images with the PET window altered to a higher upper limit allow for distinguishing the FDG-avid primary cervical malignancy *(arrowhead)* from the adjacent FDG in bladder urine.

to the cervix are stomach, colorectal, breast, and ovarian malignancies. An FDG-avid cervical mass in a patient with another primary malignancy could thus represent a primary cervical malignancy or a metastasis.

Here are a few suggestions to help optimize your interpretation of FDG PET/CT of the female pelvis:

1. Overall, FDG PET/CT is limited in its ability to evaluate the primary ovarian, endometrial, and cervical malignancy. MR will be better for T staging of these primary malignancies.

2. FDG PET/CT is often valuable for gynecologic malignancies by detection of unsuspected nodal and distant metastases (including FDG-avid subcentimeter lesions often overlooked on anatomic imaging), providing assessment of treatment response to systemic therapy and assisting detection of recurrent malignancy.

3. In premenopausal patients, FDG avidity in the endometrium and ovary is usually physiologic. In postmenopausal patients, FDG avidity in the endometrium and ovary is abnormal and should prompt further workup.

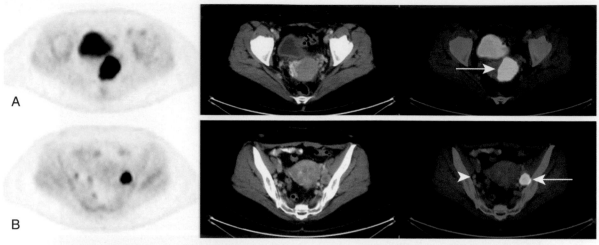

FIG. 19.20 **Detection of Additional Nodal Metastases with FDG PET/CT in a Patient with Primary Cervical Cancer.** (A) Axial PET, CT, and fused FDG PET/CT images through the cervix in a patient with known cervical cancer demonstrate the FDG-avid primary cervical malignancy *(arrow)*. (B) Axial PET, CT, and fused FDG PET/CT images of the pelvis demonstrate an enlarged FDG-avid left pelvic nodal metastasis *(arrow)* but also an FDG-avid subcentimeter right pelvic nodal metastasis *(arrowhead)* which could be overlooked on anatomic imaging alone.

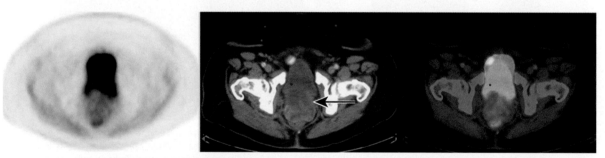

FIG. 19.21 **Non–FDG Avid Primary Cervical Malignancy in a Patient with Newly Diagnosed Cervical Cancer.** Axial PET, CT, and fused FDG PET/CT images demonstrate a low-attenuation cervical mass on CT *(arrow)*, which represents malignancy despite minimal FDG avidity.

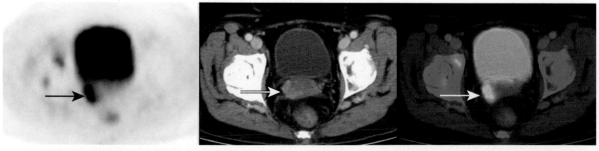

FIG. 19.22 **Cervical Metastasis.** Axial PET, CT, and fused FDG PET/CT images in a patient with mixed ductal/lobular breast cancer demonstrate an FDG-avid enhancing lateral cervical mass *(arrows)*. The differential includes a primary cervical malignancy and cervical metastasis. Biopsy revealed a cervical metastasis.

4. Beware of transposed ovaries in young women with pelvic malignancies and planned radiation therapy. Transposed ovaries may demonstrate FDG avidity in unexpected locations.

5. FDG-avid lesions in the myometrium are almost always benign leiomyomata. FDG PET/CT cannot distinguish benign leiomyomata from the rare leiomyosarcoma.

6. FDG avidity in the adjacent bowel and excreted FDG in the urinary tract may obscure FDG-avid gynecologic malignancy. Correlation with CT images will help to distinguish benign from malignant FDG-avid foci.

7. Uncertain imaging findings in the ovaries or uterus on FDG PET/CT can be further evaluated with pelvic ultrasound or MR.

SUGGESTED READINGS

Avril, et al: Prediction of response to neoadjuvant chemotherapy by sequential F-18-fluorodeoxyglucose positron emission tomography in patients with advanced-stage ovarian cancer, *J Clin Oncol* 23:7445–7453, 2005.

Bollineni, et al: High diagnostic value of 18F-FDG PET/CT in endometrial cancer: systematic review and meta-analysis of the literature, *J Nucl Med* 57:879–885, 2016.

Khiewvan, et al: An update on the role of PET/CT and PET/MRI in ovarian cancer, *Eur J Nucl Med Mol Imaging* 44:1079–1091, 2017.

Kim, et al: Incidental ovarian 18F-FDG accumulation on PET: correlation with the menstrual cycle, *Eur J Nucl Med Mol Imaging* 32:757–763, 2005.

Kitajima, et al: Diagnostic accuracy of integrated FDG-PET/contrast-enhanced CT in staging ovarian cancer: comparison with enhanced CT, *Eur J Nucl Med Mol Imaging* 35:1912–1920, 2008.

Kitajima, et al: Performance of integrated FDG-PET/contrast-enhanced CT in the diagnosis of recurrent uterine cancer: comparison with PET and enhanced CT, *Eur J Nucl Med Mol Imaging* 36:362–372, 2009.

Lee, et al: Evaluation of gynecologic cancer with MR imaging, 18F-FDG PET/CT, and PET/MR imaging, *J Nucl Med* 56:436–443, 2015.

Mohaghegh, et al: Imaging strategy for early ovarian cancer: characterization of adnexal masses with conventional and advanced imaging techniques, *Radiographics* 32:1751–1773, 2012.

Rioja, et al: Role of positron emission tomography in urological oncology, *BJU Int* 106:1578–1593, 2010.

Sala, et al: Recurrent ovarian cancer: use of contrast-enhanced CT and PET/CT to accurately localize tumor recurrence and to predict patients' survival, *Radiology* 257:125–134, 2010.

Takeuchi, et al: Utility of 18F-FDG PET/CT in follow-up of patients with low-grade serous carcinoma of the ovary, *Gynecol Oncol* 133:100–104, 2014.

Yuan, et al: Computer tomography, magnetic resonance imaging, and positron emission tomography or positron emission tomography/computer tomography for detection of metastatic lymph nodes in patients with ovarian cancer: a meta-analysis, *Eur J Radiol* 81:1002–1006, 2012.

Yun, et al: Physiologic 18F-FDG uptake in the fallopian tubes at mid cycle on PET/CT, *J Nucl Med* 51:682–685, 2010.

CHAPTER 20

Male Pelvis on FDG PET/CT

The male pelvis on 18F-fluorodeoxyglucose positron emission tomography/computed tomography (FDG PET/CT) is more straightforward than the female pelvis. The testes may demonstrate physiologic FDG avidity. FDG-avid foci within the prostate may represent benign focal prostatitis or prostate cancer.

TESTES

Physiologic FDG Avidity in the Testes

Physiologic FDG avidity is common in the testes (Fig. 20.1). There is debate over how high a testicular standardized uptake value (SUV) may be and still be considered "physiologic." If the testes are not enlarged on CT and there are no focal masses or FDG avidity in the testes, the FDG avidity is almost certainly physiologic. The testes are usually located within the scrotum; however, a testis may be located within the inguinal canal (Fig. 20.2), which could lead to confusion with the inguinal lymph node. In young men with pelvic malignancy, beware of surgically transposed testes with physiologic FDG avidity in unexpected locations. If radiation is planned for the pelvis, the testes may be surgically transposed to remove them from the radiation port, to preserve their function and fertility (Fig. 20.3).

Testicular Malignancies

Primary testicular malignancies include seminomas and nonseminomas. Testicular cancers may demonstrate lymphatic spread to lymph nodes. The gonadal lymphatics follow the testicular veins to the retroperitoneum; thus nodal metastases in the retroperitoneum may be apparent before lower pelvic nodal metastases. Alternatively, nodal metastases may be seen in the pelvis in the external iliac nodes. Internal iliac and inguinal nodes are normally not involved. Hematogenous spread to multiple organ systems, most commonly the lungs, may also occur.

The imaging technique of choice for visualizing and local staging of a primary testicular malignancy is ultrasound. There is no known clinically relevant role for FDG PET/CT in the T staging of testicular cancer. The imaging technique of choice for visualization and staging of nodal and distant metastases from testicular cancer is contrast-enhanced CT. FDG PET/CT may complement contrast-enhanced CT by detection of unsuspected FDG-avid metastases, such as nodal metastases or implants which are subcentimeter in size and thus overlooked on anatomic imaging.

The testes may be sites of involvement by lymphoma or metastases. Physiologic FDG avidity in the testes is normally homogenous, and focal areas of increased FDG avidity are suspicious for disease involvement (Fig. 20.4). In questionable cases, testicular ultrasound could be obtained for further evaluation.

Orchitis

A reminder that, as with other organ systems, increased FDG avidity can be seen with both malignant and inflammatory processes. An infected or inflamed testis may be FDG avid. Evaluation with testicular ultrasound will demonstrate hyperemia associated with orchitis (Fig. 20.5).

PROSTATE

Prostate cancer is one of the most common malignancies in males. The primary malignancy may extend directly into adjacent tissues and organs and demonstrate lymphatic spread (usually first pelvic and then later retroperitoneal lymph nodes) and hematogenous spread (most commonly to bone).

The imaging technique of choice for visualizing and local staging of a primary prostatic malignancy is magnetic resonance (MR), which most readily identifies extraprostatic spread to adjacent tissues. There is no known clinically relevant role for FDG PET/CT in the T staging of prostate cancer. An incidentally identified FDG-avid focus within the prostate may represent a previously unknown prostate cancer or focal prostatitis (Fig. 20.6). FDG PET/CT cannot distinguish between these malignant and inflammatory processes. Prostate

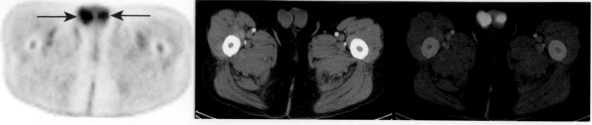

FIG. 20.1 **Physiologic Testicular FDG Avidity.** Axial PET, CT, and fused PET/CT images demonstrate FDG avidity in the bilateral testes *(arrows)* of a patient with treated lymphoma. There were no FDG-avid lesions suspicious for lymphoma in this patient. Testicular standard uptake value (SUV) was given normal testicular size, no focal testicular masses or FDG avidity, and no prior history of testicular malignancy; the testicular FDG avidity was considered physiologic. Clinical and imaging follow-up demonstrated long-term remission without evidence of lymphoma.

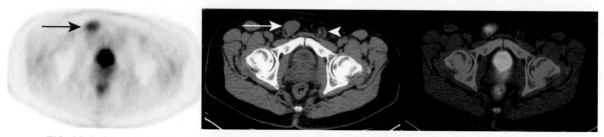

FIG. 20.2 **Testis within the Inguinal Canal.** Axial PET, CT, and fused PET/CT images demonstrate FDG-avid soft tissue in the right inguinal region *(arrows)*. In the corresponding left inguinal region is the inguinal canal containing the spermatic cord *(arrowhead)*. The FDG-avid soft tissue in the right inguinal region represents the right testis within the right inguinal canal, which may be confused with an inguinal lymph node.

MR may be considered for further evaluation. Biopsy may be needed if a new diagnosis of prostate cancer would be relevant. In a patient with widespread metastatic lung cancer, the identification of an FDG-avid focus within the prostate may not be clinically relevant. In a patient with treated lymphoma in remission, the incidental identification of an FDG-avid focus within the prostate is more likely to warrant further evaluation.

In patients with early-stage bladder cancer treated with intravesicular bacillus Calmette-Guérin immunotherapy, it is common to see FDG-avid foci within the prostate, which, when biopsied, demonstrate granulomatous prostatitis. Thus the presence of FDG-avid foci in the prostate of these patients is probably inflammatory (Fig. 20.7).

Currently, the imaging techniques of choice for visualization and staging of nodal and distant metastases from prostate cancer are nuclear bone scan and contrast-enhanced CT. Many believe that FDG PET/CT is of no use for nodal and distant metastases in patients with prostate cancer; however, this is not true. FDG PET/CT may have an effect on clinical management of some patients with prostate cancer because aggressive primary prostate tumors (Gleason score > 7) tend to be FDG avid. Following treatment of FDG-avid metastatic prostate cancers, FDG PET/CT provides good evaluation of therapy response (Fig. 20.8). Increasing sclerotic osseous lesions in a patient with prostate cancer could represent either increasing metastases or successful treatment of metastases with osseous healing, and it is difficult to distinguish these on CT. Nuclear bone scan suffers from the same limitation, with increasing tracer uptake representing either increasing metastases or osseous healing. FDG PET does not suffer from this limitation, and successful treatment response is easier to appreciate. In patients with prior prostate cancer treatment who have increasing biochemical markers such as prostate-specific membrane antigen and anatomic imaging studies which fail to localize the site of recurrence, FDG PET/CT may visualize the sites of recurrent disease, allowing for improved choice of local and systemic therapies.

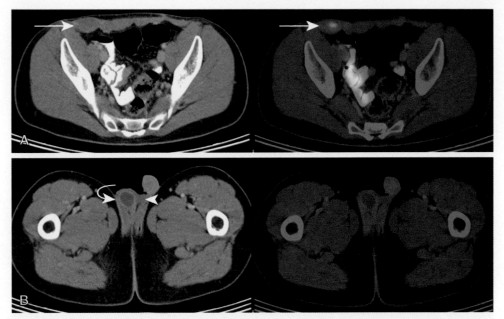

FIG. 20.3 **Physiologic FDG Avidity in a Surgically Transposed Right Testis.** (A) Axial CT and fused PET/CT images in a 20-year-old male with left paratesticular rhabdomyosarcoma post–left orchiectomy demonstrate FDG-avid soft tissue in the right inguinal region *(arrows)*. (B) Axial CT and fused PET/CT images through the scrotum demonstrate absence of the left testis due to left orchiectomy *(arrowhead)*. In the right scrotum is a fluid attenuation collection *(curved arrow)*, not the right testicle. The right testicle has been surgically transposed to the right inguinal region in (A). This patient has planned radiotherapy to the scrotum, and the remaining testis has been transposed out of the radiation port to preserve fertility. This should not be confused with a lymph node metastasis.

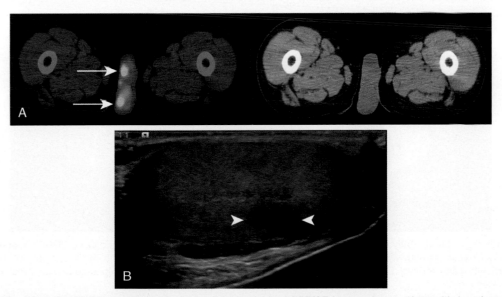

FIG. 20.4 **Testicular Lymphoma.** (A) Axial CT and fused PET/CT images in a patient with lymphoma demonstrate focal FDG-avid lesions in the bilateral testes *(arrows)*. Because testicular FDG avidity was focally increased, rather than homogenous, this was suspicious for disease involvement and ultrasound was obtained. (B) Long axis ultrasound image of the right testis demonstrates a focal hypoechoic lesion *(arrowheads)* consistent with testicular lymphoma in this patient with lymphoma.

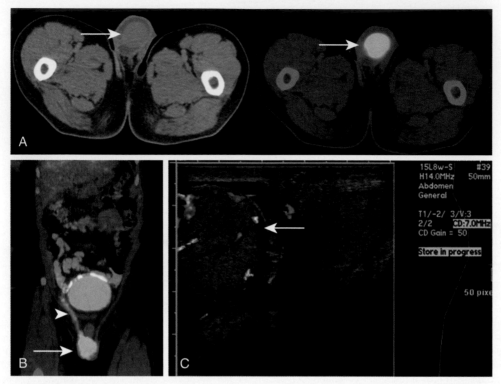

FIG. 20.5 Orchitis. (A) Axial CT and fused PET/CT images in a patient with lymphoma demonstrate an enlarged and FDG-avid right testis *(arrows)*. (B) Coronal fused PET/CT images demonstrate the enlarged and FDG-avid right testis *(arrow)* with FDG avidity extending up the spermatic cord *(arrowhead)*. (C) Short-axis color Doppler ultrasound images of the bilateral testes demonstrate increased blood flow in the right testis *(arrow)*, diagnostic of orchitis in this patient complaining of testicular pain.

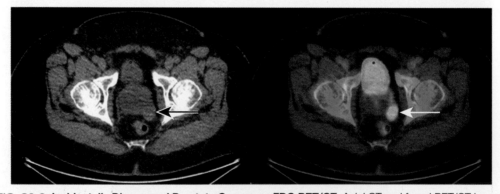

FIG. 20.6 Incidentally Discovered Prostate Cancer on FDG PET/CT. Axial CT and fused PET/CT images in a 72-year-old man with treated melanoma demonstrate FDG-avid soft tissue in the left aspect of the prostate gland *(arrows)*. Further workup and biopsy demonstrated a previously unsuspected primary prostate malignancy.

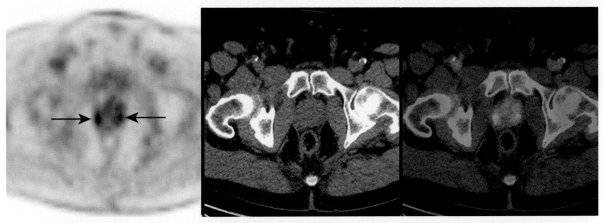

FIG. 20.7 Inflammatory FDG avidity within the prostate of a patient treated with bacillus Calmette-Guérin (BCG) immunotherapy for early-stage bladder cancer. Axial PET, CT, and fused PET/CT images in a 62-year-old man with bladder cancer treated with BCG immunotherapy demonstrate multiple FDG-avid foci in the prostate gland *(arrows)*. These foci resolved on follow-up imaging and are probably attributable to BCG immunotherapy–induced granulomatous prostatltis.

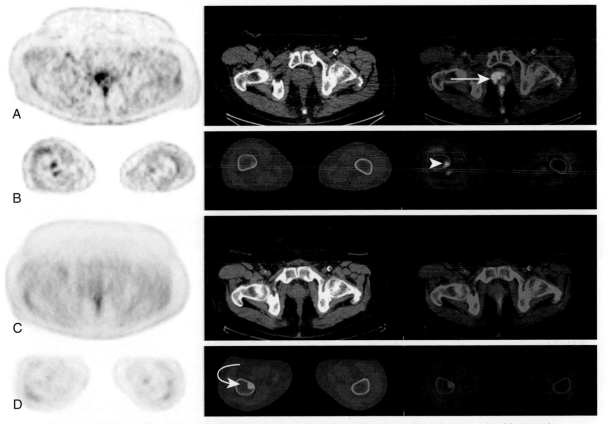

FIG. 20.8 Successful FDG PET/CT Evaluation of Treatment Response in a Patient with Metastatic Prostate Cancer. Axial PET, CT, and fused PET/CT images of the (A) prostate and (B) femurs demonstrate an FDG-avid biopsy-proven primary prostate malignancy *(arrow)* and biopsy-proven femoral osseous metastasis *(arrowhead)*. Following therapy, axial PET, CT, and fused PET/CT images of the (C) prostate and (D) femurs demonstrate resolution of FDG avidity, representing successful treatment response. The femoral lesion becomes larger and more sclerotic on CT *(curved arrow),* which could be mistaken as an increasing osseous metastasis.

Here are a few suggestions to help optimize your interpretation of FDG PET/CT of the male pelvis:

1. Overall, FDG PET/CT is limited in its ability to evaluate a primary testicular or prostate malignancy. Ultrasound is preferred for local staging of testicular malignancies and MR for local staging of prostate malignancy.

2. FDG PET/CT may be valuable for testicular and prostate malignancies by detection of unsuspected nodal and distant metastases (including FDG-avid subcentimeter lesions often overlooked on anatomic imaging) and providing assessment of treatment response to systemic therapy.

3. Testes demonstrate physiologic FDG avidity. Normal-sized testes with homogenous FDG avidity are probably physiologic.

4. Beware of transposed testes in men with pelvic malignancies and planned radiation therapy. Transposed testes may demonstrate FDG avidity in unexpected locations.

5. Uncertain imaging findings in the testis on FDG PET/CT can be further evaluated with testicular ultrasound.

6. Incidentally detected FDG-avid foci within the prostate may represent benign focal prostatitis or prostate cancer. If needed, prostate MR could be used for further evaluation. Biopsy may be needed if a new diagnosis of prostate cancer would be clinically relevant.

SUGGESTED READINGS

Hwang, et al: Is further evaluation needed for incidental focal uptake in the prostate in 18-fluoro-2-deoxyglucose positron emission tomography-computed tomography images?, *Ann Nucl Med* 27:140–145, 2013.

Jadvar: Is there use for FDG-PET in prostate cancer?, *Semin Nucl Med* 46:502–506, 2016.

Jadvar, et al: Prospective evaluation of 18F-NaF and 18F-FDG PET/CT in detection of occult metastatic disease in biochemical recurrence of prostate cancer, *Clin Nucl Med* 37:637–643, 2012.

Kim, et al: Granulomatous prostatitis after intravesical bacillus Calmette-Guérin instillation therapy: a potential cause of incidental F-18 FDG uptake in the prostate gland on F-18 FDG PET/CT in patients with bladder cancer, *Nucl Med Mol Imaging* 50:31–37, 2016.

Ozturk, et al: 18F-fluorodeoxyglucose PET/CT for detection of disease in patients with prostate-specific antigen relapse following radical treatment of a local-stage prostate cancer, *Oncol Lett* 11:316–322, 2016.

Rioja, et al: Role of positron emission tomography in urological oncology, *BJU Int* 106:1578–1593, 2010.

CHAPTER 21

Lymph Nodes on FDG PET/CT

18F-fluorodeoxyglucose positron emission tomography/computed tomography (FDG PET/CT) has become an important modality in the evaluation of lymph nodes in oncology patients, including the central role FDG PET/CT plays in managing patients with lymphoma and the ability for FDG PET to detect nodal metastases in subcentimeter nodes which may be overlooked on CT or magnetic resonance (MR). However, it is important to realize that there are multiple benign causes for FDG avidity in nodes, which must be distinguished from malignancy. The spatial distribution of the nodes, the corresponding CT findings, and the clinical history will help to distinguish benign FDG-avid nodes from malignancy.

LYMPHOMA

FDG PET/CT has become the primary imaging modality for staging and treatment response in patients with FDG-avid lymphomas. The vast majority of lymphomas are FDG avid, including the most common lymphomas, Hodgkin lymphoma (HL), diffuse large B-cell lymphoma(DLBCL), and follicular lymphoma. Some lymphomas have variable FDG avidity, including chronic lymphocytic leukemia/small lymphocytic lymphoma, lymphoplasmacytic lymphoma, and marginal zone lymphoma. FDG PET/CT would be useful in these lymphomas only if the tumor in an individual patient was proven to be FDG avid. In non–FDG avid lymphomas, contrast-enhanced CT is the standard imaging modality.

The most recent recommendations for the use of FDG PET/CT are referred to as the Lugano Classification. These guidelines were produced following an International Conference on Malignant Lymphoma held in Lugano, Switzerland. These consensus guidelines state that FDG PET/CT should be recommended for the initial staging of FDG-avid nodal lymphomas. A biopsy is needed to confirm that FDG-avid nodes represent lymphoma. The intensity of FDG avidity (the standardized uptake value max [SUVmax] of the node) cannot be used to diagnose lymphoma in lieu of a biopsy.

However, after lymphoma has been diagnosed by biopsy, the SUVmax can be used to help distinguish low-grade from high-grade lymphoma. As a rule of thumb, a pretreatment SUV of greater than 20 indicates high-grade lymphoma (see Chapter 13, Fig. 13.2), whereas SUV less than 10 is typically a low-grade lymphoma (see Chapter 13, Fig. 13.3). Values between 10 and 20 are usually high-grade lymphomas, but there is some overlap. This is valuable for patients for whom malignant transformation from a low-grade lymphoma to a more aggressive high-grade lymphoma is suspected. FDG PET/CT can identify if there are any lesions of high FDG avidity, suspicious for transformation, that have developed and can direct biopsy to an accessible highly FDG-avid lesion.

Focal FDG avidity within the bone or bone marrow is highly sensitive for osseous lymphoma in FDG-avid lymphomas. Conversely, homogenous elevation of FDG avidity in the bone marrow is usually bone marrow repopulation (see Chapter 3, Fig. 3.11). Evaluation of the osseous structures on FDG PET/CT is so sensitive for bone marrow involvement that routine bone marrow biopsy is no longer indicated for most patients with HL and DLBCL. Splenic, liver, and other organ involvement is also best evaluated by FDG PET/CT, despite physiologic activity in some organs. Only the central nervous system is described to be best evaluated by another imaging modality, MR, rather than FDG PET/CT.

Following treatment, FDG PET/CT is more accurate in determining treatment response than is CT for FDG-avid lymphomas. A five-point scale (5PS) is described in the Lugano Classification, which provides high interobserver assessment of lymphoma treatment response. The 5PS scores the greatest residual FDG avidity at a site of initial disease as follows:

1. No FDG uptake
2. Uptake less than or equal to mediastinal background
3. Uptake greater than mediastinal background but less than or equal to liver background
4. Uptake "moderately" higher than liver
5. Uptake "markedly" higher than liver or new lesions

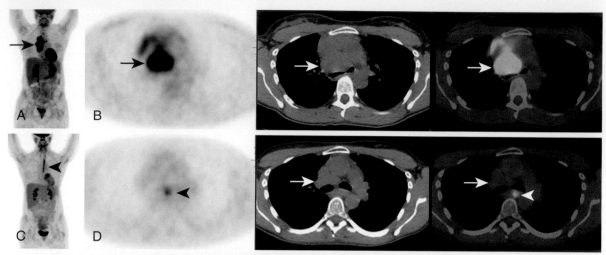

FIG. 21.1 **End of Treatment PET/CT with a Five-Point Scale (5PS) Score of 2.** (A) FDG maximum intensity projection (MIP) in a patient with lymphoma demonstrates abnormal FDG avidity in the chest *(arrow)*. (B) Axial PET, CT, and PET/CT images localize the abnormal FDG avidity to anterior mediastinal masses *(arrows)*, biopsy proven to be lymphoma. (C) FDG MIP following completion of therapy demonstrates resolution of the prior masslike FDG avidity and new linear FDG avidity over the chest *(arrowhead)*. (D) Axial PET, CT, and PET/CT images following therapy demonstrate decreased size of the masses and reduction of FDG avidity to the level of mediastinal background *(arrows, 5PS score of 2)*. The new linear FDG avidity on the MIP image corresponds with the esophagus *(arrowhead)*, representing posttherapy esophagitis. This is not FDG-avid lymphoma and is discounted when determining the 5PS score. This is considered a complete remission.

For most clinical situations, a 5PS of 1, 2, or 3 represents a complete metabolic response, without evidence of residual active lymphoma (Figs. 21.1 and 21.2). Even if there are residual masses, a complete metabolic response is considered a complete remission of lymphoma. A 5PS of 4 or 5 represents residual active lymphoma (Figs. 21.3 to 21.5). The terms "moderately" and "markedly" higher than liver are not defined, but many people interpret "markedly" to be more than twice the liver background. In general, if the SUV is decreasing, the score of 4 or 5 represents a partial metabolic response. If the SUV is without significant change, then the score of 4 or 5 represents stable metabolic disease. And if the SUV is increasing, or there are new FDG-avid lesions representing lymphoma, the score should be a 5.

There is a distinction between an "interim" scan (one that is performed in the middle of planned therapy) and an "end of treatment" scan (one that is performed after the course of therapy is finished). For an interim PET/CT, a 5PS score of 1, 2, or 3 is a highly desired result. A 5PS of 4 or 5 with decreasing SUV suggests the disease is responding, and treatment is continued. A 5PS of 5 with increasing SUV suggests treatment failure and may prompt a treatment change. For an end of treatment PET/CT, a 5PS of 1, 2, or 3 is again the desired result. But a 5PS of 4 or 5 represents a treatment failure, even if FDG avidity has decreased. That may prompt a biopsy to prove residual active malignancy and necessitate additional treatment. In most cases, for an end of treatment scan, the critical distinction is distinguishing between a 5PS score of 1 to 3 (treated disease) and 4 to 5 (residual active lymphoma), based on whether the treated lymphoma demonstrates FDG avidity less than or greater than liver background.

New sites of FDG avidity on posttherapy scans should be scrutinized to determine if the FDG avidity corresponds to a new site of lymphoma or represents a benign cause of FDG avidity. If the new FDG avidity is believed to be benign, the scan can be scored as if the benign FDG avidity does not exist (see Figs. 21.1, 21.3, and 21.4). Chemotherapy and radiation may also induce treatment-related inflammation, which may be FDG avid. To minimize posttreatment inflammation, it is recommended to wait at least 3 months following radiotherapy and 3 weeks following chemotherapy before obtaining a FDG PET/CT. Some 5PS scores of 4 may actually represent posttreatment inflammation, rather than residual active malignancy, but this is difficult to distinguish without follow-up imaging or tissue sampling.

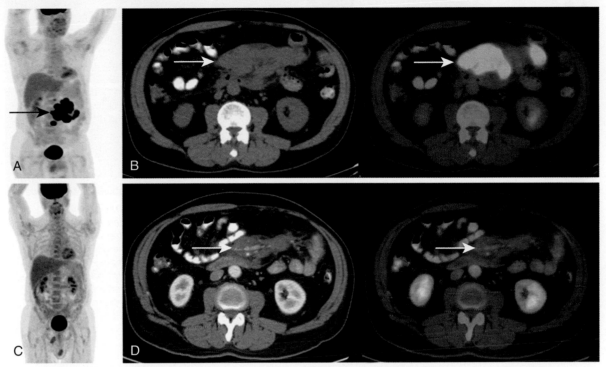

FIG. 21.2 **End of Treatment PET/CT with a Five-Point Scale (5PS) Score of 3.** (A) FDG maximum intensity projection (MIP) in a patient with lymphoma demonstrates abnormal FDG avidity in the abdomen (*arrow*). (B) Axial CT and fused PET/CT images localize the abnormal FDG avidity to mesenteric masses (*arrows*), biopsy proven to be lymphoma. (C) FDG MIP following completion of therapy demonstrates resolution of the prior abnormal FDG avidity. (D) Axial PET, CT, and PET/CT images following therapy demonstrate decreased size and FDG avidity of the masses, with residual FDG avidity greater than mediastinal but less than liver background (*arrows*, 5PS score of 3). This is considered a complete remission.

After a lymphoma patient has a complete remission, there is no evidence that routine surveillance FDG PET/CT scans provide value. If there are specific signs or symptoms of recurrence, FDG PET/CT is a value method to evaluate for recurrent lymphoma.

With the success of FDG PET/CT in patients with lymphoma, there is debate whether the CT needs to be performed with intravenous (IV) contrast. IV contrast may identify additional findings but rarely changes patient management. IV contrast is valuable for radiotherapy planning and when measurement of nodal size is needed as part of a clinical trial.

NODAL METASTASES

FDG PET/CT has the ability to detect nodal metastases in subcentimeter nodes which may be overlooked on CT or MR. This has been demonstrated throughout the body. Examples include nodal metastases arising from primary malignancies of the head and neck (see Fig. 7.22), lung, gastrointestinal tract (GI) tract, (Fig. 21.6; see Fig. 16.5), and genitourinary system (Fig. 21.7; see Fig. 18.14). Carefully inspect nodes near larger FDG-avid structures, such as the rectal malignancy in Fig. 21.6 or excreted FDG in the bladder, because the larger FDG-avid structures may obscure detection on clinically relevant FDG-avid nodes. It is important to understand the nodal drainage pathways of malignancies. Subcentimeter FDG-avid nodes along the drainage pathway of a known malignancy should raise suspicion for nodal metastases. However, subcentimeter FDG-avid nodes far removed from the primary malignancy are often benign.

BENIGN FDG-AVID NODES

The ability of FDG PET/CT to detect subcentimeter nodal metastases needs to be balanced against the relativity common occurrence of benign FDG-avid nodes,

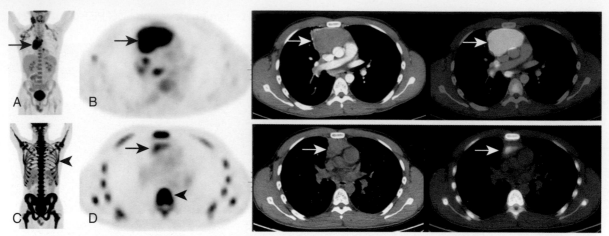

FIG. 21.3 **Interim Therapy PET/CT with a Five-Point Scale (5PS) Score of 4.** (A) FDG maximum intensity projection (MIP) in a patient with lymphoma demonstrates abnormal FDG avidity in the chest *(arrow)*. (B) Axial PET, CT, and fused PET/CT images localize the abnormal FDG avidity to thoracic masses *(arrows)*, biopsy proven to be lymphoma. (C) FDG MIP after two cycles of therapy demonstrates avidity in the bone marrow *(arrowhead)*, consistent with bone marrow repopulation. (D) Axial PET, CT, and PET/CT images following therapy demonstrate decreased size and FDG avidity of the masses, with residual FDG avidity greater than liver background *(arrows, 5PS score of 4)*. Because this is an "interim" scan, this is considered a successful response to therapy, and treatment is continued. If this had been an "end of therapy" scan, then this would be considered a treatment failure. This demonstrates the importance of the timing of the FDG PET/CT to the interpretation of the scan. The bone marrow repopulation *(arrowhead)* is not FDG-avid lymphoma and is discounted when determining the 5PS score.

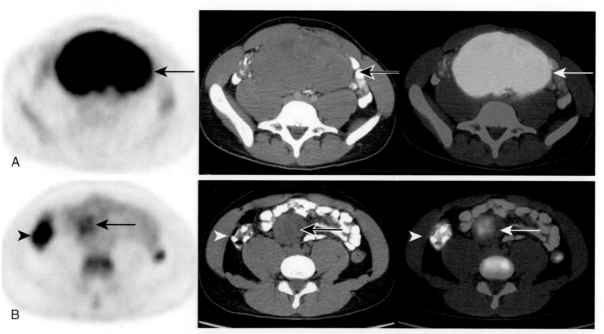

FIG. 21.4 **End of Treatment PET/CT with a Five-Point Scale (5PS) Score of 4.** (A) Axial PET, CT, and PET/CT images through the abdomen of a patient with biopsy-proven lymphoma demonstrate an FDG-avid soft tissue mass in the abdomen and pelvis *(arrows)*. (B) Following completion of therapy, axial PET, CT, and PET/CT images demonstrate decreased size of the mass and reduction of FDG avidity *(arrows)*. The standard uptake value of the mass remains greater than the background liver (not shown). This is a 5PS score of 4. The new FDG avidity corresponds with the right colon, without CT abnormality *(arrowheads)*, and is considered physiologic. This is not FDG-avid lymphoma and is discounted when determining the 5PS score.

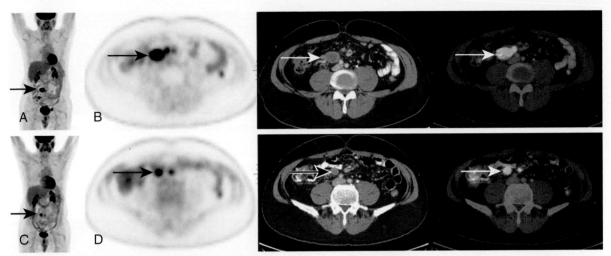

FIG. 21.5 End of Treatment PET/CT with a Five-Point Scale (5PS) Score of 5. (A) FDG maximum intensity projection (MIP) in a patient with lymphoma demonstrates abnormal FDG avidity in the abdomen *(arrow)*. (B) Axial PET, CT, and PET/CT images localize the abnormal FDG avidity to mesenteric masses *(arrows)*, biopsy proven to be lymphoma. (C) FDG MIP following completion of therapy demonstrates decreased FDG-avid lesions *(arrow)*. (D) Axial PET, CT, and PET/CT images following completion of therapy demonstrate decreased size but persistent high FDG avidity (maximum standardized uptake value of 12) in the masses *(arrows)*. This is a 5PS score of 5. This represents a partial response, but persistent active malignancy, and is considered a treatment failure.

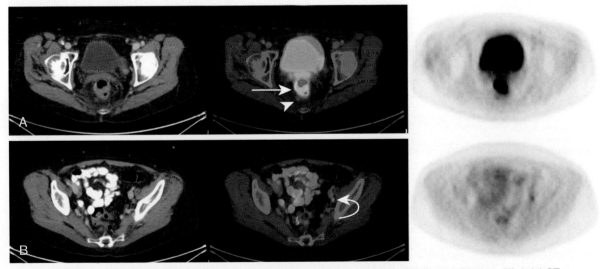

FIG. 21.6 FDG-avid Subcentimeter Nodal Metastasis in a Patient with Rectal Cancer. (A) Axial CT, fused PET/CT, and PET images through the pelvis demonstrate the FDG-avid primary rectal cancer *(arrow)*, as well a subcentimeter FDG-avid mesorectal nodal metastasis *(arrowhead)*. (B) More superior images demonstrate a subcentimeter FDG-avid left external iliac nodal metastasis *(curved arrow)*.

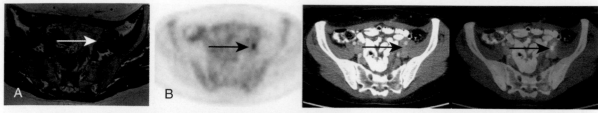

FIG. 21.7 **FDG-avid Subcentimeter Nodal Metastasis in a Patient with Cervical Cancer.** (A) Magnetic resonance (MR) image through the pelvic of a patient with newly diagnosed cervical cancer demonstrates a subcentimeter left external iliac node *(arrow)*, described an indeterminate for metastases on MR report. PET/CT was ordered for further evaluation. (B) Axial PET, CT, and PET/CT images demonstrate that the node is FDG avid *(arrows)*, consistent with a nodal metastasis.

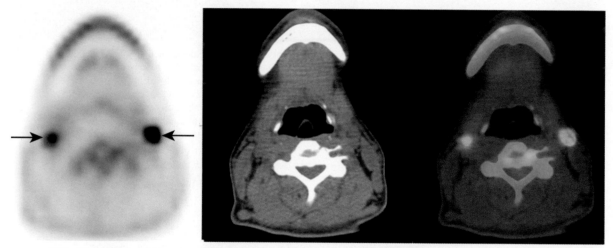

FIG. 21.8 **FDG-avid Benign Neck Nodes in a Patient with Anal Cancer.** Axial PET, CT, and FDG PET/CT images demonstrate bilateral FDG-avid neck nodes *(arrows)* in a patient with anal cancer. Because it would be unlikely for anal cancer to metastasize to neck nodes without significant malignancy elsewhere, these nodes are considered benign despite substantial FDG avidity (maximum standardized uptake value of 10).

particularly in the head and neck, where infectious organisms are processed in the nasal and oral cavities, and in the inguinal nodes, which drain the lower extremities. For example, subcentimeter FDG-avid neck nodes in a patient with an oropharyngeal squamous cell carcinoma should raise suspicion of metastases. Neck nodes with the same size and FDG avidity in a patient with anal cancer are far less likely to represent malignancy unless there is substantial malignancy elsewhere (Fig. 21.8). Likewise, subcentimeter FDG-avid inguinal nodes in a patient with anal cancer (see Chapter 16, Fig. 16.30) should raise suspicion for metastases, yet the same nodes in a patient with oropharyngeal squamous cell carcinoma are benign unless there is substantial other malignancy.

Postsurgical inflammation may also result in benign, yet enlarged or FDG-avid, nodes. Studies have shown that internal mammary nodes which are newly enlarged or FDG avid following mastectomy for breast cancer are almost always benign when tissue sampled (Fig. 21.9).

Multiple benign processes result in FDG-avid nodes, which may be markedly FDG avid. These include sarcoidosis or sarcoid-like reactions to malignancy (Fig. 21.10), amyloid, Rosai-Dorfman, and Castleman disease (Fig. 21.11). Sarcoid is a noncaseating granulomatous disease which may demonstrate multiorgan involvement mimicking widespread metastases (Fig. 21.12). Castleman disease is a rare nodal hyperplasia which may be cured by resection if disease is limited. Sometimes, these processes mimic malignancy so well that tissue sampling is needed

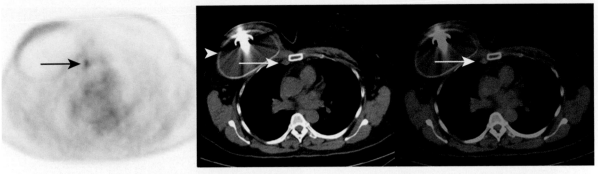

FIG. 21.9   **FDG-avid Benign Internal Mammary Node Following Mastectomy for Ductal Breast Cancer.** Axial PET, CT, and FDG PET/CT images demonstrate an enlarged and FDG-avid internal mammary node *(arrows)*. A tissue expander is seen in the mastectomy bed *(arrowhead)*. Despite enlargement and FDG avidity, it is known that new enlargement of an internal mammary node following mastectomy is usually inflammatory. This node was tissue sampled by ultrasound-guided fine-needle aspiration because of the FDG avidity and was proven to be benign.

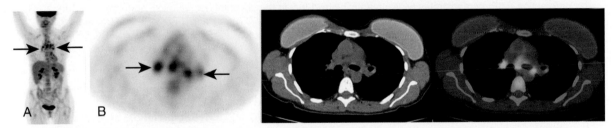

FIG. 21.10   **FDG-avid Sarcoid in a Patient with Ductal Breast Cancer.** FDG PET/CT was performed in a patient with history of ductal breast cancer and suspicion of recurrence. (A) FDG maximum intensity projection (MIP) demonstrates symmetric bilateral thoracic FDG-avid foci *(arrows)*. (B) Axial PET, CT, and PET/CT localize the FDG-avid foci to normal-sized symmetric bilateral hilar and mediastinal nodes *(arrows)*. Because it would be highly unusual for breast cancer to skip the axillary and internal mammary nodes to metastasize in this pattern, this should be recognized as almost certainly benign. Unfortunately, a PET/CT report (at an outside hospital, of course) called these nodes suspicious for malignancy, and this patient underwent a mediastinoscopy to biopsy these nodes. The biopsy diagnosed sarcoid. The patient suffered a left vocal cord paralysis from the biopsy, a complication which could have been prevented by recognizing these FDG-avid nodes as benign on the PET/CT.

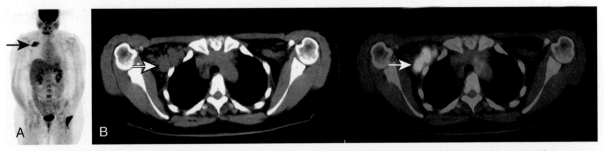

FIG. 21.11   **FDG-avid Castleman Disease.** (A) FDG maximum intensity projection (MIP) in a patient presenting with lymphadenopathy demonstrates FDG-avid foci overlying the right chest *(arrow)*. (B) CT and PET/CT localize the FDG avidity to enlarged right axillary nodes *(arrows)*, suspicious for nodal metastases from an unknown primary. However, biopsy diagnosed Castleman disease.

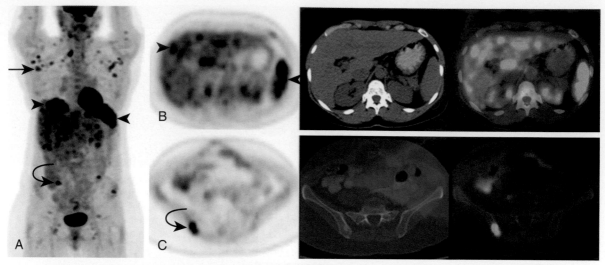

FIG. 21.12 **Multiorgan System Sarcoid Mimicking Widespread Metastases.** (A) FDG maximum intensity projection (MIP) demonstrates widespread FDG-avid foci in the chest (nodes, *arrows*), abdomen (liver and spleen, *arrowheads*), and pelvis (bone, *curved arrow*). (B) PET, CT, and fused FDG PET/CT through the abdomen localize the FDG-avid liver and spleen lesions *(arrowheads)*. (C) PET, CT, and fused FDG PET/CT through the pelvis localize an FDG-avid osseous lesion *(curved arrow)*. Biopsy of a node and bone both returned a diagnosis of sarcoid.

to diagnose the benign process. Other times, such as with sarcoid and sarcoid-like reactions, the distribution of the FDG-avid nodes may reveal its benign nature and avoid an unnecessary biopsy. For example, most malignancies would not result in symmetric bilateral hilar and mediastinal nodal metastases. When this distribution of FDG avidity is encountered, a benign sarcoid-like process should be strongly considered. This could prevent unnecessary biopsies and biopsy complications.

A wide range of infectious and inflammatory processes may also cause enlarged or FDG-avid nodes. Mycobacterial infections, such as tuberculous, may be markedly FDG avid. Viral infections, including mononucleosis, herpes, and HIV may cause more mildly FDG-avid enlarged nodes. HIV may cause mildly avid and enlarged lymph nodes that are benign, particularly during active AIDS (Fig. 21.13). This must be carefully evaluated against the possibility of AIDS-related malignancies such as lymphoma and Kaposi sarcoma. Inflammatory processes, such as lupus and inflammatory pseudotumors, may be FDG avid, and several medications may cause nodal enlargement.

Following allogeneic stem cell transplantation, there may be mildly enlarged FDG-avid nodes which are benign on biopsy (Fig. 21.14). This possibly represents a graft-versus-host phenomenon, eliciting inflammation in host nodes. These benign FDG-avid nodes may persist for some time following an allogeneic stem cell transplant.

Indeed, there is a large and diverse differential for enlarged and/or FDG-avid nodes which can complicate FDG PET/CT interpretation. In a patient with a known malignancy, and FDG-avid nodes in an expected drainage pattern, nodal metastases are the leading differential; otherwise, other etiologies should be entertained.

Other physiologic processes may obscure FDG-avid nodes on FDG PET/CT. Brown fat may be FDG avid and, if extensive enough or if found in areas of expected nodal drainage from a malignancy, could complicate FDG PET/CT interpretation. Brown fat is indistinguishable from energy storing white fat on CT but contains many brown-pigmented mitochondria used for heat production. Common sites of brown fat include the neck, supraclavicular, axillary, mediastinal, and paravertebral regions (Fig. 21.15). When extensive, brown fat may be found in the diaphragmatic, retrocrural, or retroperitoneal regions. Brown fat is more common in children, but extensive brown fat may still be found in adults. When brown fat is encountered, careful correlation with the CT is prudent. It may be very difficult to distinguish FDG-avid brown fat from FDG-avid malignancy on the PET; however, the CT distinguishes fat attenuation brown fat from soft tissue attenuation FDG-avid malignancy (Fig. 21.16). When a patient demonstrates a propensity to have FDG-avid brown fat on their FDG PET/CT, and this may interfere with FDG PET/CT

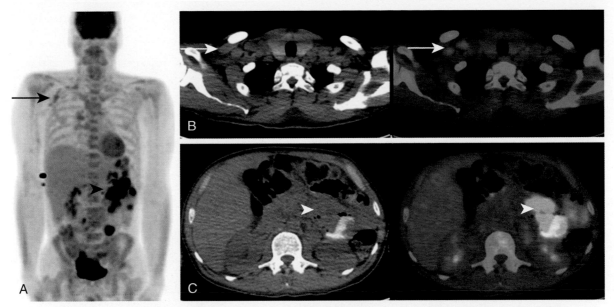

FIG. 21.13 Mildly FDG-avid Nodes and Markedly FDG-avid Lymphoma, Both Related to HIV/AIDS.
(A) FDG maximum intensity projection (MIP) demonstrates mildly FDG-avid foci overlying the neck and chest
(arrows), as well as more markedly FDG avidity in the abdomen *(arrowhead)*. (B) Axial CT and fused FDG
PET/CT through the upper chest localize the mildly FDG-avid foci to mildly enlarged neck and chest nodes
(arrows). These were biopsied and shown to be benign, probably reactive to HIV/AIDS. (C) Axial CT and
fused FDG PET/CT through the abdomen localize the more marked FDG avidity to bowel soft tissue masses
(arrowheads). On pathology, this was lymphoma, probably AIDS-associated lymphoma.

interpretation, measures can be taken during FDG uptake
to minimize the appearance of FDG-avid brown fat on
scans. This may be as simple as providing warm blankets
to the patient before and during FDG uptake, to phar-
macologic interventions such as beta-blockers, which
have been shown to reduce brown fat.

If FDG is extravasated at the injection site, the FDG
will infiltrate the adjacent fat and soft tissues. Some
FDG will be picked up by the lymphatic system and
transit to draining nodes. This may result in an FDG-avid
node with very benign morphology on CT (Fig. 21.17).
This is not necessarily a malignant node, rather it is a
sentinel node draining the injection site, usually the
arm. Again, if the primary malignancy is remote from
the site of primary malignancy, small FDG-avid nodes
will usually have a benign etiology.

Here are a few suggestions to help optimize your
interpretation of FDG PET/CT of lymph nodes:

1. FDG PET/CT is the image modality of choice for
FDG-avid lymphomas. Current recommendations for
the use of FDG PET/CT in patients with lymphoma are
referred to as the Lugano Classification.

2. Lymphoma response to therapy is graded on a 5PS.
In most cases, for an end of treatment scan, the critical
distinction is distinguishing between a 5PS score of 1 to
3 (treated disease) and 4 to 5 (residual active lymphoma),
based on whether the treated lymphoma demonstrates
FDG avidity less than or greater than liver background.

3. FDG PET/CT often provides greater sensitivity than
does CT or MR to detect subcentimeter nodal metastases.
This ability must be weighed against the relativity
common occurrence of benign FDG-avid small nodes,
particularly in the head/neck and inguinal regions. It is
important to understand the nodal drainage pathways
of malignancies. Subcentimeter FDG-avid nodes along
the drainage pathway of a known malignancy should
raise suspicion for nodal metastases. However, subcentimeter FDG-avid nodes far removed from the primary
malignancy are often benign.

4. The presence of FDG-avid brown fat does not preclude
synchronous FDG-avid malignancy. When brown fat is
suspected, use the CT images to confirm that the FDG
avidity corresponds to fat attenuation (usually brown
fat) or soft tissue attenuation (something else).

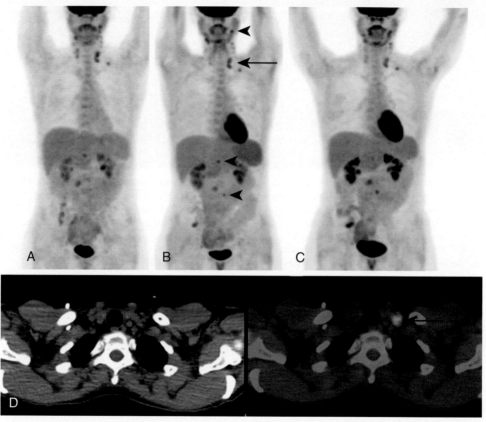

FIG. 21.14 **Benign FDG-avid Nodes in a Patient with Lymphoma Following Allogeneic Stem Cell Transplant.** (A), (B), and (C) serial FDG maximum intensity projection (MIP) images following allogeneic stem cell transplant demonstrate evolving FDG-avid foci which correspond to nodes in the neck, chest, and abdomen (*arrow* and *arrowheads*). (D) CT and fused FDG PET/CT through the upper chest localize FDG avidity to a mildly enlarged node in the thoracic inlet *(arrow).* Benign FDG-avid nodes may be encountered following allogeneic stem cell transplant, possibly a graft-versus-host reaction.

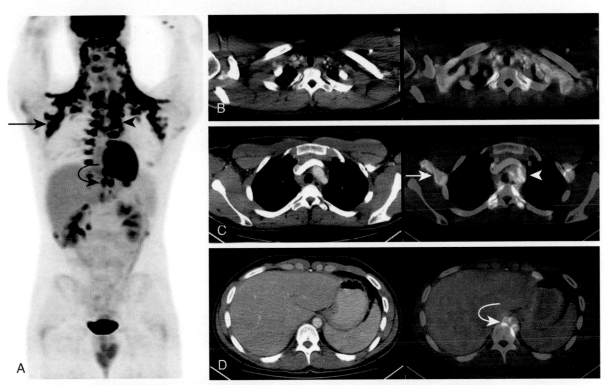

FIG. 21.15 **Extensive FDG-avid Brown Fat.** (A) FDG maximum intensity projection (MIP) image in a patient being followed for lymphoma demonstrates extensive symmetric FDG avidity in the neck and chest (*arrow*, *arrowhead*, and *curved arrow*). Axial CT and FDG PET/CT images demonstrate FDG avidity corresponding to fat in the (B) thoracic inlet, (C) axillary *(arrow)*, mediastinal *(arrowhead)*, and paravertebral regions, and (D) retrocrural *(curved arrow)* and diaphragmatic regions. Extensive brown fat such as this could obscure underlying FDG-avid nodes; however, no corresponding nodes are seen on this CT.

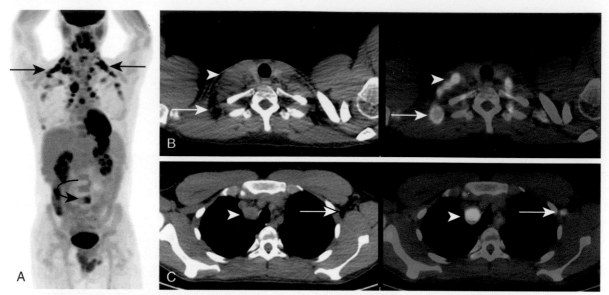

FIG. 21.16 FDG-avid Brown Fat and FDG-avid Lymphoma in the Same PET/CT Scan. (A) FDG maximum intensity projection (MIP) image in a patient with lymphoma demonstrates extensive FDG avidity in the neck and chest *(arrows)*. (B) Axial CT and fused FDG PET/CT images through the lower neck demonstrate both FDG-avid brown fat that correlates with fat on CT *(arrows)* and FDG-avid lymphoma that correlates with soft tissue on CT *(arrowheads)*. (C) Axial CT and fused FDG PET/CT images through the chest neck demonstrate both FDG-avid brown fat that correlates with fat on CT *(arrows)* and FDG-avid lymphoma that correlates with soft tissue on CT *(arrowheads)*. The presence of FDG-avid brown fat does not preclude synchronous FDG-avid malignancy. An FDG-avid lesion was also seen in the spine *(curved arrow* in (A)).

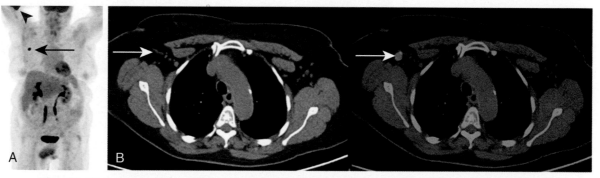

FIG. 21.17 Extravasation of FDG at the Injection Site Resulting in FDG Avidity in a Benign Draining Node. (A) FDG maximum intensity projection (MIP) image in a patient with vulvar cancer demonstrates an FDG-avid focus overlying the right chest *(arrow)*. (B) Axial CT and fused FDG PET/CT images through the chest demonstrate that the FDG avidity localizes to a benign-appearing node on CT *(arrows)*. Scrutiny of the MIP reveals the extravasation of FDG at the injection site in the right arm *(arrowhead* in (A)), which has resulted in drainage of FDG to a benign right axillary node. The fact that the primary malignancy is remote from the node and no other disease is visible provides assurance that this node is benign.

SUGGESTED READINGS

Barrington, et al: Role of imaging in the staging and response assessment of lymphoma: consensus of the International Conference on Malignant Lymphomas Imaging Working Group, *J Clin Oncol* 32:3048–3058, 2014.

Cheson, et al: Recommendations for initial evaluation, staging, and response assessment of Hodgkin and non-Hodgkin lymphoma: the Lugano classification, *J Clin Oncol* 32: 3059–3068, 2014.

El-Galaly, et al: Routine bone marrow biopsy has little or no therapeutic consequence for positron emission tomography/ computed tomography-staged treatment-naive patients with Hodgkin lymphoma, *J Clin Oncol* 30:4508–4514, 2012.

Fuster, et al: Is there a role for PET/CT with esophagogastric junction adenocarcinoma? *Clin Nucl Med* 40:e201–e207, 2015.

Johnson, et al: Imaging for staging and response assessment in lymphoma, *Radiology* 276:323–338, 2015.

Khiewvan, et al: An update on the role of PET/CT and PET/ MRI in ovarian cancer, *Eur J Nucl Med Mol Imaging* 44: 1079–1091, 2017.

Malibari, et al: PET/computed tomography in the diagnosis and staging of gastric cancers, *PET Clin* 10:311–326, 2015.

Numan, et al: Peri- and postoperative management of stage I-III non small cell lung cancer: which quality of care indicators are evidence-based? *Lung Cancer* 101:129–136, 2016.

Olsen, et al: Clinical end points and response criteria in mycosis fungoides and Sézary syndrome: a consensus statement of the International Society for Cutaneous Lymphomas, the United States Cutaneous Lymphoma Consortium, and the Cutaneous Lymphoma Task Force of the European Organisation for Research and Treatment of Cancer, *J Clin Oncol* 29:2598–2607, 2011.

Ulaner, et al: False-positive [18F]fluorodeoxyglucose-avid lymph nodes on positron emission tomography-computed tomography after allogeneic but not autologous stem-cell transplantation in patients with lymphoma, *J Clin Oncol* 32:51–56, 2014.

CHAPTER 22

Measuring Treatment Response on FDG PET/CT

Currently, the most common method of measuring treatment response in malignancy uses size measurements on computed tomography (CT) and magnetic resonance (MR). However, metabolic changes in tumors, measurable by 18F-fluorodeoxyglucose positron emission tomography (FDG PET)/CT, are often more rapid and more profound than anatomic changes measurable on CT or MR. Although changes in size following effective treatment may take months to manifest on CT or MR, reductions in FDG avidity are often apparent after days or weeks. And for some tumors, such as gastrointestinal stromal tumors, there may even be an increase in size following effective therapy. Thus decreases in FDG avidity may be far more accurate than tumor sizes for assessment of treatment effectiveness. As this knowledge becomes more widespread, the use of FDG PET/CT for determining response or progression during treatment is rapidly growing.

It is important to have a framework for how response to treatment is measured on FDG PET/CT. For lymphoma, the Lugano Classification and its five-point scale are described in Chapter 21. This has been widely accepted and used in clinical practice and clinical trials. Measuring treatment response with FDG PET/CT in solid tumors is somewhat less clear. There is significant variability in the extent of FDG avidity reduction needed to predict successful outcomes for different solid tumors. Nevertheless, some standardization is needed. The current standard is PERCIST—Positron Emission Tomography Response Criteria in Solid Tumors.

PERCIST defines four categories of treatment response, overly simplified here:

1. Complete metabolic response (CMR)
    A. Decrease in FDG avidity of all tumor lesions to background AND
    B. No new tumor lesions
2. Partial metabolic response (PMR)
    A. Decrease in FDG avidity of 30% or more from baseline measurements AND
    B. No new tumor lesions

3. Stable metabolic disease (SMD)—not CMR, PMR, or progressive metabolic disease (PMD).
4. PMD
    A. Increase in FDG avidity of 30% or more from baseline measurements OR
    B. Increase in extent of FDG avidity (bigger tumor) OR
    C. New tumor lesions

How is FDG avidity measured in PERCIST? Standard in PERCIST is SULpeak, which is the standardized uptake volume (SUV) normalized by lean body mass in a sphere with 1 cm^3 volume in the most avid portion of the tumor. However, PERCIST criteria could be used with other quantitative measurements, such as the more commonly used SUVmax, the SUV normalized by body weight for the single most avid voxel within the region of interest (ROI). Lean body mass provides less variance of measurement than body weight in patients if their weight is changing. The peak 1 cm^3 sphere provides less variance than does SUVmax when there is more noise in the images. However, SUVmax is so highly reproducible and easy to calculate that it is currently the most commonly used measure of FDG avidity in clinical practice.

How many lesions are measured? PERCIST is designed for use of the single, most avid lesion in each scan, although up to five lesions may be measured. If multiple lesions are selected, PERCIST does not define how to combine the data from multiple lesions.

Does a CMR mean that SUV reduces to zero? No. Remember that normal body structures such as the blood pool and liver have an SUV above zero; thus it is highly unlikely that a tumor will reduce to an SUV of zero. A reduction in the SUV of tumors to equal to or less than the level of a normal structure background, either the liver or local blood pool background, is adequate for a CMR.

Is a 30% reduction or 30% increase representative of a change in the tumor? To the best of our knowledge, the answer is yes. SUV is not as precisely reproducible as size measurements and thus is often referred to as "semiquantitative" (see Table 2.2). If you perform an FDG

PET/CT in the same patient on 2 consecutive days, you may get slightly different SUVs. Biologic and technical factors often result in a 10% to 20% difference in SUV even if there is no change in the tumor. Thus a 30% change in SUV between two scans appears highly likely to represent a true change in the tumor metabolism.

Do all FDG-avid findings represent tumor? No. As we have seen throughout this book, there are multiple FDG-avid findings that are benign. Benign findings may be more FDG avid than the malignancy on an FDG PET/CT scan. Thus it is critical to carefully distinguish malignancy from the multiple FDG-avid physiologic and inflammatory processes that may complicate an FDG PET/CT.

It takes some practice to apply PERCIST criteria in daily practice. Examples of CMR are shown in Chapter 3, Figs. 3.6 and 3.7. In both of these cases there are FDG-avid lesions at baseline which decrease to local background following treatment. Fig. 3.6 is particularly impressive because this may be interpreted as new osseous lesions by CT and thus progressive disease; however, the reduction of FDG avidity to background demonstrates this is much better classified as a CMR by PERCIST. Note that in both of these examples the FDG avidity did not decrease to zero. There is some residual FDG avidity that is indistinguishable from background. For example, in Fig. 3.7, SUVmax values for osseous metastases before treatment were up to 14 and after treatment reduced to 1.2. The residual SUVmax of 1.2 was equal to background, and thus this represents a CMR. These are excellent examples of how tumor response measurement by FDG PET/CT may be far superior to measurement by CT.

An example of PMR is demonstrated in Fig. 22.1. This patient with metastatic ductal breast cancer has a dominant sternal mass with extension into the

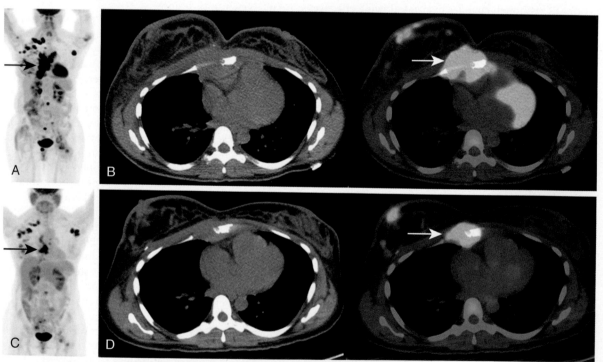

FIG. 22.1 **Partial Metabolic Response (PMR) by Positron Emission Tomography Response Criteria in Solid Tumors (PERCIST).** (A) FDG maximum intensity projection (MIP) in a patient with metastatic ductal breast cancer demonstrates multifocal abnormal FDG avidity with a dominant focus overlying the chest *(arrow)*. (B) Axial CT and PET/CT images localize the dominant FDG focus to a sternal/parasternal mass *(arrow)*. Standardized uptake value (SUV) of the mass was calculated to be 22. (C) FDG MIP following completion of therapy demonstrates decreased FDG-avid foci, including the dominant focus *(arrow)*. (D) Axial CT and PET/CT images following therapy demonstrate decreased extent of the FDG-avid sternal/parasternal mass *(arrow)*. SUV of the mass is now 14. The calculated percentage reduction is (22 − 14)/22 × 100% = 36%, enough for a PMR by PERCIST.

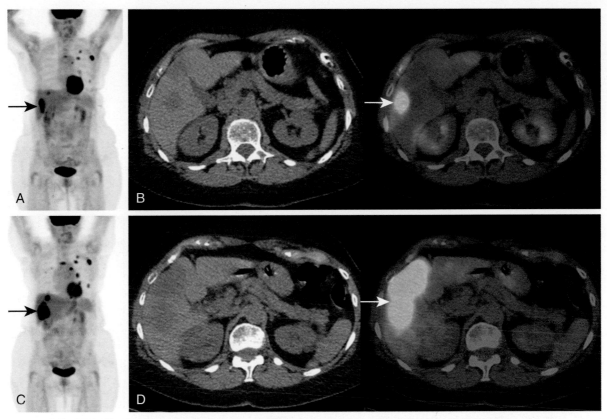

FIG. 22.2 Progressive Metabolic Disease (PMD) by Positron Emission Tomography Response Criteria in Solid Tumors (PERCIST). (A) FDG maximum intensity projection (MIP) in a patient with metastatic ductal breast cancer demonstrates multifocal abnormal FDG avidity with a dominant focus overlying the right abdomen *(arrow)*. (B) Axial CT and PET/CT images localize the dominant FDG focus to a liver metastasis *(arrow)*. Standardized uptake value (SUV) of the mass was calculated to be 7. (C) FDG MIP following completion of therapy demonstrates increased FDG-avid foci, including the dominant focus *(arrow)*. (D) Axial CT and PET/CT images following therapy demonstrate increased extent of the FDG-avid liver metastasis *(arrow)*. SUV of the mass is now 14. The calculated percentage increase is (14 − 7)/7 × 100% = 100%, representing a PMD by PERCIST.

parasternal soft tissues. Following therapy, the SUV of this mass decreased by 36%, consistent with a PMR.

An example of PMD is demonstrated in Fig. 22.2. This patient with metastatic ductal breast cancer has a dominant liver metastasis. Following therapy, the SUV of this mass increased by 100%, consistent with a PMD. The lesion has also increased in extent (become bigger); thus it could qualify for PMD even if the SUV had stayed the same. PERCIST does not define exactly how much larger an FDG-avid lesion must become to qualify for PMD.

It is uncommon for malignancy to demonstrate discordance between FDG avidity and size (decrease in FDG avidity while increasing in size, or increasing in FDG avidity while decreasing in size). When this happens, there can be considerable confusion about whether the tumor has progressed or responded to therapy (Fig. 22.3). As discussed, this may occur with gastrointestinal stromal tumors, which may increase in size following effective therapy, and in cases such as these the FDG PET is usually the better measure of response. Additional possibilities include hemorrhage into a tumor or cystic changes which artificially increase the size of a tumor, and again FDG PET will be the better measure of response. Care must be taken to analyze the time course of the imaging studies and treatment changes. For instance, if there has been a treatment change between two FDG PET/CT scans, there may have been increasing

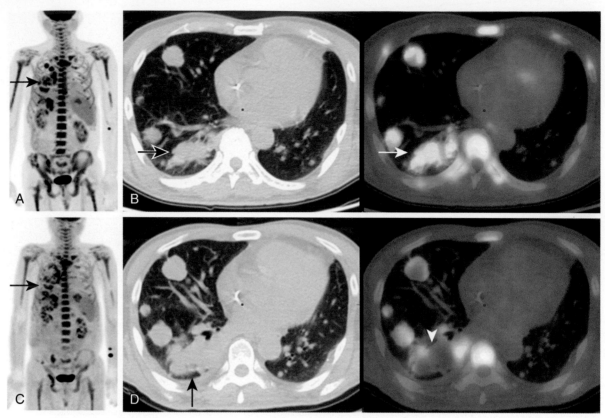

FIG. 22.3 **Discordance Between Changes in Size and FDG Avidity.** (A) FDG maximum intensity projection (MIP) in a patient with metastatic colon cancer demonstrates multifocal abnormal FDG avidity including a focus overlying the right chest *(arrow)*. (B) Axial CT and PET/CT images this focus to a lung metastasis *(arrows)*. This patient also has liver, bone, and node metastases. (C) FDG MIP following completion of therapy demonstrates decreased FDG avidity in the abnormal foci *(arrow)*. (D) Axial CT and PET/CT images following therapy demonstrate increased size of metastases *(arrow)* but decreased standardized uptake value (SUV) measurements *(arrowhead)*. This discordance between changes in size and FDG avidity could have many factors, including failing to perform FDG PET/CT scans in a manner that would minimize variability between scans, as well as the timing between treatment changes and PET/CT scans. In this case, there had been a treatment change between the two PET/CT scans. This probably represents growth of the lesions before the treatment change, then quicker decrease in FDG avidity than in size following change to a more effective treatment. Care must be taken to analyze treatment response, particularly when there is discordance between changes in size and changes in FDG avidity.

size of the tumor before the therapy change, then quick reduction of FDG avidity after the treatment change, complicating interpretation. Similarly, if the baseline FDG PET/CT was performed significantly before therapy began, there could have been tumor growth before therapy, then quick reduction of FDG avidity after therapy began. Knowledge of the patient's schedule of therapies may make a large difference in how scans are interpreted.

Here are a few suggestions to help optimize your interpretation of treatment response in solid tumors by FDG PET/CT:

1. PERCIST provides a framework for measuring treatment response in solid tumors by FDG PET/CT. In brief, reduction of FDG avidity to background is a CMR, reduction of more than 30% is a PMR, and an increase of more than 30% is a PMD. An increase in the size of

an FDG-avid malignancy or a new focus of FDG-avid malignancy may also cause PMD. SMD is when the change does qualify for CMR, PMR, or PMD.

2. Care must be taken in selecting FDG-avid tumor lesions, because many FDG-avid foci are benign. Mistaking a benign focus for malignancy will cause a big problem when calculating treatment responses and deciding if there has been response or progression.

3. Measurement of FDG avidity is semiquantitative, and many biologic and technical factors can produce changes in FDG avidity when there is no change in the underlying lesion. Care must be taken to perform FDG PET/CT in a manner that minimizes variation between scans.

SUGGESTED READINGS

Avril, et al: Prediction of response to neoadjuvant chemotherapy by sequential F-18-fluorodeoxyglucose positron emission tomography in patients with advanced-stage ovarian cancer, *J Clin Oncol* 23:7445–7453, 2005.

Barrington, et al: Role of imaging in the staging and response assessment of lymphoma: consensus of the International Conference on Malignant Lymphomas Imaging Working Group, *J Clin Oncol* 32:3048–3058, 2014.

Cheson, et al: Recommendations for initial evaluation, staging, and response assessment of Hodgkin and non-Hodgkin lymphoma: the Lugano classification, *J Clin Oncol* 32:3059–3068, 2014.

O, et al: Practical PERCIST: a simplified guide to PET response criteria in solid tumors 1.0, *Radiology* 280:576–584, 2016.

Wahl, et al: From RECIST to PERCIST: evolving considerations for PET response criteria in solid tumors, *J Nucl Med* 50(Suppl 1):122S–150S, 2009. PMID: 19403881.

Weber, et al: Prediction of response to preoperative chemotherapy in adenocarcinomas of the esophagogastric junction by metabolic imaging, *J Clin Oncol* 19:3058–3065, 2001.

CHAPTER 23

Artifacts on FDG PET/CT

All imaging modalities may be compromised by artifacts which obscure malignancy or mimic malignancy. 18F-fluorodeoxyglucose positron emission tomography/computed tomography (FDG PET/CT) may be compromised by a multitude of artifacts, primarily associated with technical performance of PET/CT scanners and unexpected biodistribution of FDG. A few of the more common artifacts on FDG PET/CT are discussed here.

MOTION

Patient motion during acquisition of PET/CT images may introduce multiple artifacts which need to be recognized. The PET/CT scanner is composed of separate PET and CT imaging elements. Thus, although we refer to PET/CT images, it is important to remember that separate PET and CT images are obtained and then fused together. Under idealized conditions we expect there to be perfect alignment of the PET and CT images; however, this is virtually never the case. Motion of the patient between acquisition of the CT images and the PET images will result in misregistration of the combined PET/CT images, which may obscure an otherwise appreciable malignancy. This is common in the head and neck, if the head is not immobilized. This will also produce incorrect attenuation correction maps from the CT images and lead to incorrect calculation of standardized uptake values (SUVs).

Even if voluntary muscular motion of the head/neck and extremities is perfectly controlled for, involuntary motion will invariably affect PET/CT images. Motion of the diaphragm will cause misregistration between CT and PET images in the lower lungs and upper abdomen, sometimes quite significantly. This could result in artifactual placement of liver lesions over the lung on PET (Fig. 23.1), or vice versa. Incorrect localization of photons and suboptimal attenuation correction maps from diaphragmatic motion will artifactually lower SUVs

for lesions near the diaphragm. In the extreme, this problem may cause lesions in the lower lungs or upper abdomen to artifactually disappear from PET images (Fig. 23.2). Careful evaluation of the CT images near the diaphragm is important to prevent these errors.

ATTENUATION CORRECTION ARTIFACTS

Structures with fat, water, and bone cause relatively similar attenuation of CT x-rays and PET 511 KeV photons. However, at high densities, such as metal or contrast, there is greater attenuation of lower-energy CT x-rays than higher-energy PET 511 KeV photons. Because the CT is used for attenuation correction, overcorrection of attenuation can produce artifactual foci of elevated FDG avidity at sites of metal or contrast on CT (Fig. 23.3). If an attenuation correction artifact is suspected, the key is to examine the corresponding non–attenuation-corrected PET images. If the focus is not present on the non–attenuation-corrected images, an attenuation correction artifact is likely. Attenuation correction artifacts are currently much less common compared with those 10 years ago because updated computer software has compensated for the errors in attenuation correction which would otherwise occur. Metal implants may also lead to streak artifacts on CT images which then generate incorrect attenuation correction maps and cause artifacts on attenuation-corrected PET images.

PARTIAL VOLUME EFFECT ARTIFACTS

FDG photons counted by PET/CT scanners are categorized into voxels of space. Smaller lesions may not fully cover a voxel; thus calculated SUVs may be artifactually lower in small lesions. You may notice that smaller lung or liver lesions have lower calculated SUVs than do larger lesions in the same patient. The larger lesion may have more metabolically active tumor cells, but it is just as

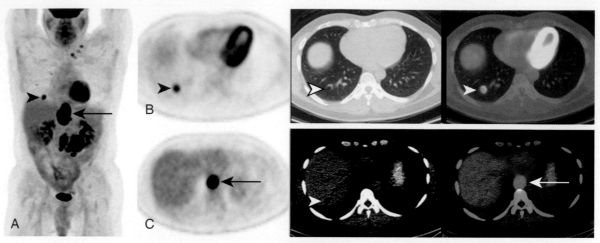

FIG. 23.1 Diaphragmatic Motion Causing Mislocalization of a Liver Metastasis on to the Lung. (A) FDG maximum intensity projection (MIP) in a patient with metastatic paraganglioma demonstrates substantial abnormal FDG avidity overlying the midline abdomen *(arrow)* and an abnormal focus overlying the lower right chest *(arrowhead)*. (B) Axial PET, CT, and fused FDG PET/CT images demonstrate the focus overlying the chest localizes to the right lung; however, no lung abnormalities are apparent of CT *(arrowheads)*. (C) Axial PET, CT, and fused FDG PET/CT images over the upper abdomen demonstrate the primary malignancy *(arrows)* and the liver metastasis on CT *(arrowhead)*, which is mislocalized onto the lung on the PET images.

likely that partial volume effect artifacts are resulting in smaller lesions having apparently lower SUVs.

BIODISTRIBUTION OF FDG

In the perfect scenario, all of the administered FDG travels through the bloodstream to predictable sites of physiologic and pathologic uptake. However, suboptimal FDG biodistribution may lead to multiple artifacts. If there is extravasation of FDG at the injection site, FDG may travel through local lymphatics and cause an FDG-avid node in the drainage pathway of the injection site (usually the axilla after an arm injection), which should not be confused with a nodal metastasis (see Chapter 21, Fig. 21.17). If a substantial proportion of the FDG was extravasated, this would leave less FDG to be taken up by tumor tissues and could result in artifactually lower SUVs for lesions. If an FDG is trapped within a small clot of blood during FDG administration, the clot will likely lodge in the lung capillaries, causing an artifactual FDG-avid focus in the lung, without correlate on CT (see Chapter 8, Fig. 8.18). The resulting FDG tracer embolus should be distinguished from a lung metastasis or a clinically relevant central pulmonary embolus. Patients with high blood glucose levels or patients who have recently eaten may have high blood insulin levels that redistribute glucose and FDG to muscle (see Chapter 4, Fig. 4.7). The high uptake of FDG in muscle will reduce the available FDG for uptake in tumors and cause artifactually lower SUVs for lesions.

"BLOOMING" OF HIGHLY CONCENTRATED FDG

When FDG is highly concentrated, it may appear to fill a larger volume than it actually does. This blooming artifact is most commonly encountered in the kidneys, ureters, and bladder because excreted FDG may accumulate in very high concentrations in the urinary tract. Highly concentrated FDG in a normal urinary tract could be mistaken for an obstructed, hydronephrotic system (Fig. 23.4). Correlation with CT images will demonstrate the caliber of the urinary tract and help to prevent overcalling this artifact.

Here are a few suggestions to help optimize your interpretation of artifacts on FDG PET/CT:

1. Motion is a source of multiple artifacts on PET/CT. Involuntary motion cannot be prevented; however, proper patient positioning on the scanner and instructions on breathing can help to minimize motion artifacts.

2. Multiple artifacts can artifactually lower the SUVs calculated for a lesion. These artifacts should be considered when evaluating changes in SUV between scans.

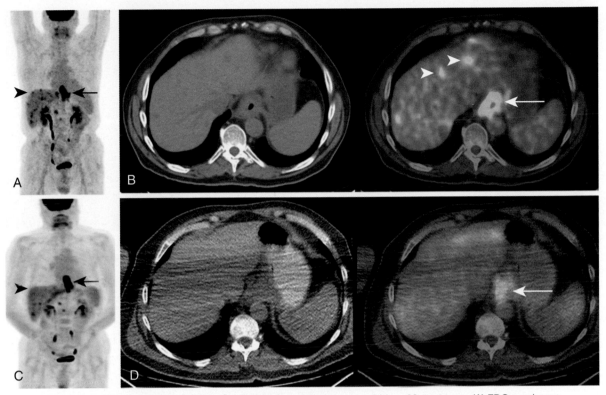

FIG. 23.2 Diaphragmatic Motion Contributing to "Disappearing" Liver Metastases. (A) FDG maximum intensity projection (MIP) in a patient with primary esophageal cancer demonstrates the FDG-avid primary esophageal malignancy *(arrow)* and abnormal FDG foci overlying the liver *(arrowhead)*. (B) Axial CT and fused FDG PET/CT images demonstrate the primary esophageal malignancy *(arrow)* and FDG-avid liver metastases *(arrowheads)*. (C) FDG MIP in the same patient on a repeat baseline FDG PET/CT performed for requirements of a clinical trial. No therapy in the interim. The primary esophageal malignancy *(arrow)* in unchanged, but metastases in the superior portion of the liver have disappeared *(arrowhead)*. Note the flattening of the superior surface of the liver near the arrowhead, which is a clue to the problem on PET. (D) Axial CT and fused FDG PET/CT images also demonstrate the primary esophageal malignancy is unchanged *(arrow)* but the superior liver metastases have disappeared. Motion at the diaphragm between CT and PET images, and the arms-down positioning, has contributed to obscuring the metastases that should be seen on the superior aspect of the liver.

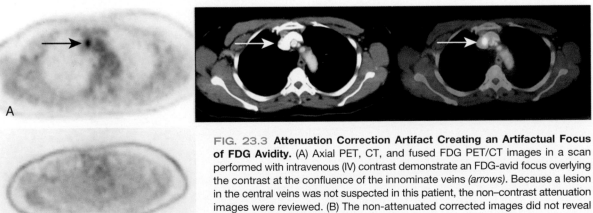

FIG. 23.3 Attenuation Correction Artifact Creating an Artifactual Focus of FDG Avidity. (A) Axial PET, CT, and fused FDG PET/CT images in a scan performed with intravenous (IV) contrast demonstrate an FDG-avid focus overlying the contrast at the confluence of the innominate veins *(arrows)*. Because a lesion in the central veins was not suspected in this patient, the non–contrast attenuation images were reviewed. (B) The non-attenuated corrected images did not reveal a focus of increased FDG avidity. It is likely that IV contrast led to an attenuation correction artifact.

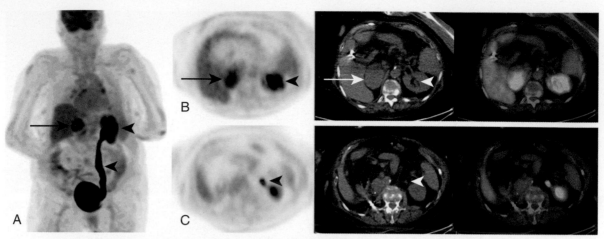

FIG. 23.4 Blooming Artifact from Highly Concentrated FDG in the Urinary Collecting System. (A) FDG maximum intensity projection (MIP) in a patient with a right kidney carcinoid post-resection and recurrence demonstrates an abnormal focus of FDG avidity in the right upper abdomen *(arrow)*, as well as a very prominent left kidney collecting system *(arrowheads)*. (B) Axial PET, CT, and fused FDG PET/CT through the left kidney demonstrate the FDG-avid tumor in the right nephrectomy bed *(arrows)*. The prominent FDG in the left kidney collecting system correlates with a normal-appearing collecting system on CT *(arrowheads)*. (C) Axial PET, CT, and fused FDG PET/CT through the left ureter demonstrate that the prominent left ureter on PET correlates with a normal-sized ureter on CT *(arrowheads)*. Blooming of concentrated FDG in the left urinary collecting system on PET could be mistaken for left-sided obstruction and hydronephrosis, but the corresponding CT images reveal this is only a PET artifact.

SUGGESTED READINGS

Boellaard, et al: FDG PET/CT: EANM procedure guidelines for tumour imaging: version 2.0, *Eur J Nucl Med Mol Imaging* 42:328–354, 2015.

Corrigan, et al: Pitfalls and artifacts in the use of PET/CT in oncology imaging, *Semin Nucl Med* 45:481–499, 2015.

Delbeke, et al: Procedure guideline for tumor imaging with 18F-FDG PET/CT 1.0, *J Nucl Med* 47:885–895, 2006.

Even-Sapir, et al: Imaging the normal and abnormal anatomy of the female pelvis using (18)F FDG-PET/CT, including pitfalls and artifacts, *PET Clin* 5:425–434, 2010.

Hojgaard, et al: Head and neck: normal variations and benign findings in FDG positron emission tomography/computed tomography imaging, *PET Clin* 9:141–145, 2014.

Zukotynski, et al: Abdomen: normal variations and benign conditions resulting in uptake on FDG-PET/CT, *PET Clin* 9:169–183, 2014.

CHAPTER 24

Radiotracers Other Than FDG for Oncologic PET/CT

The development and use of positron emission tomography (PET) radiotracers has tremendous potential for the advancement of oncologic imaging. There has been preclinical development on hundreds of PET radiotracers, and the most promising have advanced into clinical trials. As of 2018 the US Food and Drug Administration (FDA) has approved five PET radiotracers which are used for oncologic imaging:

1. 18F-fluorodeoxyglucose (FDG)
2. 18F-sodium fluoride (Na18F)
3. 18F-anti-1-amino-3-18F-fluorocyclobutane-1-carboxylic acid (18F-FACBC, also known as fluciclovine and by the brand name Axumin)
4. ^{11}C-choline
5. ^{68}Ga-DOTA-octreotate (^{68}Ga-DOTATATE, also known by the brand name NETSPOT)

The majority of this book was dedicated to FDG. This final chapter introduces the other four FDA-approved oncologic imaging radiotracers, as well as one of the many radiotracers targeting the prostate-specific membrane antigen (PSMA) protein, which are currently in clinical trials. Although FDG has by far been the most commonly used radiotracer for oncologic PET/computed tomography (CT) imaging, continued research and development into PET radiotracers could profoundly alter the usage of radiotracers in oncology, as well as multiple other disciplines of medicine.

This brief introduction is not intended to help master these complex PET/CT radiotracers, each of which could be the basis of its own textbook. Rather, this is to demonstrate the versatility of PET/CT as a platform for the development of novel imaging studies. Although it is common to hear clinicians discuss ordering a "PET/CT," they are actually ordering an FDG PET/CT, a Na18F PET/CT, or a ^{68}Ga-DOTATATE PET/CT. Each study has its own uses, advantages, and limitations.

18F-SODIUM FLUORIDE (NA18F)

Intravenous administration of Na18F leads to incorporation of 18F into bone at sites of altered osteogenesis.

Because tumors involving the bone often lead to altered osteogenesis, Na18F can be used to detect malignancy involving the bone. Na18F was approved by the FDA in 1972 and became the first "bone scan" for detection of osseous metastases in the 1970s. The development of less expensive Tc-99m pertechnetate (99mTc)-labeled bisphosphonate agents and Anger gamma cameras optimized for imaging the 140-KeV photons from 99mTc led to Na18F bone scans being replaced by 99mTc radiotracers such as Tc-99m medronate (MDP). Decades later, the development of PET and then PET/CT scanners has led to resurgence in the use of Na18F bone scans. Na18F PET/CT allows for higher spatial resolution and improved image quality compared with MDP planar and single-photon emission computed tomography (SPECT)/CT imaging. Na18F also has higher lesion-to-background signal and more rapid blood clearance than does MDP, allowing for shorter tracer injection to scanning times. These technical advantages have clinical implications because Na18F PET/CT has been shown to have greater sensitivity and specificity for the detection of osseous metastases than does MDP imaging. The major drawbacks of Na18F PET/CT are cost, given that MDP can be performed inexpensively, and radiologist time, because interpretation of the thousands of images in a Na18F PET/CT takes significantly longer than most MDP studies.

Because Na18F targets sites of osteogenesis, the skeleton is the dominate finding on a normal Na18F study (Fig. 24.1). Na18F is excreted by the kidneys, thus the kidneys, ureter, and bladder may be visualized. In contrast to FDG, which accumulates in the tumor itself, it is important to recognize that Na18F does not image the tumor itself but rather the osteogenic reaction to tumor causing bone destruction (you image the bone, not the tumor). The osteogenic reaction to tumor may be substantial, and thus Na18F may demonstrate extensive osseous malignancy (Fig. 24.2). Depending on the extent of the osteogenic reaction and the metabolism of the tumor, more osseous metastases may be visualized by Na18F than by FDG. Unfortunately, many

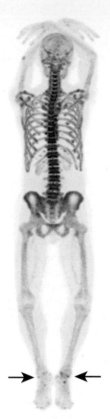

FIG. 24.1 Normal Na18F Maximum Intensity Projection (MIP). MIP Image from a Na18F PET/CT Demonstrates the Osseous Structures. The kidneys are faintly visualized. Almost all "normal" Na18F studies will have focal uptake at sites of mechanical stress or degenerative changes, as seen in this patient's bilateral ankles *(arrows)*.

benign processes also elicit osteogenesis. Na18F uptake will be seen at sites of arthritis, trauma, and metabolic abnormalities, as well as at areas of bone remodeling caused by Paget disease and fibrous dysplasia and by benign bone tumors such as osteoid osteomas. Benign processes may be more Na18F avid than malignancies; thus the standardized uptake value (SUV) cannot reliably differentiate benign from malignant processes. The morphology of the Na18F avidity, such as linear avidity at vertebral endplates, may help to classify uptake as degenerative and thus benign. Often, the corresponding CT images will help to distinguish benign from malignant Na18F avidity (Fig. 24.3). In general, Na18F foci within the bone, not associated with the joint surface, and without a benign correlate on CT (such as fracture, degenerative changes, or benign bone tumor), are suspicious for osseous malignancy.

Because you are imaging the bone, not the tumor, increasing Na18F avidity following therapy presents a conundrum. Just as increasing MDP avidity following therapy may represent either increasing metastases or decreasing metastases with "flare response" from osseous healing, the same can be seen with Na18F.

68GA-DOTATATE

Neuroendocrine tumors (NETs) arise from cells of the nervous and endocrine systems. They are most common in the small bowel, pancreas, and lung. They may also be found in the thyroid, thymus, pituitary, adrenal gland, and many other organs. Small bowel and lung NETs are often referred to as carcinoids. NETs of the pancreas arise in the pancreatic islet cells. Merkel cell carcinomas are a NET of the skin. Pheochromocytomas/paragangliomas are NETs of the adrenal glands and sympathetic nervous system. These diverse neoplasms share common features, such as production of polypeptide hormones and expression of somatostatin receptors (SSTRs).

There are multiple radiotracers that target SSTRs, allowing for SSTR imaging. ^{68}Ga-DOTATATE is a molecule that predominantly targets SSTR2, radiolabeled with the positron emitter [68]Ga. In 2016 the FDA approved ^{68}Ga-DOTATATE for PET localization of SSTR-positive NETs. Well-differentiated NETs often express relatively high levels of SSTR and are ^{68}Ga-DOTATATE avid. Poorly differentiated NETs often lose SSTR expression and are not well imaged by ^{68}Ga-DOTATATE. Poorly differentiated NETs may have high metabolism and be visualized by FDG. Thus well-differentiated NETs are often well visualized by ^{68}Ga-DOTATATE but poorly visualized by FDG, whereas poorly differentiated NETs demonstrate the reverse imaging characteristics. Of course, there is a spectrum of ^{68}Ga-DOTATATE and FDG avidity among NETs, and some may be visualized by both radiotracers or by neither.

SSTR imaging with ^{68}Ga-DOTATATE PET/CT has been found to be more sensitive than SSTR imaging with [111]indium-penteoctreotide (Octreoscan), as well as anatomic imaging with magnetic resonance (MR) or CT for the detection of many primary and metastatic NETs. ^{68}Ga-DOTATATE PET/CT is also superior to Octreoscan SPECT/CT due to improved image quality and spatial resolution, reduced patient radiation dose, and the ability to perform same day imaging. Given the many strengths of ^{68}Ga-DOTATATE PET/CT, it is likely to increasingly replace Octreoscan SPECT/CT for imaging of NETs.

Physiologic ^{68}Ga-DOTATATE avidity is found in multiple organs which express SSTR (Fig. 24.4). Intense ^{68}Ga-DOTATATE signal is seen in the spleen and kidneys, with somewhat less intense uptake in the liver. The pituitary, salivary, thyroid, and adrenal glands are also often ^{68}Ga-DOTATATE avid. The bladder may be seen

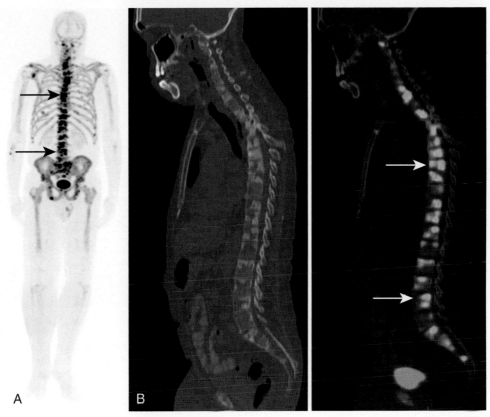

FIG. 24.2 **Osseous Metastases on Na18F PET/CT.** (A) Na18F maximum intensity projection (MIP) in a 70-year-old man with prostate cancer demonstrates widespread foci, greatest in the spine and pelvis *(arrows)*. This is a distribution typical of osseous metastases. (B) Sagittal CT and fused Na18F PET/CT images demonstrate the widespread Na18F-avid sclerotic osseous metastases *(arrows)*. In this patient, excreted Na18F can be seen in the bladder.

due to renal excretion. The pancreas may contain areas of ^{68}Ga-DOTATATE avidity, particularly in the uncinate process, and this avidity may be confused with neoplasm.

^{68}Ga-DOTATATE may be used in the initial staging of a newly diagnosed NET because it often depicts the extent of disease better than other imaging modalities (Fig. 24.5). It may also be used in cases of metastatic NET of unknown primary, to identify the primary tumor site. ^{68}Ga-DOTATATE avidity may also be used to gauge the likelihood of a NET to respond to SSTR-targeted radiotherapies such as [177]lutetium DOTATATE, a beta particle–emitting agent which has been shown to improve survival in patients with some NETs.

Unfortunately, many benign processes are ^{68}Ga-DOTATATE avid, including infections, inflammatory processes such as sarcoid, and benign lesions such as hemangiomas. Thus careful correlation with the clinical history and CT scan are needed to distinguish benign from malignant ^{68}Ga-DOTATATE avidity.

The remaining three tracers in this chapter have application in patients with prostate cancer. Although FDG has been greatly successful in a large number of malignancies, it did not have the same success with detection of prostate cancer. Although some high-grade prostate cancers are FDG avid, FDG is insensitive for many prostate malignancies. Thus there has been emphasis on the development of radiotracers with greater utility for the detection of prostate cancers. To date, two have been FDA approved (^{11}C-choline and fluciclovine), and one class of radiotracers currently demonstrates substantial potential (PSMA-targeted agents).

[11]C-CHOLINE

Choline, an important component of phospholipids in cell membranes, demonstrates increased uptake in several malignancies, including brain and prostate cancers. Several radiolabeled choline analogues have

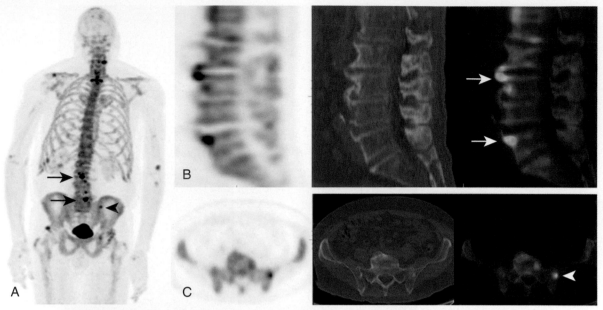

FIG. 24.3 Degenerative Changes and an Osseous Metastasis on Na18F. (A) Na18F maximum intensity projection (MIP) in a 75-year-old man with prostate cancer multiple foci, greatest in the spine and pelvis *(arrows and arrowhead)*. (B) Sagittal PET, CT, and fused Na18F PET/CT images demonstrate the Na18F-avid benign osteophytes at the anterior aspect of the lumbar spine *(arrows)*. (C) Axial PET, CT, and fused Na18F PET/CT images of the pelvis demonstrate a Na18F-avid sclerotic osseous metastasis in the left ilium *(arrowhead)*. This patient has both benign and malignant foci of Na18F avidity, best differentiated with the assistance of the corresponding CT images.

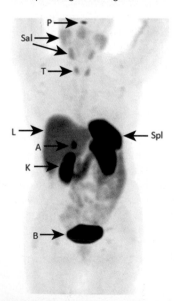

FIG. 24.4 Normal 68Ga-DOTATATE Maximum Intensity Projection (MIP). MIP image from a 68Ga-DOTATATE PET/CT demonstrates the greatest signal in the spleen *(Spl)* and kidneys *(K)*. Avidity is also seen in the pituitary *(P)*, salivary glands *(Sal)*, thyroid *(T)*, liver *(L)*, and adrenal *(A)*. Excreted tracer is seen in the bladder *(B)*.

been synthesized to image choline uptake in disease. 11C-choline is choline radiolabeled with the positron emitter 11C. In 2012 the FDA approved 11C-choline for PET imaging of patients with suspected prostate cancer recurrence based on elevated prostate-specific antigen (PSA) levels but undetectable disease on bone scan, CT, or MR.

Physiologic 11C-choline avidity is found in the liver, spleen, kidneys, and exocrine glands such as the pancreas and salivary glands (Fig. 24.6). Urinary excretion may be seen in the ureters and bladder, particularly on delayed images (11C-choline PET/CT).

11C-choline may detect recurrence in the prostatectomy bed, metastatic nodes overlooked on anatomic imaging because they are subcentimeter, osseous metastases with or without a CT correlate, and other sites of metastases (Fig. 24.7). 11C-choline has been found to localize the site of prostate cancer recurrence at a higher rate than FDG PET/CT.

False-positive 11C-choline avidity has been found in benign nodes, attributed to hyperplasia, as well as benign skeletal lesions such as in Paget disease. As with other PET tracers, careful correlation with the clinical history and CT scan is needed for high-accuracy assessment of 11C-choline

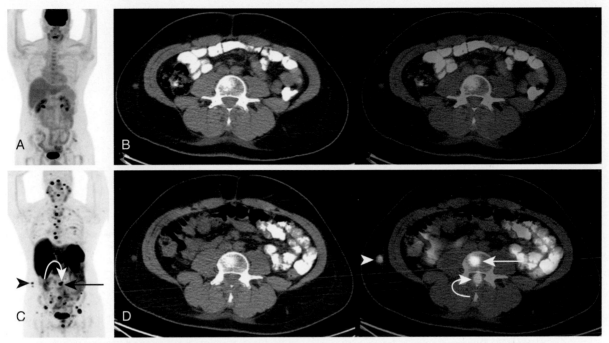

FIG. 24.5 **^{68}Ga-DOTATATE PET/CT Demonstrates More Malignancy than Does FDG PET/CT in a Patient with Metastatic Lung Carcinoid.** (A) FDG maximum intensity projection (MIP) and (B) axial CT and fused FDG PET/CT in a patient with known metastatic lung carcinoid do not demonstrate FDG-avid lesions. (C)^{68}Ga-DOTATATE MIP and (D) axial CT and fused ^{68}Ga-DOTATATE PET/CT in the same patient demonstrate widespread ^{68}Ga-DOTATATE-avid malignancy, including osseous *(arrows)*, subcutaneous *(arrowheads)*, and spinal canal *(curved arrows)* lesions. This demonstrates that different PET radiotracers may be more valuable in different clinical scenarios.

PET/CT. It is important to remember that prostate cancer normally involves the pelvic nodes before involvement of inguinal or high retroperitoneal nodes. Thus, in the absence of pelvic nodal disease, be wary of diagnosing metastases in inguinal or high retroperitoneal nodes. An advantage of ^{11}C-choline over FDG and Na18F in the bones is that degenerative osseous lesions are usually not ^{11}C-choline avid but often FDG and Na18F avid.

FLUCICLOVINE

Amino acid transport is upregulated in multiple malignancies, including brain and prostate cancers. Several radiolabeled amino acid analogues have been synthesized to evaluate amino acid metabolism. Fluciclovine is a synthetic amino acid analogue, radiolabeled with 18F, which is transported into cells via specific amino acid transporters. In 2016 the FDA approved fluciclovine for PET imaging of patients with suspected prostate cancer recurrence based on elevated PSA levels following prior treatment.

Physiologic fluciclovine avidity is seen in the liver, pancreas, and skeletal muscle (Fig. 24.8). There is negligible uptake in kidneys and bowel. Urinary excretion is delayed; thus early imaging results in little physiologic uptake in the pelvis, where most prostate cancer recurrences are found.

Detection of local recurrences in a treated prostate is confounded by fluciclovine uptake in benign prostate processes such as prostatic hypertrophy and inflammation. Outside of the prostate, fluciclovine has a high positive predictive value, allowing detection of recurrence in a prostatectomy bed, metastatic nodes overlooked on anatomic imaging because they are subcentimeter, and osseous metastases with or without a CT correlate, as well as other sites of metastases (Fig. 24.9). Because uptake in sclerotic osseous metastases may be low, a bone scan may be indicated in addition to a fluciclovine PET/CT.

Fluciclovine avidity has been seen in other malignancies, such as brain and breast cancers, as well as multiple benign processes, such as infections, inflammation, meningiomas, and osteomas. Similar to ^{11}C-choline,

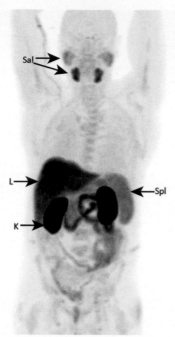

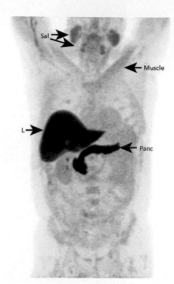

FIG. 24.6 Normal ¹¹C-Choline Maximum Intensity Projection (MIP). MIP image from a ¹¹C-choline PET/CT demonstrates signal in the liver *(L)*, kidneys *(K)*, spleen *(Spl)*, and salivary glands *(Sal)*. Excreted activity can be seen in the proximal bowel.

FIG. 24.8 Normal Fluciclovine Maximum Intensity Projection (MIP). MIP image from a fluciclovine PET/CT demonstrates signal in the liver *(L)*, pancreas *(Panc)*, skeletal muscle *(Muscle)*, and salivary glands *(Sal)*.

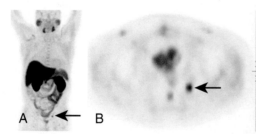

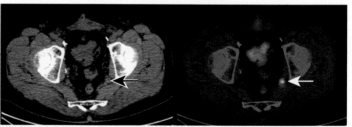

FIG. 24.7 ¹¹C-Choline PET/CT Demonstrates Metastatic Disease in the Pelvis. (A) ¹¹C-choline maximum intensity projection (MIP) in a patient with prostate cancer post-prostatectomy and pelvic nodal dissection with increasing prostate-specific antigen demonstrates a focus of avidity in the left pelvis *(arrow)*. (B) Axial CT and fused ¹¹C-choline PET/CT localize the avidity to a left pelvic side wall nodal metastasis *(arrows)*.

fluciclovine avidity is not usually seen in degenerative bone lesions.

⁶⁸GA-PSMA-11

PSMA is a transmembrane protein which is markedly overexpressed in approximately 90% of prostate malignancies, making it an excellent target for imaging prostate cancer. There is currently an FDA-approved anti-PSMA antibody used for gamma camera imaging, ProstaScint; however, poor tumor-to-background signal has limited

its use. More recently, several small molecule inhibitors of PSMA have been radiolabeled for use as imaging agents, including agents labeled with ⁶⁸Ga and 18F, which are in clinical trials. The PSMA inhibitor ⁶⁸Ga-PSMA-11 was developed in 2011 and to date is the most widely used PSMA-targeting radiotracer in clinical trials.

Physiologic ⁶⁸Ga-PSMA-11 avidity is seen in the kidneys, lacrimal and salivary glands, liver, and spleen (Fig. 24.10). Excreted activity is expected in the ureters, bladder, and bowel. Excreted tracer in the bladder may limit visualization of lesions adjacent to the bladder. There is little

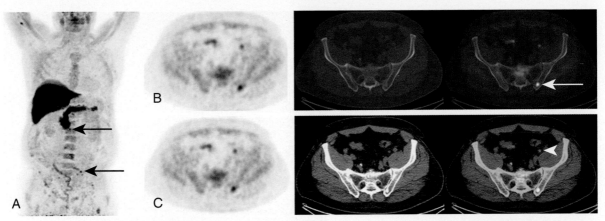

FIG. 24.9 Fluciclovine PET/CT Demonstrates Osseous and Nodal Metastases. (A) Fluciclovine maximum intensity projection (MIP) in a patient with prostate cancer post-prostatectomy with increasing prostate-specific antigen demonstrates multiple abnormal foci in the abdomen and pelvis *(arrows)*. (B) Axial PET, CT, and fused fluciclovine PET/CT on a bone CT window localize one focus to a small sclerotic metastasis in the left ilium *(arrow)*. (C) The same images on a soft tissue CT window localize another focus to a subcentimeter left pelvic nodal metastasis *(arrowhead)*.

background uptake in benign nodes and bones, which are the most common sites of prostate cancer metastases.

^{68}Ga-PSMA-11 improves detection of metastatic nodes overlooked on anatomic imaging because they are subcentimeter, osseous metastases, and other sites of disease (Fig. 24.11). Multiple publications report ^{68}Ga-PSMA-11 has higher detection rates for primary, metastatic, and recurrent prostate cancer than do other radiotracers used for prostate cancer imaging. ^{68}Ga-PSMA-11 also has been able to visualize the site of prostate cancer recurrence at lower PSA levels than can other radiotracers. This is important because salvage therapies, such as radiation and surgery, are most successful with low-volume disease. PSMA-targeting agents may also be labeled with radiotherapeutics, such as the beta-emitting [177]lutetium. Thus PSMA-targeting agents could be used for both diagnostic imaging and radiotherapy, part of the growing field of "theranostics."

PSMA is found on a number of tissue types; thus the protein is not "prostate specific," despite the name. There are many benign and malignant lesions that demonstrate ^{68}Ga-PSMA-11 uptake. Benign uptake in sympathetic ganglia may be mistaken for nodal metastases. Multiple infectious and inflammatory processes are ^{68}Ga-PSMA-11 avid, including granulomatous inflammation such as sarcoid, benign osseous lesions such as fractures, Paget, fibrous dysplasia, and hemangiomas, and benign neoplasms such as meningiomas and schwannomas. In addition, approximately 10% of prostate cancers do not overexpress PSMA, limiting the value of PSMA-targeting agents in these patients. For example, prostate cancers with

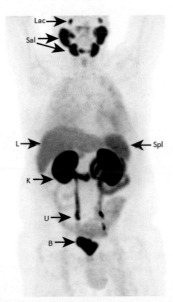

FIG. 24.10 Normal ^{68}Ga-PSMA-11 Maximum Intensity Projection (MIP). MIP image from a ^{68}Ga-PSMA-11 PET/CT demonstrates signal in the lacrimal glands *(Lac)*, salivary glands *(Sal)*, liver *(L)*, spleen *(Spl)*, and kidney *(K)*, ureters *(U)*, and bladder *(B)*.

neuroendocrine differentiation are often not visible with ^{68}Ga-PSMA-11.

PSMA-targeted agents have also been radiolabeled with 18F. One 18F-labeled PSMA ligand, 18F-DCFPyL, has demonstrated very high levels of uptake in primary

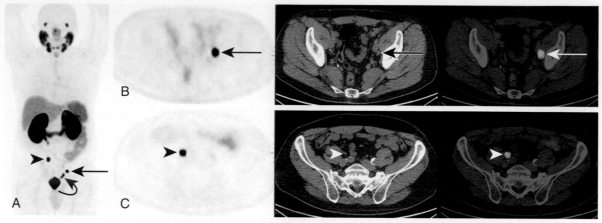

FIG. 24.11 **⁶⁸Ga-PSMA-11 PET/CT Demonstrates Subcentimeter Nodal Metastasis.** (A) ⁶⁸Ga-PSMA-11 maximum intensity projection (MIP) in a patient with prostate cancer post-prostatectomy with increasing prostate-specific antigen demonstrates multiple abnormal foci in the pelvis (*arrow, arrowhead,* and *curved arrow*). (B) Axial PET, CT, and fused ⁶⁸Ga-PSMA-11 PET/CT localize one focus to a subcentimeter left pelvic node, subsequently proven to be a nodal metastasis *(arrows)*. This demonstrates the ability of targeted metabolic imaging to visualize disease that would be overlooked on anatomic imaging. (C) Axial PET, CT, and fused ⁶⁸Ga-PSMA-11 PET/CT images higher in the pelvis localize another focus to the right ureter *(arrowheads)*, representing benign tracer excretion. The curved arrow on the MIP image localized to the left ureter. This demonstrates the importance of anatomic imaging to the proper interpretation of metabolic images.

and metastatic prostate cancer and has better tumor-to-background ratios than does ⁶⁸Ga-PSMA-11. Future development of 18F-labeled PSMA ligands is greatly expected.

CONCLUSION

FDG has to date been by far the most commonly used radiotracer for oncologic PET/CT imaging and continues to be of remarkable importance for the care of patients with cancer. Research into novel PET radiotracers demonstrates the versatility of PET/CT as a platform for the development clinically useful imaging studies. Although this textbook focuses on oncologic imaging with PET/CT, the modalities of PET, PET/CT, and PET/MR represent imaging modalities with tremendous potential in a wide range of medical specialties.

SUGGESTED READINGS

Barrio, et al: The Impact of somatostatin receptor-directed PET/CT on the management of patients with neuroendocrine tumor: a systematic review and meta-analysis, *J Nucl Med* 58:756–761, 2017.

Bastawrous, et al: Newer PET application with an old tracer: role of 18F-NaF skeletal PET/CT in oncologic practice, *Radiographics* 34:1295–1316, 2014.

Deppen, et al: ⁶⁸Ga-DOTATATE compared with 111In-DTPA-octreotide and conventional imaging for pulmonary and gastroenteropancreatic neuroendocrine tumors: a systematic review and meta-analysis, *J Nucl Med* 57:872–878, 2016.

Giovacchini, et al: PET and PET/CT with radiolabeled choline in prostate cancer: a critical reappraisal of 20 years of clinical studies, *Eur J Nucl Med Mol Imaging* 44:1751–1776, 2017.

Langsteger, et al: ¹⁸F-NaF-PET/CT and 99mTc-MDP bone scintigraphy in the detection of bone metastases in prostate cancer, *Semin Nucl Med* 46:491–501, 2016. PMID: 27825429.

Maurer, et al: Current use of PSMA-PET in prostate cancer management, *Nat Rev Urol* 13:226–235, 2016.

Mick, et al: Molecular imaging in oncology: (18)F-sodium fluoride PET imaging of osseous metastatic disease, *AJR Am J Roentgenol* 203:263–271, 2014.

Rauscher, et al: ⁶⁸Ga-PSMA ligand PET/CT in patients with prostate cancer: how we review and report, *Cancer Imaging* 16:14, 2016.

Savir-Baruch, et al: Imaging of prostate cancer using fluciclovine, *PET Clin* 12:145–157, 2017.

Sheikhbahaei, et al: Pearls and pitfalls in clinical interpretation of prostate-specific membrane antigen (PSMA)-targeted PET imaging, *Eur J Nucl Med Mol Imaging* 2017. [Epub ahead of print].

Virgolini, et al: Current knowledge on the sensitivity of the (68)Ga-somatostatin receptor positron emission tomography and the SUVmax reference range for management of pancreatic neuroendocrine tumours, *Eur J Nucl Med Mol Imaging* 43:2072–2083, 2016.

Index

Page numbers followed by "*f*" refer to illustrations; page numbers followed by "*t*" refer to tables; page numbers followed by "*b*" refer to boxes.

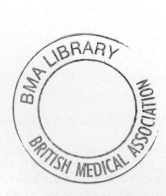